Advances in Immunity
and Cancer Therapy

Advances in Immunity and Cancer Therapy

Series Editor: P.K. Ray

Advances in Immunity and Cancer Therapy

Volume 1

With 25 Figures

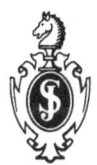

Springer-Verlag
New York Berlin Heidelberg Tokyo

P.K. RAY
Director, Industrial Toxicology
  Research Centre
Mahatma Gandhi Marg, Post Box 80
Lucknow - 226001 - India

ISSN: 0178-2134

Typeset by Bi-Comp, Incorporated, York, Pennsylvania.

9 8 7 6 5 4 3 2 1

ISBN-13: 978-1-4612-9549-5   e-ISBN-13: 978-1-4612-5068-5
DOI: 10.1007/978-1-4612-5068-5

Preface

The rapid and continuous upsurge of interesting data in the subject of tumor immunology necessitates the publication of an annual series to furnish the updated materials to the students, researchers, and clinicians in this rapidly advancing field. Concepts and methodologies are ever changing. Also, current research in tumor immunology promises to offer breakthroughs in the future. Important is the need to communicate to the right people the exact role of immunodiagnostic methods and immunological intervention in cancer prevention and treatment. The role of immunotherapy in combination with conventional modalities of treatment needs to be understood in its proper perspective. Oncogene, interferon, lymphokines, monoclonal antibodies, natural killer cells, platelet-mediated cytotoxicity of antibody-coated target cells, suppressor cells, platelet-derived factors, plasma-blocking factors, control of suppressor cell function, abrogation of plasma-blocking factors, etc., are some of the areas that are continually advancing. Progress in these areas will have implication in cancer therapy. Further, it is already understood that if immunocompetence of the host can be maintained at a reasonably good level, there exists the potential to increase the therapeutic indexes of conventional modalities of treatment. This series will attempt to present updated information in all these areas based on contributed and solicited articles.

P.K. Ray
July 1985

Contents

Contributors

HENRIC BLOMGREN
Stockholm County Microbiology
   Laboratory
Karolinska Hospital
Stockholm, Sweden

PETER D. COOPER
Department of Microbiology
John Curtin School of Medical
   Research
Australian National University
Canberra, Australia

MICHAEL G. HANNA, JR.
Litton Institute of Applied
   Biotechnology
Litton Bionetics, Inc.
Kensington, Maryland, U.S.A.

HERBERT C. HOOVER, JR.
Department of Surgery
Division of Surgical Oncology
State University of New York
Stony Brook, New York, U.S.A.

MARC E. KEY
Department of Surgery
Division of Surgical Oncology
State University of New York
Stony Brook, New York, U.S.A.

KENNETH J. MCCORMICK
Otolaryngology—Head & Neck
   Surgery
The University of Chicago
   Medical Center
Chicago, Illinois, U.S.A.

CLAUDIO OGIER
Department of Medical Pathology
University of Ferrara
Ferrara, Italy

BJORN PETRINI
Karolinska Hospital
Stockholm County
Microbiology Laboratory
Stockholm, Sweden

T.B. PODUVAL
Biomedical Group
Bhabha Atomic Research Centre
Bombay, India

P.K. RAY
Industrial Toxicology Research
   Centre
Lucknow, India

PETER REIZENSTEIN
Division of Hematology
   and Radiumhemmet
Karolinska Hospital
Stockholm, Sweden

M. SHESHADRI
Biomedical Group
Bhabha Atomic Research Centre
Bombay, India

PAUL H. SUGARBAKER
Public Health Service
National Institutes of Health
Bethesda, Maryland, U.S.A.

JERZY WASSERMAN
Stockholm County Microbiology
   Laboratory
Karolinska Hospital
Stockholm, Sweden

Chapter 1

Cells Responsible for Tumor Surveillance in Man: Effects of Radiotherapy, Chemotherapy, and Biologic Response Modifiers*

PETER REIZENSTEIN, CLAUDIO OGIER, HENRIC BLOMGREN, BJORN PETRINI, AND JERZY WASSERMAN

Contents

---

* Supported by Swedish Cancer Research Foundation.

The immunologic response in tumor patients is affected both by the tumor itself and by the chemotherapy and radiotherapy given (1–3). The effects of chemotherapy and radiotherapy on the biologic response is dealt with here. In addition, cells responsible for antigen-dependent and independent mechanisms of tumor surveillance are discussed.

In addition to treatment aimed directly at the tumor cell, therapeutic attempts to influence the biologic and immunologic response of the patient have been made, using bacteria and bacterial and fungal extracts, some peptides derived from immunoglobulin, thymus extracts, and a few synthetic drugs. This chapter concentrates on the relatively well-studied examples of Bestatin in bladder and prostatic cancer and of BCG in acute myeloid leukemia.

Tumor Surveillance

Tumor-Specific and Associated Antigens

During the past decade, many studies of immunomodulation, immunotherapy, and tumor immunology have attempted to reproduce, in spontaneous tumors in man, the findings from animal studies. In animals, T-cell-mediated, tumor-specific antigen-dependent cytotoxicity is seen in transplantable experimental tumors or against virus-infected cells. Initially, various techniques of confronting lymphocytes with autologous or allogeneic tumor cells were used. It was frequently possible to obtain a lymphocyte response in allogeneic systems (5–8), but this could have been secondary to human leukocyte antigen (HLA) II differences.

It is still controversial whether patients with lymphocytes responding to autologous tumor cells have any better prognosis than patients without such lymphocytes (9–11). Patients with blastogenesis, incomplete remission lymphocytes stimulated by autologous leukemic cells, had no better prognosis than patients without blastogenesis in such cells. Patients with osteosarcoma, soft tissue sarcoma, or lung cancer, on the other hand, whose lymphocytes were cytotoxic to autologous tumor cells obtained during operation, did have a better prognosis than patients without such lymphocytes (11,12). It remains to be seen whether the contradiction is caused by different methods of studying lymphocytes (blastogenesis *vs* cytotoxicity), by differences between the tumors studied, or by immunosuppression in patients who still have an appreciable tumor load after operation. This experimental model thus neither proves nor excludes the possibility that cross-reactive, tumor-specific antigens may occur in human tumor cells.

Immunoheterogeneity of Tumors

The later development of hybridomas led to the use of literally hundreds of monoclonal antibodies, both to leukemic and other tumor cells, such as melanoma, oat-cell carcinoma, and a number of gastrointestinal tumors

(4). Most of these antibodies were initially hoped to be tumor specific, but further study usually showed cross reactivity with embryonal cells, other tumor cells, and activated states of normal cells. One of the first described, and thus one of the best studied antigens in this category was the common acute lymphatic leukemia antigen against which a number of monoclonal antibodies have been produced. These are bound, however, not only to acute lymphatic leukemia cells, but also to more mature B cells in chronic lymphatic leukemia and non-Hodgkin's lymphoma, to embryonal kidney cells, to certain leukemic cells from patients with acute myeloid leukemia, and to cells in certain nonmalignant, nonfetal tissues (13). It cannot be concluded, therefore, that this technique has succeeded in demonstrating tumor-specific antigens on the surface of human malignant cells.

What the technique has succeeded in confirming, however, is the tumor immunoheterogeneity first described with other methods by Miale et al (14). He found wide variations in tumor cell antigenicity and in the presence of HLA II antigens on tumor cells. The latter findings have been confirmed with monoclonal antibodies (15). Similar findings have been made by Olsson and Mathé (16) in animal tumors and for several antigens in human acute myeloid leukemia (17). This immunoheterogeneity is very pronounced, and the percentages of cells expressing even apparently fundamental surface structures like HLA II or insulin receptors may vary between 0 and 100. This immunoheterogeneity, which may be considered to correspond to the classical morphologic polymorphism of malignant cells, can be regarded as an additional indication against tumor-specific antigen-dependent immune surveillance, as it would make such surveillance quite inefficient.

Antigen-Independent Biologic Response

Defense against tumors may contain cytostatic and cytotoxic elements. The hyposideremia and hypofolatemia (4) characteristically seen in patients with malignant tumors form a part of so-called nutritional immunity, depriving tumor cells of necessary nutrients. This may have a cytostatic effect. So may certain hormonal, coagulational, and vascular disturbances in tumor patients (4).

Cytotoxic effects may be humorally or cellularly mediated. Tumor necrosis factor (13) and certain cytokines (14,15) are examples of humorally mediated, antigen-independent cytotoxicity.

Macrophages

Cells mediating antigen-independent cytotoxicity are macrophages, natural killer (NK) cells, certain stimulated T-cell subpopulations, and possibly certain granulocytes (Table 1-1, refs. 19,22–23,25–39,43,48,89, 151,152). It has been notoriously difficult to demonstrate that so-called immunotherapy, using for instance BCG, can stimulate T-cell responses

Table 1-1. Cell-mediated in vitro cytotoxicity.

Effector cells	Mechanisms of cytotoxicity	Examples of triggering and enhancing factors	Reference
Macrophages	Phagocytosis	BCG	21,22
	ADCC	Gamma-IFN	23
		Lipopolysaccharide (LPS)	43
	Antigen (Ag)-independent nonspecific cytotoxicity (cyt)	Endotoxin	19
NK cells	Ag-independent cyt (target recognized by NK receptor)	Gamma-IFN	25–27
		Levamisole	28
		C parvum	29
		Lymphotoxin	30
		BCG	31,48
		Protein A	32
K cells	ADCC		89
In vitro-generated cytotoxic cells (GCC)			
1. Lectin-GCC	Ag-independent cyt (NK-like)	PHA	33,34,
2. IL-2 and interferon (IFN)-GCC		IL-2 gamma-IFN	151,152
3. (MLC)-GCC	Ag-dependent MHC-restricted (CTL) and Ag-independent (NK-like) cyt	Allogeneic lymphocyte	35–37
Cytotoxic T lymphocytes (CTL)	MHC-restricted Ag-dependent		39
Polymorphonuclear cells (PMN)	ADCC	CSF alpha, beta	39

in general. In fact, inhibition of T-cell responses to lectins is seen (40), which seems unrelated to increased T-suppressor or macrophage suppressor cell functions.

In contrast, similar immunotherapy does stimulate certain macrophage functions and NK cell activity. Moreover, there are many indications that macrophage activation plays an important and central role in the general biologic response to tumors (4). In vitro, the macrophage activating factor (MAF) induces human blood monocytes to present a cytotoxicity that discriminates between normal and tumorigenic target cell lines (41). Monocytes from cancer patients exhibit signs of activation such as an increased expression of Fc-receptors (42,43) and proliferation (44). Cytotoxic macrophages can be induced both by MAF-producing lymphocytes after a major histocompatibility complex (MHC) restricted recognition of the antigen (45) and by Fc receptor binding of antibodies in antibody-dependent, cell-mediated cytotoxicity (ADCC) (46). After binding of murine monoclonal antibodies of the G2a subclass against human tumor-associated antigens (TAAS), human macrophages can kill tumor cells in vitro (47). There are, thus, more indications in human tumors for an involvement of the macrophages than for that of the antibody- or antigen-dependent cytotoxic T cells.

Natural Killer Cells

The NK function, an antibody-independent, relatively rapid cytotoxicity measurable mainly in vitro with cell-lines resembling K 562 or Chang, but not with viable human tumor cells as targets, seems to be expressed by a cell population that includes large granular lymphocytes, cells with T-cell markers, and other cells with macrophage markers, as shown in Table 1-2. The activity or number of NK cells is increased by interferons (19–21), lectins (20), protein A (26), and probably immunomodifiers like BCG (31,48) and *Corynebacterium parvum,* and inhibited by the corticosteroid-induced granulocyte-produced phospholipase lipomodulin (49) and by an NK-inhibiting substance isolated from rat peritoneum (50). Interferon seems to induce the expression of the OKM1-marker (27). Despite the intriguing sharing of myelomonocyte and T antigens (Table 1-3) (51–63), NK cells probably are a T-cell subpopulation, maturing along a T-independent pathway (64). NK cells are nonadherent and have a much faster cytotoxicity than macrophages. The K 562 line was originally isolated from the pleural effusion of a patient with chronic myelocytic leukemia (65).

Rather than only an in vitro finding, the NK phenomenon probably constitutes in vivo surveillance of at least lymphomas, which are frequently seen in NK-deficient beige mice and Chediak-Higashi-patients

Table 1-2. Markers of cytotoxic effectors.

	Adherence	E-rec	Fc-gamma rec	T10	T3	T4	T8	M1
Macrophages	+	−	+	−	−	−	−	+
NK	−	+	+	+/−	+/−	−	+/−	+
K	−	+/−	+	+/−	+/−	−	+/−	+/−
In vitro generated cytotoxic cells	+/−	+	+/−	+/−	+	−	+	−
Cytotoxic T lymphocytes	−	+	−	−	+	+/−[a]	+	−
Polymorphonuclear cells	+	−	+	−	−	−	−	−

[a] Some T4-positive cytotoxic lymphocyte clones have been isolated which seem to recognize MHC-related antigens different from those recognized by T8-positive lymphocyte clones.

Table 1-3. Membrane markers found on NK activity-exhibiting cells.

| | Cross-reactivity with | | | |
	Polymorphonuclear cell	Macrophages	T cells	Reference
General Markers:				
E-receptor (low affinity)	−	−	+	51
Fc-gamma-receptor	+	+	±	52
Monoclonal Antibodies:				
Leu 7 (HNK-1Ag)	−	−	−	53
OKM 1	+	+	±	54
MO1	+	+	−	55
B 43.4	+	+	−	56
B 73.1	+	+	−	57
NKP-15	+	+	±	58
H-25	−	+	±	59
H-366	−	+	±	59
OKT 8 } <50%	−	−	+	60
Leu 2a	−	−	+	60
OK 11 A	−	−	+	61
9.6	−	−	+	61
OKT 10	−	−	±	62
OKT 3	−	−	+	63
Human leukocyte antigen (HLA)-II 25%	−	+	±	63

(66,67). Changes in NK activity are also seen in nonmalignant conditions (Table 1-4, refs. 68–78).

NK-like and Mixed Lymphocyte Culture (MLC)-Generated Cytotoxic Cells

Even NK-cell-depleted lymphocytes can be stimulated by allogeneic lymphocytes, lectins, or interleukin 2 to recruit cytotoxic cells. Interferon can amplify cell clones cytotoxic to both autologous and allogeneic tumor cells (80,81). Preincubation with a transitional cell carcinoma cell line (82) or with autologus tumor cells is sometimes enough to induce cytotoxic cells (8,11,12). When peripheral lymphocytes from cancer patients are strongly stimulated in an MLC, OKM1-negative cells are generated with cytotoxicity not only to K 562, but also to less NK-susceptible cell lines (so-called NK-like cytotoxicity) and even to fresh allogeneic and autologous tumor cells (35–37,83).

Unlabeled K 562 cells could completely inhibit autologous tumor cell lysis when effected by stimulated interleukin 2 (IL 2), but only partially when effected by allo-stimulated lymphocytes (37). This suggests that different receptors, different effectors, or effectors at various differentiation stages are probably involved.

Table 1-4. Diseases associated with changes in NK activity.

		Disease	Reference
	Malignancies	Preleukemia	68
		Leukemia[a]	69
		Melanoma	70
		Non-Hodgkin's lymphoma	71
		Others	72
Low activity[b]		Autoimmune diseases	73
		Severe combined immunodeficiency	74
		Multiple sclerosis	75
		Infectious mononucleosis	
		Chediak-Higashi	67
High activity		Chronic alcoholism	76
		Rheumatoid arthritis	77
		Hodgkin's involved tissues[c]	78

[a] The mechanism of the reduced NK activity appears to be a reduced recycling capacity of NK effectors rather than a decrase in their number since cells with NK-associated phenotype are normal.
[b] NK suppressing cells, one of several possible explanations of low NK activity, are medium-sized, high-density, Fc-receptor-positive lymphocytes (96).
[c] NK cells are normally present in lymphoid tissues HNK−1+ cells are found in follicular centers and they are T 3+, Leu 1+ but M1−; while in the red pulp HNK−1+ cells are also M1+, and this phenotype is associated to a higher NK activity than the M5 one. (79).

Even monoclonal T cells can be induced to show NK-like activity (84). Clones killing either autologous cells alone (35,36), or these cells as well as Daudi cells (36), have been isolated. These findings suggest that strongly stimulated T cells seem to express the Fc-receptor and to be able to attack, for instance, K 562 cells. These cells are called NK-like. If they are less strongly stimulated, they seem able to attack only autologous tumor cells (35,37,85). Several of the cytotoxic cells discussed here seem to show a continuous increase in cytotoxicity related to their differentiation. For instance, NK activity goes up when cell size and granulation and Fc-receptors increase and adherence and affinity for sheep erythrocytes decrease (27) (Fig. 1-1).

Tumor Surveillance and Autoreactivity

It is not yet known if and why NK cells, NK-like cells, and possibly autologous cytotoxic T lymphocytes attack tumors rather than normal cells. NK target structures have been suggested, which might be recognized also by the antibody-dependent killer cells (86). Several other glycolipids, glycoproteins, and monosaccharides have been shown to be possible targets for NK activity (87). Undifferentiated cells appear to be more sensitive to cytotoxicity than more mature ones. When Garson, for exam-

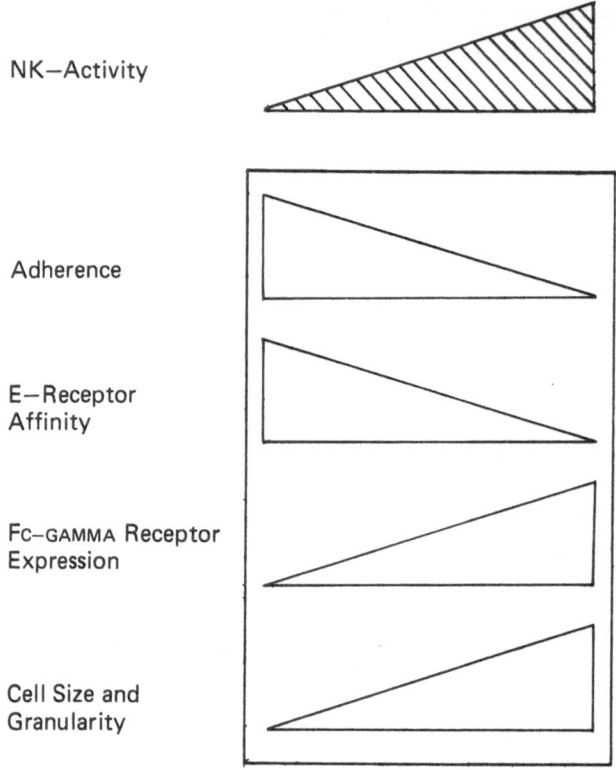

Figure 1-1. Gradient of NK activity in relation to expression of different cell markers: as NK activity increases, so do Fc-gamma receptors, cell size and granularity, while adherence and E-receptors decrease.

ple (88), induced K 562 cells to mature, they became NK resistant. Humoral factors could sensitize tumor cells, as, for example, Wright's NK cytotoxic factor (89), lymphotoxin (20), and some protease-like activities (90). A relationship between IL-2 production and NK activity has been reported in cancer patients (91), which might, in part, be accounted for by IL-2 capacity to boost gamma-interferon production (92). No information is yet available as to whether the regulatory effect, expressed by NK cells on some normal cells as well (93–95), is also mediated through a recognition step involving the NK receptor. Normal cells might protect themselves with NK inhibitors like the NK-inhibitory substance isolated from rat peritoneum (50) or lipomodulin (49). Similar mechanisms for escaping NK surveillance might also be used by tumor cells, or they could surround themselves with nonadherent, medium-sized, heavy, Fc-receptor positive, OKT3-positive, OKM1-negative NK-suppressing lymphocytes

(96,97). Fibrin deposition could also be a protective mechanism (98), as could prostaglandin production (99).

It is also possible that tumor cells require more iron than normal cells, and thus have more transferrin receptors that could target certain cytotoxic cells and form a basis for nutritional immunity (148). Another possibility is that membrane defects—perhaps associated with oncogen-coded, membrane-associated protein kinases or glycoproteins or with a membrane deficiency of neuraminic acid—make malignant cells more vulnerable (149).

It is also possible that alloantigens cross react with TAAs, and thus induce cells that are cytotoxic to autologous tumors, but neither to the allogeneic normal cells nor to K 562. This supports the hypothesis above, that tumor cells are more sensitive than normal ones. Another explanation is that a very small population of in vivo TAA-sensitized T cells exists, which is possibly amplified by release of IL 2 into mixed lymphocyte cultures. However, Taylor could preinduce cytotoxic lymphocytes even in HLA-identical siblings (150). A third explanation would be that an NK-like, TAA-independent effect is seen, although this may perhaps not be supported by Parmiani's and Taylor's failure to absorb the autocytotoxic effect with K 562 cells (pers. comm.).

It is thus possible that the immunologic abnormality of tumor cells is caused not only by asynchrony of differentiation antigens and infidelity of tissue antigens, but also by TAAs. The demonstrated weakness of TAAs may be caused by their presence on few of the tumor cells or by the sensitization of few T cells, which could hypothetically be amplified and reach a detectable level of cytotoxicity (37). This might explain the cytotoxicity to fresh and cultured autologous but not allogeneic tumor cells by cancer patient lymphocytes strongly stimulated with allogeneic cells (Table 1-5).

Modulation of the Biologic Response in Cancer Patients

Radiotherapy- and chemotherapy-treated cancer patients are at high risk for developing not only early infectious complications but also second malignancies. This might, in part, be due to radiotherapy- and chemotherapy-induced modifications of immune surveillance. Therefore, the possibility of preventing or restoring this iatrogenic paraneoplastic immunodeficiency by various natural and synthetic compounds is of great interest. In addition, the effect of chemotherapy might be mediated not only by its direct cytotoxic effect on cancer cells but also by changes in the immunologic effector mechanisms. In the next two sections of this chapter the effects of radiotherapy and chemotherapy on the lymphocyte subpopulations of breast cancer patients are presented.

Table 1-5. Spontaneous and in vitro induced cytotoxicity, to tumor and normal cells studied in direct and cold target inhibition assays.

Effector cells	Fresh or cultured target cells	Active on:					Reference
		Autologous tumor cells	Allogeneic tumor cells	Autologous an allogeneic unstimulated, or lectin-stimulated lymphocytes	K 562	Anibody[a] sensitized nucleated or not nucleated target cells	
1. Macrophages	Both	−	−	−	−	+	43
2. NK	Cultured	−	−	−	+	−[b]	51, 87
3. K	Both	−	−	−	−	+	
4. Lymphocytes from tumor patients							
(A) SLMC (spontaneous lymphocyte-mediated cytotoxicity)[d]	Fresh	±[c]	−	−	+	+	11, 12, 37, 150
(B) IL-2 and interferon (IFN)-generated generated cytotoxicity	Cultured	+	+	−	+	+	82
	Fresh	+	+	−	+	+	37, 151, 152
(C) MLC-generated cytotoxicity	Fresh	+	±[e]	−	±[c]	+	33, 35, 36, 37, 149

[a] Antibody-sensitized sheep or human red blood cells or tumor cell lines.
[b] Operational definition of overlapping cell populations.
[c] Tumor patients ranging from 10% to 40% have lymphocytes with SLMC to autologous tumor cells.
[d] Includes NK and other T cells.
[e] In contrast to IL-2 generation cytotoxicity, two different autologous tumor cytotoxic effectors seem to be generated in MLC-stimulated cultures—one absorbed by K562 cells and the other not. Vose was able to isolate allo-stimulated clones cytotoxic to autologous tumor cells but not to K 562 or allogeneic-stimulated lymphoblasts or to allogeneic tumor cells.

Radiotherapy

Radiotherapy affects lymphocyte reactivity in breast cancer patients given 45 Gray postoperatively with a 6- to 9-meV electron beam and ^{60}Co. Lymphocyte subsets as identified by different surface markers were determined before and at intervals during the 28 months following radiotherapy. Lymphocyte numbers were reduced to approximately 30% at completion of radiation, but there was a significant difference between the pattern of depletion and repopulation of T lymphocytes (E rosette-forming cells) and non-T lymphocytes (EAC cells, cells with receptors for C3) (Fig 1-2). These non-T cells, mainly B cells, were reduced to a greater extent than T cells. On the other hand, T cells were less swiftly replaced than non-T cells.

T-cell Subpopulations

T cells with Fc-receptors for IgG (Tg cells, active as suppressor cells in certain experimental systems) were reduced to a higher relative extent than T cells with Fc-receptors for IgM (Tm cells, helper cells in certain experimental systems) (100). The proportion of T-suppressor and T-helper cells as determined by monoclonal antibodies against lymphocyte antigens (Leu 2A and Leu 3A, respectively) on the other hand were largely unchanged (100). One year after radiation there was a significant recovery of both types of suppressor cells (Tg cells and Leu 2A cells), whereas this was not the case for both types of helper cells (Tm cells and Leu 3A cells) (101).

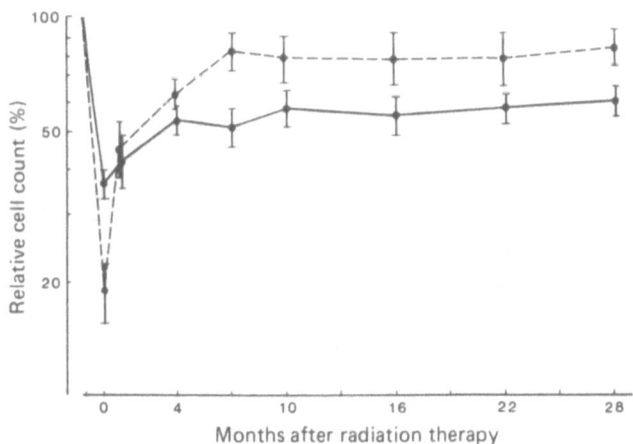

Figure 1-2. Relative changes of blood lymphocyte subpopulations in 24 patients treated with radiation for mammary carcinoma. E receptor positive cells (—), EAC cells (---).

Total lymphocyte and T-cell counts were significantly lower in breast cancer patients 10 years after radiation than in patients treated by mastectomy only. There was a persisting significant reduction of Leu 3A-binding cells (helper cells), but not of suppressor cells in the irradiated patients, who had 631 T-helper cells/μl blood on an average. Nonirradiated patients had 1,128 cells ($P < .001$). No significant change was found in T-suppressor cells at this time.

The above results clearly demonstrate that although all T cells examined were markedly reduced at the end of radiotherapy, the radiosensitivity and the repopulation pattern were not the same for different subsets. The helper cells, as identified by two different markers, were depleted to about the same extent, whereas the suppressor cells with Fc-receptors for IgG were more depleted than suppressor cells identified by Leu 2A antibodies. The reason for these apparently contradictory findings is probably an incomplete overlapping of these two suppressor subpopulations (100), which display different degrees of radiosensitivity (102). Another possibility could be an increased shedding of Fc-receptors due to radiotherapy. This could make a proportion of Tg cells undetectable. Of special interest in this context is the finding that both Tg and Leu 2A cells were significantly repopulated 15 months after radiation whereas Tm and Leu 3A cells were not (101). This indicates that T-suppressor cells, as identified both by Fc-receptors for IgG and by lymphocyte antigens, are probably relatively short-lived cells with a rapid turnover, whereas T-helper cells appear to be long-lived lymphocytes with a slow turnover.

The reduced total lymphocyte numbers one decade after radiation appear to reflect a depletion of approximately half of the helper T cells, revealing a long-term effect of radiation treatment in breast cancer.

T-cell Functions

Although the above-mentioned phenotype markers have been correlated to some extent to functions, the correlations have sometimes been inconsistent, and little is known about the stability of certain surface markers. In view of what has been observed about changing phenotypes during activation of T cells with Fc-receptors for IgG, this particular marker might express an activation stage rather than a functional status. Therefore it is appropriate to supplement all markers studied by functional tests.

The proliferative response to PPD (103) was markedly decreased at the end of the treatment and partially recovered during the following 6 months. After this time the increase of the response was slower and the reactivity was totally restituted in approximately 2 years (103–105). The allo-reactivity was also strongly reduced but was restored after 3 months (106). The response to phytohemagglutinin (PHA) varied. The depression of proliferative responses of lymphocytes from irradiated patients could be due to involvement of suppressor T lymphocytes or monocytes. It is less likely that the T lymphocytes were implicated, as it was shown that at least some suppressor T cells were more radiosensitive than T-helper cells (107). Moreover, lymphocytes treated by concanavalin in A, which increases the inhibitory activity of T-suppressor lymphocytes, reduced the mitogenic response to the same extent before and after radiotherapy (100a). Finally, depletion of adherent and phagocytic cells largely prevented the radiation-induced decrease of lymphocyte proliferation. (106, 108). Therefore, it is possible that radiation therapy induces nonspecifically immunosuppressive monocytes, or abnormal lymphocyte sensitivity to these cells. This hypothesis is supported by additional experimental findings. Radiation treatment increases the oxidative metabolism of blood monocytes as measured by reduction of nitroblue tetrazolium (109), and both silica (toxic for monocytes) and indomethacin increase lymphocyte responses (110).

T-cell Cytotoxicity

At the completion of radiation there was a distinct decrease in the ADCC by blood lymphocytes (111). Three to 4 years later this cytotoxic activity was significantly increased in irradiated patients (112). On the other hand, there was no change in lectin-dependent cellular cytotoxicity (LDCC) of lymphocytes after radiation therapy (111). NK activity of the irradiated patients' lymphocytes against K 562 cells was reduced at the completion of radiation and restituted approximately 3 months later, remaining on the same level thereafter (113). The cytotoxicity against Chang cells on the other hand did not decrease after radiation but rather increased 3 to 4 months later, remaining elevated for at least 2 years (113).

These changes in cytotoxic functions observed after radiation correlate fairly well with the shifts in the proportions of lymphocyte subsets which induce these reactions. Thus, the frequencies of total lymphocytes with Fc-receptors for IgG (113) and of T cells with these receptors decreased at the completion of radiation therapy well below pretreatment values. Furthermore, both these cell types were repopulated rather swiftly in contrast to T cells of helper phenotype. This can very well explain the increase of certain cytotoxic functions either in relation to pretreatment values or to the activity in nonirradiated patients.

Immunoglobulin Production

The examination of pokeweed mitogen (PWM)-stimulated Ig synthesis in vitro by nonfractionated lymphocytes following radiation therapy showed a significant decrease of both IgG and IgM production (114). These results can be seen in Fig. 1-3. Several kinds of cells interact in this particular experimental system and are known to be affected by radiation selectively to a varying extent. B cells, which are known to be radiosensitive, are the

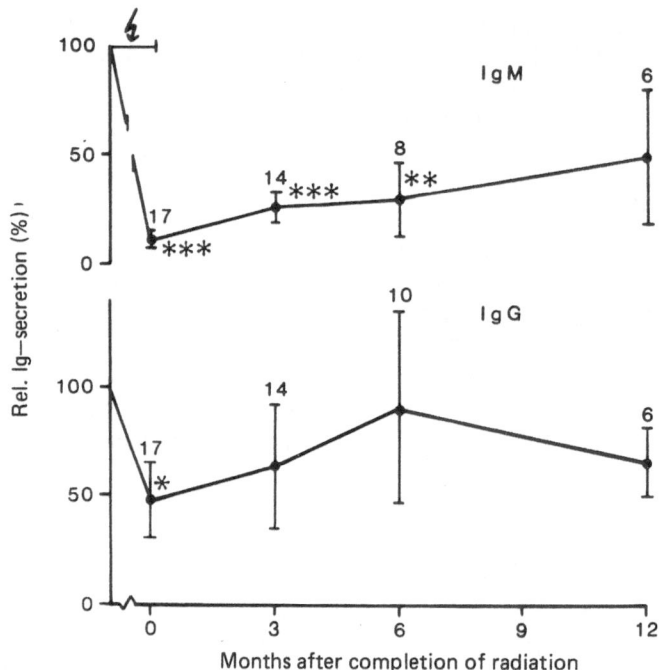

Figure 1-3. Relative IgG and IgM production in vitro by lymphocytes in presence of PWM (means ±SE). Number of patients is shown for each test. Statistical significance is expressed as * (P < .05), ** (P < .001). Time of radiation therapy is indicated by ♮ .

foremost candidates for radiation injury leading to a decrease of Ig synthesis. However, a possibility of an effect on T cells, which have both suppressor and helper functions, as well as on monocytes must be taken into account. The following experiments were performed to elucidate this question. PWM-induced, in vitro Ig synthesis was measured in co-cultures of B lymphocytes from healthy controls and of T lymphocytes from breast cancer patients collected before and after radiation treatment, respectively (102a). As the amounts of IgG and IgM were the same in these two types of cultures, the influence of T lymphocytes on the decrease of Ig synthesis is less likely. However, the role of monocytes in the postradiation inhibition of PWM-induced Ig synthesis could not be excluded.

No Prognostic Implications

No correlation could be demonstrated between the pretreatment number of lymphocytes and lymphocyte stimulation on one hand and the clinical course of the disease on the other hand (115). Also, no correlation whatsoever was found between the radiation-induced lymphopenia, postradiation PHA and PPD responses, and the recurrence of breast cancer during 4.5 to 7 years (116).

The recovery rate of the peripheral lymphocyte population of the patients who developed distant metastases was the same as that of those who remained disease-free during this period (105). Thus the observed disorders in the immunologic reactivity appeared to stay below the threshold of a clinical effect.

Chemotherapy

Cytostatics

Adjuvant combination chemotherapy was recently introduced in the management of relatively advanced operable breast cancer (117). Initially chlorambucil, methotrexate, and 5-fluorouracil were combined (LMF treatment), but later chlorambucil was replaced by cyclophosphamide (CMF). LMF consisted of 12 cycles, each with 600 mg/m^2 of 5-fluorouracil, 50 mg/m^2 of methotrexate, and 15 mg/m^2 of chlorambucil. CMF consisted of 12 cycles, each with 600 mg/m^2 of 5-fluorouracil, 40 mg/m^2 of methotrexate, and 100 mg/m^2 of cyclophosphamide by mouth.

Lymphocyte Subpopulations

Cyclic treatment with cytostatic drugs reduced the blood lymphocyte population by approximately 40% within a few cycles, and lymphocyte counts remained at this level during the whole treatment. An incomplete repopulation started when therapy was finished, but lymphocyte counts were still decreased several months thereafter. Non-T cells, defined by EAC or ME (mouse erythrocyte) rosette formation, were somewhat more reduced than T cells forming E rosettes (118). Lymphocytes with Fc-receptors for IgG (EA cells) were reduced in a similar way. Blood lymphocyte counts and numbers of EA-cells in blood were normalized 4 to 6 years following adjuvant cyclic chemotherapy for breast cancer (119). T-helper and T-suppressor lymphocyte subsets determined with monoclonal antibodies against lymphocyte differentiation antigens (120) showed different kinetics during CMF treatment. T-helper-cell counts were much more reduced than T-suppressor-cell counts, which were only slightly affected. The differential depletion of the two subsets resulted in a reduced T-helper/T-suppressor ratio persisting still 2 to 3 years after CMF therapy. This ratio was 2.4 on an average prior to chemotherapy and 1.1 to 1.6, on an average, during the first year after chemotherapy.

Lymphocyte Functions

Responses to stimulation with PHA, PPD, or allogeneic lymphocytes (MLC reaction) were reduced to a varying extent during chemotherapy (Fig. 1-4) and were not substantially restituted within 15 months after

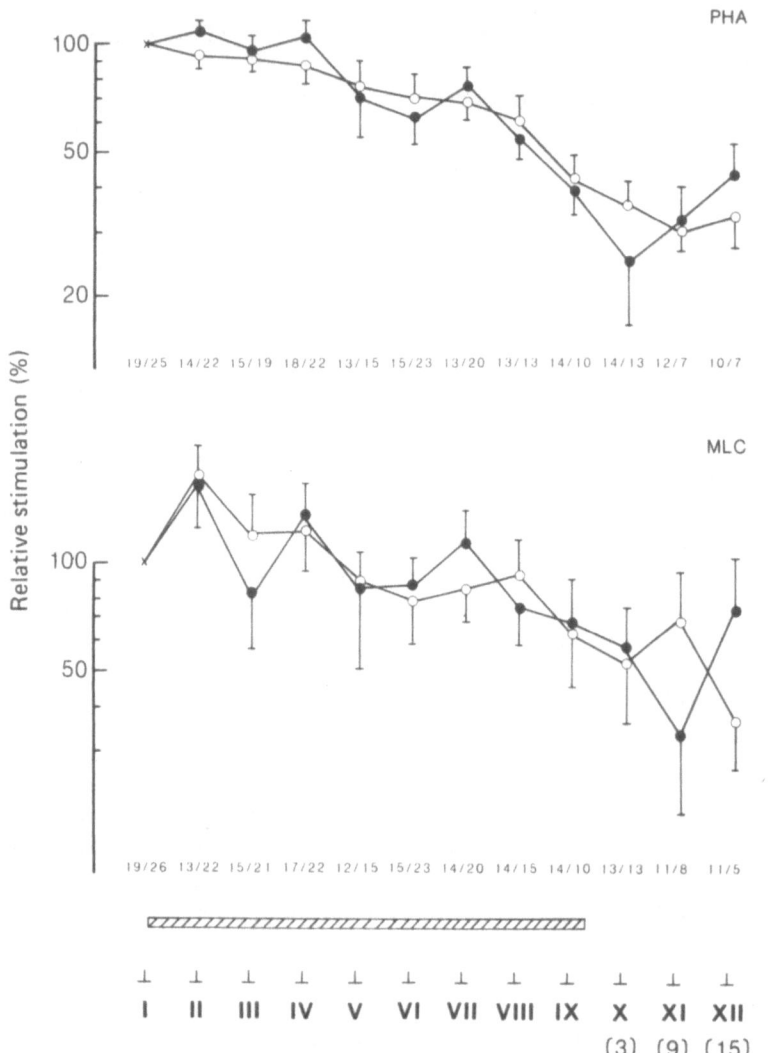

Figure 1-4. PHA and MLC reactivity during and after LMF chemotherapy for patients free of disease 4.5–6 years after LMF treatment and patients who relapsed. Mean values ±SE are given. Arabic numbers at bottom of each diagram indicate number of disease-free relapsed patients. Total period of chemotherapy is indicated by ▨.

Sample numbers are given with Roman numerals at bottom of figure. Arabic figures in brackets indicate time period in months after completion of chemotherapy. Differences between means were statistically nonsignificant (122).

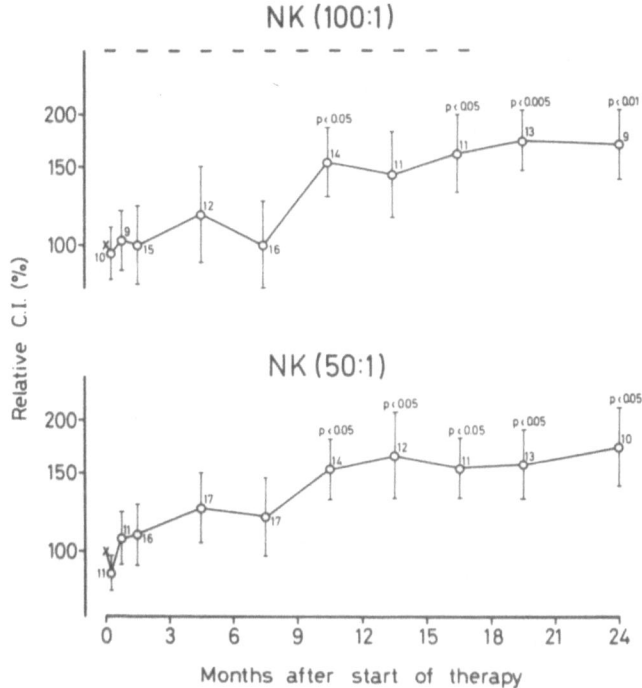

Figure 1-5. Changes of relative NK activity of blood lymphocytes against Chang cells during and after CMF therapy. Mean values ±SE are given, and number of patients are shown at the symbols. Statistically significant changes are indicated by *P* values (154).

completion of chemotherapy. Spontaneous cytotoxicity (NK activity) for 51Cr labeled Chang cells increased during CMF therapy and remained elevated thereafter despite the fact that EA cells, capable of exerting NK activity, were reduced (Fig. 1-5). NK activity was the only lymphocyte function shown to exhibit a relative increase during therapy with cytostatic drugs. Four to 6 years following treatment, relative NK activity was still moderately elevated, whereas PHA stimulation and MLC reactivity were restituted to levels of healthy, age-matched women (119).

Prognostic Implications

The prognostic significance of clinical and immunologic variables assessed after surgery but before the start of chemotherapy was evaluated statistically in a group of 45 operated breast cancer patients who had undergone surgery and who had received LMF or CMF chemotherapy. It was confirmed that the tumor stage and doses of cytostatic drugs had prognostic significance, whereas various immunologic parameters had not (121).

The relation between recurrent disease and various lymphocyte sub-populations and reactivity was examined in patients who had received LMF 4.5 to 6 years previously (122). The patients were divided into those who had remained disease-free and those who relapsed during the period of follow-up. There were no differences between the two patient groups in the immunologic parameters during chemotherapy or in the repopulations thereafter (Figs. 1-4, 1-5).

Bestatin

There is an array of agents that are tested for their immunopotentiating properties in animals and man. Some of these such as mycobacterial ethanol residue (MER), biostim, lipopolysaccharides, and picibanil are derived from bacteria whereas others such as glucans, levan, schizphyl-lan, and Bestatin are derived from fungi. There is also much interest in substances like thymic hormones and various lymphokines, which are natural substances of mammals known to affect the maturation of lymphocytes and to regulate immune responses. In addition, a number of chemically synthesized compounds are being tested for their immunopotentiating properties. Among these are levamisole, cimetidine, indomethacin, and inositil.

Most immunopotentiating agents seem to affect several functions of both lymphocytes, monocytes, and granulocytes, and it is difficult or impossible to predict which agent would be most adequate in different clinical situations. Bestatin has been selected here as a good example of such agents because it is orally active, chemically defined, and relatively nontoxic.

Animal Studies

In 1976 (2S, 3R)-3-amino-2-hydroxy-4-phenylbutanoyl L-leucine (Bestatin) was discovered in the culture broth of *Streptomyces olivoreticuli* (123). This compound was observed to be a potent, competitive inhibitor of the enzymes aminopeptidase B and leucine aminopeptidase, which are known to be associated with the outer membrane of most mammalian cells, including the lymphoid (124,125). The agent was, therefore, tested for its possible immunomodulatory activity.

Administration of Bestatin to rodents augmented delayed-type hypersensitivity reactions (126,127). This effect was most pronounced in immunosuppressed animals (128). Treatment of mice with Bestatin also increased the generation of splenic antibody-forming cells following immunization with SRBC (126,127). In addition, prolonged treatment of old mice with Bestatin reversed the age-dependent change of ADCC activity in the spleen (127).

In a series of experiments it was shown that treatment of mice with Bestatin alone or in combination with certain cytotoxic drugs rendered them more resistant to transplantable tumors (124,128,129). It was also observed that Bestatin treatment diminished the incidence of tumors in methylcholantrene-treated animals (128). Moreover, chronic treatment of mice with Bestatin significantly reduced the spontaneous tumor development (127), possibly in part because of an activation of tumoricidal macrophages by this agent (127,25).

Immunomodulatory Activity of Bestatin in Human Systems

The mitogenic responses of human blood lymphocytes to specific antigens or polyclonal mitogens in vitro are not affected by Bestatin. This conclusion was drawn from experiments in which the cells were either pretreated with the compound or present during mitogen exposure (130). However, the release of mitogenic factors from PHA-pulsed human lymphocytes was strongly enhanced by Bestatin (131). Treatment of human lymphocytes with Bestatin also increased the NK activity of the cells and possibly also the lectin-dependent cellular cytotoxicity (130). There was no indication, however, that human monocytes become cytotoxic after Bestatin exposure in vitro (11). In addition to its effects on lymphocytes, Bestatin exposure of human granulocytes and monocytes in vitro significantly enhanced their phagocytic activity (132,133). Treatment of patients with advanced cancer with Bestatin increased the frequency of lymphocytes forming rosettes with SRBC, augmented the NK activity, and enhanced the phagocytic activity of granulocytes and monocytes (132,134,135). In addition, the phagocytic activity of granulocytes from patients with furunculosis, which was shown to be significantly impaired, was increased after oral Bestatin treatment (136). Mitogenic responses were not changed (134).

The biologic effects observed could possibly be due to Bestatin-induced changes in the cell membranes, as in vitro exposure of lymphocytes to the drug increased their capacity to form rosettes with SRBC (137) and interfered with the turnover of cell-membrane-associated Fc-receptors for IgG (138).

Clinical Trials with Bestatin

A number of prospective trials have been started during recent years to assess the clinical value of adjuvant Bestatin treatment in various types of cancer. In one ongoing Japanese trial, patients with melanoma Stages Ib and II are randomized into two treatment groups following chemotherapy and surgery: 30 mg daily of oral Bestatin or no further treatment. The last interim report showed a significantly improved survival of the Bestatin-treated group (139). Improved survival has also been reported in patients receiving Bestatin as an adjunct to chemotherapy in acute nonlymphocytic leukemia (140).

Two trials have been started in Sweden to assess the clinical value of adjuvant Bestatin treatment in cancer: one in prostatic carcinoma (141) and one in urinary bladder carcinoma (142). The latter will be described briefly since most of the patients who enter this trial are being monitored with respect to some hemopoietic and immunologic parameters.

Eligible patients must have biopsy-proven transitional cell carcinoma of the urinary bladder. After local radiation therapy (64 Gy) half of the patients, stratified according to T-category, receive 10 mg of oral Bestatin three times daily for at least 1 year. The other patients do not receive any further treatment. The blood lymphocyte counts of both patient groups are reduced to approximately 40% at completion of treatment. Currently there is no indication that repopulation of lymphocytes or any other cell type in the blood proceeds faster in the Bestatin-treated patients. A striking difference between the two groups, however, is that the frequency of lymphocytes forming rosettes with SRBC is significantly higher in the Bestatin-treated patients 1 month after start of treatment (62% *vs* 50%, $P < .01$). Thereafter the frequency of these cells declines, and at 3 months it approaches the level of the nontreated group.

Some of the bladder cancer patients were also examined with respect to NK activity against Chang liver cells using a 4 h 51Cr-release assay. The results obtained show that the NK activity is only increased in those

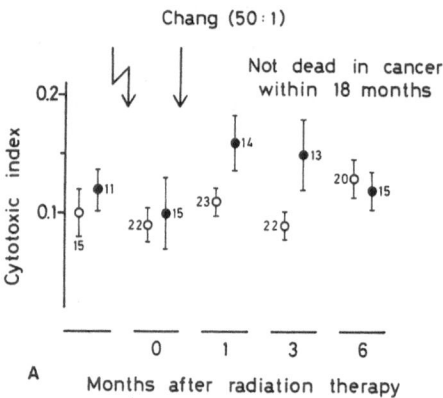

Figure 1-6A. Relative NK activity for Chang cells at a lymphocyte: Target cell ratio of 50 : 1 expressed as an index, or pui ified blood lymphocytes obtained from patients with bladder cancer before and at various times after local radiation therapy (indicated by ꜝ). At completion of irradiation some of the patients received daily oral Bestatin treatment (indicated by ↓). Patients who were allocated to Bestatin treatment are symbolized by ● and those without Bestatin by ○. M ±SE are presented and figures at the symbols show number of patients tested. Data presented are obtained from patients with a relatively good prognosis. Note increased NK activity after 1 and 3 months of Bestatin treatment ($P < .02$ and $P < .01$, respectively)

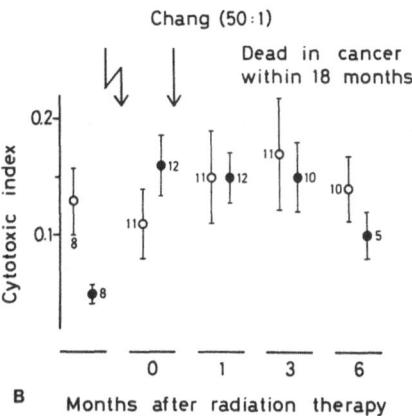

Figure 1.6B. Data analogous to those presented in Fig. 1-6A except that the patients had a relatively poor prognosis. Note that Bestatin treatment did not increase NK activity compared to non-Bestatin treated group.

Bestatin-treated patients who did not die of cancer within 18 months. This is illustrated in Fig. 1-6A, which shows that the NK activity was significantly augmented after 1 and 3 months of Bestatin administration, but there was no difference at 6 months. Bestatin treatment did not increase NK activity in patients who died of cancer within 18 months (Fig. 1-6B).

The results described above suggest that at least some of the immunopotentiating properties of Bestatin become exhausted after prolonged administration. This raises the question of whether Bestatin should be given intermittently rather than continuously. The observation that NK activity was not increased in patients with a relatively poor prognosis further suggests that the Bestatin dose should be increased. Despite these uncertain factors, the preliminary clinical results look promising. There is a trend toward an improved disease-free survival in patients treated with Bestatin (142). This also seems to be the case in patients with carcinoma of the prostate who receive Bestatin as an adjunct to radiation therapy (141).

Clinical Trials with BCG in Acute Myeloid Leukemia

A relatively large number of early immunotherapy trials in acute myeloid leukemia (AML) have been summarized (143–146). Conclusions are cautious becauses of differences in trial design. Some trials were randomized, others were not. Some used only so-called nonspecific immunotherapy with BCG or levamisol, others tried hopefully more specific approaches, including irradiated or nonirradiated, usually allogeneic leukemic cells.

Patient numbers in many of the trials were limited. The general impression, however, is that many well-designed early trials showed a statistically significant but relatively limited prolongation of survival and, in some cases, of duration of the first remission. This impression is supported by our own results (146,147) and by the composite statistical analysis of the best trials by Vogler. Almost all studies yielding not significant difference between the treatment groups showed a trend in favor of immunotherapy. This is true also of the Medical Research Council trial, where significant results were found in some analyses, but not in others.

Later, however, several trials were published where no statistically significant difference was found, and Vogler even found an apparently harmful effect of immunotherapy in one trial. Several of these negative studies were performed by the same groups, with presumably the same skill and care, which had previously found statistically significant effects. It was suggested that patient groups with more than 49% complete remissions did not show any statistically significant effects of immunotherapy in contrast to groups with lower remission frequencies. Since advances in combination chemotherapy and in maintenance treatment have continuously increased remission frequencies in acute leukemia, this could explain why earlier results seemed better than the later ones. One could also speculate that patients who achieved remission with earlier, moderately efficient chemotherapy had leukemias that were more immunotherapy sensitive.

Summary

Currently, the most probable theory of tumor surveillance is neither the existence of any tumor-specific, antigen-dependent, T-cell-mediated cytotoxic effect that could eliminate spontaneous tumors in man and that could be used for some kind of vaccination against tumors, nor the complete absence of any surveillance or defense systems against tumors. What is probable is the cooperation of a number of antigen-independent, relatively weakly cytotoxic or possibly only cytostatic humoral and cellular effects, including nutritional immunity, tumor necrosis factor, certain cytokines, and the cytotoxic effects mediated by macrophages, NK cells, NK-like cells, and certain stimulated T-cells.

One question remaining to be solved is why these antigen-independent effects do not attack normal cells. A number of plausible hypotheses are discussed.

The hypothetical surveillance system is modulated both by traditional cancer treatment and by attempts at immunomodulation. Radiotherapy reduced the T-helper cell function for almost a decade, but not those of macrophages or NK cells. T-cell changes have no prognostic implication, supporting, perhaps, the suggestion of a major role for macrophages and NK cells.

Cyclic adjuvant chemotherapy reduces the peripheral lymphocyte population and several lymphocyte functions but not NK activity. Most of the parameters were normalized some years following treatment, but NK activity remained elevated and Th/Ts cell ratio was still decreased. This might possibly be taken to support the surveillance role of NK cells.

Bestatin increases the frequency of lymphocytes forming rosettes with sheep red blood cells (but not their mitogenic responses), enhances NK activity, and augments the phagocytic capacity of granulocytes and monocytes (but not their cytotoxic activity). Improved survival with Bestatin treatment following chemotherapy has been observed in patients with melanoma Stages 1b and II and in patients with acute nonlymphatic leukemia, where BCG also seems active, although possibly only in patient groups with less than 49% complete remissions.

References

1. Ogier C., Sjögren A.M., Reizenstein P.: *Cancer Immunol. Immunother.* 12:241, 1982.
2. Braun P.B., Harris J.E.: *Cancer Immunol. Immunother.* 15:165, 1983.
3. Ray P.K.: *Immunobiology of Transplantation, Cancer and Pregnancy* (ed. P.K. Ray), Pergamon Press, 1983.
4. Olsson L., Mathé G., Reizenstein P.: *Clinical Chemotherapy 3: Antineoplastic chemotherapy* (ed. Karrer), Grune and Stratton Inc., New York.
5. Herberman R.B.: *Adv. Cancer Res.* 1920:7, 1974
6. Gutterman J.V., Hersch E.M., Mavligit G.M., Freireich E.J., Rossen R.D., Butler W.T., McCredie K.B., Bodey G.P., Rodriguez V.: *Natl. Cancer Inst. Monogr.* 37:163, 1973.
7. Vanky F., Stjärnsvärd C.: *In Vitro Methods in Cell Mediated and Tumor Immunity*, Vol II.
8. Uden A.M., Lindemalm C., Pauli C., Vanky F., Reizenstein P.: *Cancer Immunol Immunother.* 4:239, 1978.
9. Pauli C., Vanky F., Hast R., Lindemalm C., Uden A.M., Reizenstein P.: *Cancer Immunol. Immunother.* 5:1, 1978.
10. Esaki K., Hersch E.M., Keating M., Dyre S., Hollinshead A., McGredie K.B., Mavligit G.M., Gutterman J.V., 1978.
11. Vanky F., Willems J., Kreichbergs A., Aparisi T., Andreen M., Broström L.A., Nilsonne V., Klein E., Klein G.: *Cancer Immunol. Immunother.* 16:11, 1983.
12. Vanky F., Peterfly A., Böök K., Willems J., Klein K., Klein G.: *Cancer Immunol. Immunother.* 16:17, 1983.
13. Canon C., Ogier C., Reizenstein P., Goutner A., de Vassal F., Mathé G.: *Biomedicine and Pharmacotherapy* 37:90, 1983.

14. Miale T.D., Stenke Å.L., Lindblom J.B., Sjögren A.M., Reizenstein P., Uden A.M., Lawson D.L.: *Acta Haemat.* 68:3, 1982.
15. Biberfeld P., Christensson B., Beran M., Hast R., Reizenstein P., Skoog L., Öst Å., Olsson L.: First International Workshop on Human Leukocyte Differentiation Antigens. Paris, 1982.
16. Olsson L., Mathé G.: *Cancer Res.* 37:1743, 1977.
17. Biberfeld P., Christensson B., Beran M., Hast R., Reizenstein P., Skoog L., Öst Å., Olsson L.: Correlative studies on differentiation patterns and clinical behavior of ANLL. In First International Workshop on Human Leukocyte Differentiation Antigens. Paris, 7-11/11, 1982.
18. Reizenstein P.: *Hematologic Stress Syndrome,* Praeger, New York, 1983.
19. Carswell E.A., Old L.J., Kassel R.L., Green S., Fiore N., Williamson B.: *Proc. Natl. Acad. Sci., USA* 72:3666, 1975.
20. Granger G.A., Hiserodt J.C., Ware C.F.: *Biology of the Lymphokines.* Cohen S., Pick E., Oppenheim J.J. (eds.), Acad. Press., New York, p. 141.
21. Schultz R.M., Papamatheakis J.D., Chirigos M.A.: *Science* 197:674, 1977.
22. Hibbs J.B.: In the macrophage in neoplasia (ed. K.M.A. Fin), Acad. Press, New York, p. 83, 1976.
23. Shen L., Guyre P.M., Fanger M.G.: *Molecular Immunology,* 21:167, 1984.
24. Schorlemmer H.V., Bosslet K., Sedlace K.H.H.: *Cancer Res.* 43:4148, 1983.
25. Santoli D., Trinchieri G., Moretta L., Zmijewski C., Korrowski M.H.: *Clin. Exp. Imm.* 33:309, 1978.
26. Masucci G., Masucci M.G., Bejarano M.T., Klein E.: *J. Immunol. Methods* 63:57, 1983.
27. Salata R. A., Schacter B.Z., Ellner J.J.: *Clin Exp. Immunol.* 52:185, 1983.
28. Shau H., Dawson J.K.: *Cancer Immunol. Immunother.* 13:24, 1982.
29. Flexman J.P., Shellam G.R.: *Brit. J. Cancer* 42:41, 1980.
30. Ransom J.H., Pintus C., Evans C.H.: *Int. J. Cancer* 32:93, 1983.
31. Mandeville R., Sombo F.M., Rocheleau N.: *Cancer Immunol. Immunother.* 15:17, 1983.
32. Olinescu A., Hristescu S., Sjöquist J., Ghetie V.: *Immunology Letters* 6:231, 1983.
33. Mazumder A., Rosenstein M.: *Proc. Am. Assoc. Cancer Res.* 23:833, 1983.
34. Grimm E.A., Wilson D.J., Rosenberg S.H.: *Proc. Am. Ass. Cancer Res.* 23:835, 1983.
35. Vose B.M., White W.: *Cancer Immunol. Immunother.* 15:227, 1983.
36. De Vries J.E., Spits H.: *J. Immunol.* 132:510, 1984.
37. Parmiani G., Balsari A., Fossati G., Taramelli D., Storchi I., Cascinelli N.: *Proceedings of the Sanrocco 83. Meeting on Biological Response Modifiers* (in press).
38. Mitsuya H., Matis L.A., Megson M., Bunn P.A., Murray C., Mann D.L., Gallo R.C., Broder S.: *J. Exp. Med.* 158:994, 1983.
39. Vadas M.A., Nicola N.A., Metcalf D.: *J. Immunol.* 130(2):795, 1983.
40. Reizenstein P., Ogier C., Sjögren A.M.: *Recent Results in Cancer Research* 75:29, 1980.
41. Kleinerman E.S., Fidler I.J.: *Proc. Am. Assoc. Cancer* 23:842, 1983.
42. Rhodes J., Bishop M., Benfield J.I.: *Science* 203:179, 1979.

43. Ralph P., Williams N., Nakoinz I., Jackson H., Watson J.D.: *J Immunol.* 129(1):427, 1982.
44. Schmitt E., Meuret G., Waldermann F., Hoffmann G.: *Nuklearmedizin* 21(2):49, 1982.
45. Pels E., Deweger R.A., Den Otter W.: *Immunobiol.* 166:84, 1984.
46. Espevik T., Ammerström J.: *Acta Path. Immunol. Scand.* 91:211, 1983.
47. Steplewsky Z., Lubeck M.D., Koprowski H.: *Science* 221:865, 1983.
48. Arends-Merino A., Sjögren A.M., Reizenstein P.: *Anticancer Res.* 3:239, 1983.
49. Hattori T., Hirata F., Hoffman T., Hizuta, Herberman R.B.: *J. Immunol.* 131:662, 1983.
50. Lichtenstein A., Mickel R., Zighelboim J.: *Cellular Immunology* 80:66, 1983.
51. Timonen T., Ortaldo J.R., Herberman R.B.: *J. Exp. Med.* 153:569, 1981.
52. West W.H., Cannon G.B., Kay H.D., Bonnard G.C., Herberman R.B.: *J. Immunol.* 118:355, 1977.
53. Abo T., Balch C.M.: *J. Immunol.* 127:1024, 1981.
54. Zarling J.M., Eskra L., Borden E.C., Horoszewicz J., Carter W.A.: *J. Immunol.* 123:63, 1979.
55. Todd R.F. III., Van Agthoven A., Schlossman S.F., Terhorst C.: *Hybridoma* 1:329, 1982.
56. Perussia B., Trinchieri G., Lebman D., Jauchiewicz, Lange B., Rovera G.: *Blood* 59:382, 1982.
57. Perussia B., Acuto O., Terhorst C. et al: *J. Immunol.* 130:2127, 1983.
58. Phillips J.H., Babcock G.F.: *Immunology Letters* 6:143, 1983.
59. Bai Y., Beverley P.C.L., Knowles R.W., Bodmer W.F.: *Eur. J. Immunol.* 13:521, 1983.
60. Perussia B., Fanning V., Trinchieri G.: *J. Immunol.* 131:223, 1983.
61. Fast L.D., Hansen J.A., Newman W.: *J. Immunol.* 127:448, 1981.
62. Terhorst C., Van Aghtoven A., LeClair K., Snow P., Reinherz E., Schlossman S.: *Cell* 23:771, 1981.
63. Abo T., Cooper M.D., Balch C.M.: *J. Immunol.* 129:1752, 1982.
64. Herberman R.B.: *Immunobiology of Transplantation Cancer and Pregnancy* (ed. P.K. Ray), Pergamon Press, New York, 1983.
65. Lozzio C.B., Lozzio B.B.: *Blood* 45:321, 1975.
66. Roder J.C., Duwe A.: *Nature* 279:451, 1979.
67. Lauzon R.J., Haliotis T., Roder J.C.: *Pathophysiological Aspects of Cancer Epidemiology* (eds. Mathé G., Reizenstein, P.), Pergamon Press (in press).
68. Anderson R.W., Volsky D.J., Greenberg B., Knox S.J., Bechtold T., Kuszynski C., Harada S., Purtilo D.T.: *Leukemia Research* 7:389, 1983.
69. Matera L., Giancotti: *Acta Haemat.* 70:158, 1983.
70. Hersey P., Edwards A., Honeyman M., McCarthy W.H.: *Brit. J. Cancer* 40:113, 1975.
71. Neri A., Brugiatelli M., Ozger T.V., Astaldi G: *Boll Ist Sieroter* 60:394, Milan, 1981.
72. Balch C.M., Tilden A.B., Dougherty P.A., Cloud G., Abo T.: *Proc. Am. Assoc. Cancer Res.* 23:905, 1983.
73. Oshini K., Gonda N., Sumiya M., Kano S.: *Clin. Exp. Immunol.* 40:83, 1980.

74. Koren H.S., Amos D.B., Buckley R.H.: *J. Immunol.* 120:796, 1978.
75. Benczur M., Petranyi C.Gy., Palffy Gy., Varga M., Talas M., Kotsy B., Foldes I., Hollan S.R.: *Clin. Exp. Immunol.* 39:657, 1980.
76. Saxena Q.B., Mezey A., Alder W.H.: *Int. J. Cancer* 26:413, 1980.
77. Faure G., Bene M.C., Tamisier J.N., Thomas P.: *Arthritis and Rheumatism* 26:1173, 1983.
78. Ruco L.P., Procopio A., Uccini S., Marcorelli E., Baroni C.D.: *Cancer Res.* 42:2063, 1982.
79. Banarjee D., Thibert R.F.: *Nature* 304:270, 1983.
80. Moore M., Taylor G.M., White W.J.: *Cancer Immunol. Immunother.* 13:56, 1982.
81. Zarling J.M., Kung P.C.: *Nature* 288:394, 1980.
82. Hansson Y., Paulie S., Larsson Å., Lunblad M.L., Perlmann P., Näslund I.: *Cancer Immunol. Immunother.* 16:23, 1983.
83. Mazumder R.W., Grimm E.A., Rosenberg S.A.: *Cancer Immunol. Immunother.* 15:1, 1983.
84. Brooks C.G.: *Nature* 305:155, 1983.
85. Vanky F., Gorsky T., Gorsky Y., Masucci M.G., Klein E.: *J. Exp. Med.* 155:83, 1982.
86. Ullberg M., Jondal M.: *Clin. Exp. Immunol.* 53:101, 1983.
87. Obexer G., Rumpold H., Kraft D.: *Immunbiol.* 165:15, 1983.
88. Garson D., Dokhelar M.C., Vainchenker W., Tursz T.: *Cellular Immunology,* 78:400, 1983.
89. Wright S.C., Weitzen M.L., Kahle R., Granger G.A., Bonavida B.: *J. Immunol.* 130:2479, 1983.
90. Gundersen S., Funderud S., Bloom B.R., Godal B.R.: *Acta Path. Microbiol. Immunol. Scand.* Sect C. 91:137, 1983.
91. Rey A., Klein B., Zagury D., Thierry C., Serroui B.: *Immunology Letters* 6:175, 1983.
92. Kawase I., Brooks C.G., Kuribayashi K., Olabuenaga S., Newman W., Gillis S., Henney C.S.: *J. Immunol.* 131:288, 1983.
93. Aria S., Yamamoto H., Itoh K., Kumagai K.: *J. Immunol.* 131:651, 1983.
94. Mangan K.F., Winkelstein A., Hartnett M.E., Matis S.A.: *Clin. Res.* 30:773A, 1982.
95. Pistoia V., Nocera A., Perata A., Leprini A., Ghio R., Ferrarini M.: *Surv. Synth. Path. Res.* 2:47, 1983.
96. Tarkkanen J., Saksela E., von Willebrand E., Lehtonen E.: *Cellular Immunol.* 79:265, 1983.
97. Herberman R.B., Ortaldo J.R.: *Science* 214:24, 1981.
98. Gorelik E., Bere W.W., Herberman R.B.: *Int. J. Cancer:*33:87, 1984.
99. Droller M.J., Schneider M.U., Perlman P.: *Cell Immunol.* 39:165, 1978.
100. Petrini B., Wasserman J., Glas U., Blomgren H.: *Eur. J. Cancer Clin. Oncol.* 18:921, 1982.
100a. Petrini B., Wasserman J., Blomgren H., Glas U., Baral E., Strender L.E.: *Int. Arch. Allergy Appl. Immunol.* 67:57, 1982.
101. Petrini B., Wasserman J., Blomgren H., Glas U.: *Cancer Letters* 19:27, 1983.
102. Wasserman J., Petrini B., Blomgren H.: *J. Clin. Lab. Immunol.* 7:139, 1982.

102a. Wasserman J., Petrini B., van Stedingk L.V., Blomgren H., Juhlin I.: *J. Clin. Lab. Immunol.* 11:33, 1983.

103. Glas U., Wasserman J.: *Acta Radiol.* 13:83, 1974.

104. Baral E., Blomgren H., Petrini B., Wasserman J.: *Int. J. Radiat. Oncol. Biol. Phys.* 2:289, 1977.

105. Blomgren H., Wasserman J., Wallgren A., Baral E., Petrini B., Ideström K.: *Int. J. Radiat. Oncol. Biol. Phys.* 6:471, 1980.

106. Blomgren H., Wasserman J., Wallgren A., Ideström K., Baral E., Petrini B.: *Int. J. Radiat. Oncol. Biol. Phys.* 5:49, 1979.

107. Wasserman J., von Stedingk L.V., Biberfeld G., Petrini B., Blomgren H., Baral E.: *Clin. Exp. Immunol.* 38:366, 1979.

108. Blomgren H., Wasserman J., Baral E, Petrini B.: *Int. J. Radiat. Oncol. Biol. Phys.* 4:249, 1978.

109. Jarstrand C., Petrini B., Wasserman J., Blomgren H., Strender L.E.: *Anticancer Research* 2:209, 1982.

110. Blomgren H., Rotstein S., Petrini B., Wasserman J., Baral E.: *Radiother. Oncology,* 1:255, 1984.

111. Wasserman J., Melén B., Blomgren H., Glas U., Perlmann P.: *Clin. Exp. Immunol.* 22:230, 1975.

112. Wasserman J., Petrini B., Baral E., Blomgren H., Perlmann P.: *J. Clin. Lab. Immunol.* 1:73, 1978.

113. Blomgren H., Strender L.E., Petrini B., Wasserman J.: *Eur. J. Cancer Clin. Oncol.* 18:637, 1982.

114. Strender L.E., Blomgren H., Wasserman J., Forsgren M., von Stedingk L.V., Petrini B., Wallgren, A.: *Anticancer Research* 3:41, 1983.

115. Baral E., Blomgren H., Petrini B., Wasserman J., Ogenstad S., Silfverswärd C.: *Acta Radiol. Oncol.* 16:417, 1977.

116. Baral E., Blomgren H., Ideström K., Ogenstad S., Petrini B., Silfverswärd C., Wallgren A., Wasserman J.: *Acta Radiol. Oncol.* 18(4):313, 1979.

117. Bonadonna G., Valagussa B.S.: *N. E. J. Med.* 304:10, 1981.

118. Strender L.E., Petrini B., Blomgren H., Wasserman J., Wallgren A., Baral E.: *Acta Radiol. Oncol.* 21:217, 1982.

119. Blomgren H., Rotstein S., Petrini B., Wasserman J.: *Acta Radiol. Oncol.,* in press.

120. Engleman E.G., Benlike C.J., Glickman E., Evans R.L.: *J. Exp. Med.* 153:193, 1981.

121. Rotstein S., Blomgren H., Nilsson B., Petrini B., Wasserman J., Baral E.: To be published.

122. Petrini B., Rotstein S., Blomgren H., Wasserman J., Baral E.: *Anticancer Res.,* in press.

123. Umezawa H., Aoyagi T., Suda., Hamada M., Takeuchi T.: *J. Antibiot,* 29:97, 1976.

124. Aoyagi T., Ishizuka M., Takeuchi T., Umezawa H.: *J. Antibiot.* 30:1221, 1977.

125. Aoyagi T., Suda H., Nagai M., Ogawa K., Suzuki J., Takeuchi T., Umezawa H.: *Biochim. Biophys. Acta* 452:131, 1978.

126. Umezawa H., Ishizuka J., Aoyagi T., Takeuchi T.: 24:857, 1976.

127. Bruley-Rosset M., Florentin I., Kiger N., Schultz J., Mathé G.: *Immunology* 38:75, 1979.

128. Ishizuka M., Masuda T., Kanbayashi N., Fukasawa S., Takeuchi T., Aoyagi T., Umezawa H.: *J. Antibiot.* 33:642, 1980.

129. Umezawa H.: *Antibiot. Chemother.* 24:9, 1978.

130. Blomgren H., Strender L.E., Edsmyr F.: *Small Molecular Immunomodulators of Microbial Origin. Fundamental and Clinical Studies of Bestatin* (ed. Umezawa H.), Japan Scientific Press, 1981, p. 71.

131. Blomgren H.: *Biomedicine* 34:188, 1981.

132. Jarstrand C., Blomgren H.: *J. Clin. Lab Immunol.* 9:193, 1982.

133. Jarstrand C., Blomgren H.: *J. Clin. Lab. Immunol.* 5:67, 1981.

134. Blomgren H., Strender L.E., Edsmyr F.: *Biomedicine* 32:178, 1980.

135. Jarstrand C., Blomgren H.: *J. Clin. Lab. Immunol.* 7:115, 1982.

136. Mattson L., Blomgren H., Holmgren B., Jarstrand C.: *Infection* 11:205, 1983.

137. Blomgren H., Wasserman J.: *Cancer Letters* 11:303, 1981.

138. Blomgren H.: *Human Lymphocyte Differentiation* 1:159, 1981.

139. Ikeda S., Ishihara, K.: 13th International Congress of Chemotherapy. *Proceedings* (eds. Spitzy K.H. and Karrer K.), 1983, p. 204/21.

140. Ota K.: 13th International Congress of Chemotherapy. *Proceedings* (eds. Spitzy K.H., Karrer K.), 1983, p. 204/31.

141. Edsmyr F., Esposti P.L., Andersson L., Näslund I., Blomgren H.: 13th International Congress of Chemotherapy. *Proceedings* (eds. Spitzy K.H., Karrer K.), 1983, p. 245/5.

142. Blomgren H., Edsmyr F., Espositi P.L., Näslund I., Blomgren H.: 13th International Congress of Chemotherapy. *Proceedings* (eds. Spitzy K.H., Karrer K.), 1983, p. 204/44.

143. Reizenstein P., Miale T.: Concluding remarks: Immunotherapy of acute myeloid leukemia in man. In *Immunotherapy of Malignant Diseases* (ed. H. Rainer), F.K. Schattauer Verlag, Stuttgart-New York, 441, 1978.

144. Vogler W.R.: *Cancer Immunol. Immunother.* 9:15, 1981.

145. Urbanitz D., Bückner Th., Pielken H., van de Loo J.: *Klin. Wochenschr.* 61:947, 1983.

146. Reizenstein P. et al: in *Immunotherapy of Cancer: Present Status of Trials in Man* (eds. Terry W.D., Windhorst D.), New York, Raven Press, 1978.

147. Reizenstein P. et al: in *Immunotherapy of Human Cancer* (eds. Terry W.D. and Rosenberg S.A.), Excerpta Medica, New York, 1982.

148. Vodinelich L.: *Hamatol. Bluttransf.* 28:472, 1983.

149. Kennett R.H., Johak Z.L., Byrd R.: In *Methods in Cancer Research,* Vol. XX:355, 1982.

150. Taylor G.M., Bradley B.A.: *Cancer Immunol. Immunother.* 15:39, 1983.

151. Vilien M., Troye-Blomberg M., Perlmann P., Wolf H., Rasmussen F.: *Cancer Immunol. Immunother.* 14:137, 1983.

152. Masucci G., Masucci M.G., Klein E.: *Cell. Immunol.* 69:21, 1982.

153. Vanky F., Masucci M.G., Bejarano M.T., Klein E.: *Int. J. Cancer* 133:185, 1984.

154. Blomgren H. et al: *Chemotherapia* 1:402, 1982.

Chapter 2

Immunity and Its Role in Conventional Cancer Therapy

P.K. Ray, M. Seshadri, and T.B. Poduval

> Drugs can only repress symptoms. They cannot erradicate the
> disease. The true remedy for all diseases is nature's remedy. . . .
> Nature has provided, in the white corpuscles as you call them—in
> the phagocytes as we call them—a natural means of devouring and
> destroying all disease germs. There is at bottom only one genu-
> inely scientific treatment for all diseases, and that is to stimulate
> the phagocytes. Stimulate the phagocytes . . . they devour the
> disease, and the patient recovers. Unless, of course, he's too far
> gone.
>
> George Bernard Shaw
> Sir Bloomfield Bonnington in "The Doctor's Dilemma"
> Royal Gold Theatre, London
> 20 November 1906

Contents

(continued)

Cancer Therapy and the Immune Process

During the last several decades the therapeutic management of cancer has been practiced, with some success, through surgery, chemotherapy, and radiation therapy. Complete eradication of the disease, however, has proved an elusive goal. Surgical success has been attributed to the physical removal of the tumor mass; success with radiotherapy has been attributed to the direct killing of tumor cells by means of ionizing radiation; and success with chemotherapy is due to either the killing of tumor cells using cytotoxic drugs, or to controlling their proliferation using cytostatic drugs.

Little attention has been paid to the fact that underlying these successes might be a common factor, the functioning of the patient's immune system.

There is abundant literature about conventional modalities of therapy having immunosuppressive effects in the host. Such suppression may counter the therapeutic effect because it may aid the process of metastasis. To the extent that cures have been achieved, immunosuppression may have greatly compromised that benefit. In this chapter we review the evidence that circumvention of immunosuppression does, in fact, take place under certain circumstances and that when it does, the chances for success of conventional modalities of treatment are enhanced. As the number of pertinent references is overwhelmingly voluminous, we ask for understanding if we have not been entirely exhaustive in our citations of the literature.

Whereas chemotherapy is resorted to whenever a tumor is nonresectable and whenever there is a likelihood of dissemination, surgery or radiotherapy is used to treat localized disease. Mortality in most cancers is due to dissemination of tumors from a primary site to distant sites, where proliferation occurs. Our present understanding of the defense mechanisms in the tumor-bearing host suggests that the immune system has an important role in the control of metastatic spread and growth of tumors. The usefulness of an active immune response in a host bearing a progressive tumor is equivocal. Therefore, the aim of any approach to controlling cancer should be to utilize optimally the immune mechanisms operative in the tumor-bearing host to achieve maximal therapeutic benefit.

Effector Cells in Antitumor Immunity: In Vitro and In Vivo Relevance

The effector cells involved in antitumor activity include effector T cells, killer cells, macrophages, nonspecific natural killer cells, and cells mediating antibody-dependent cell-mediated cytotoxicity (ADCC). The activity of these cells is dependent on the helper and suppressor lymphocytes and on the lymphokines produced by the various cells involved in the immune function. Thus, immune reactions involve a complex network of interacting factors and are ultimately dependent on the antigenicity and immunogenicity of the tumor. There is growing evidence that malignant cells contained in primary tumors may be heterogeneous with regard to a number of their characteristics, including metastatic potential, chemotherapeutic responsiveness, radiosensitivity, metabolic properties, growth rate, hormone receptors, pigment production, and immunogenicity (1–3).

Contact between an antigen and a lymphocyte receptor can have any one of a number of outcomes, including activation, tolerance induction, blockade of receptors, induction of helper activity, induction of suppression, or none of these, depending on a multitude of operational variables. The persistence of tumor cells bearing new antigens within a living animal with an intact immune system is no longer seen as an impossible flouting of immunologic dogma (4). Impairment of cell-mediated immunity and macrophage function has been found in patients with various tumors by a number of investigators (5–20). However, it is difficult to generalize the findings and to pinpoint a defect in the immune system because of a number of factors. These include the tissue of origin of the tumor, site of the tumor, degree of differentiation, and the varied nature of tests employed. Because most of our knowledge has come from a variety of in vitro studies wherein it was observed that various effector cells are reactive to some extent, it is difficult to ascribe a dominant role to any one of them. It is likely that some systems seemingly operative in vitro may be totally ineffective in vivo or may be of minimal importance. The functional differences between in vivo and in vitro systems could be due to a number of reasons; some of the following seem especially worth mentioning. In vitro, effector cells and target cells are brought into close proximity for the determination of cytotoxicity, and a much higher concentration of effector cells is used than may be achievable in vivo. Some of the effector cells that are very efficient in vitro may not have the ability to migrate to the tumor site. These cells may have more reactive capability for controlling metastatic spread to a remote site rather than having control at the primary site of the tumor. In vitro, some of the restricting factors operative in the microenvironment of the tumor may be eliminated by careful manipulation, or else unknowingly.

In experimental tumor immunology, effector cells are usually obtained from lymph nodes and spleen, whereas in clinical studies the source of effector cells is usually peripheral blood lymphocytes or, when available, the draining lymph node. In the recent past the importance of immune cells sequestered within the milieu of the tumor has been recognized, and these cells have been investigated for their immune potential (21–28). Haskill et al (29) showed that the nature of effector cells found within the tumor mass may vary from tumor to tumor and that the action of those found within the tumor mass may or may not correlate with the action of those found in spleen, peripheral lymph nodes, or blood of the same tumor-bearing animal. Immunocytes derived from the tumor mass may possess greater antitumor immunity, both specific and nonspecific, than the cells derived from systemic organs (22,26,29–33) or they may have less activity (34). There is also evidence that such immunocytes may exert a negative influence on resistance (35). We still are not fully informed about (a) the mechanisms that control accumulation of effector cells in the tumor site, (b) the relative contribution of the local tissue environment, (c) the different capabilities of cells derived from a general pool, or from a regional lymphoid organ, to mediate cytotoxic reaction, (d) the variation in the expression of antigenic property by the tumor, and (e) the relative immunoresistance of the cells in different regions of the body. Future research may reveal more about these areas so that the tumor-host relationship will become more understandable.

Histologic investigations of tumors and their invasive zones have yielded useful information, but the method limits us to identifying cell types in broad categories without giving any information about the functional nature of the cells. Use of immunologic markers, such as cell surface markers mediating different functions, and antibodies directed against different lymphokines may help to study the immune response. Even with broad identification of cells, three categories of interaction among immunocompetent cells have been distinguished in the invasive zones of carcinoma of the uterine cervix (36). Lymphocyte-macrophage association and blastogenic transformation of lymphocytes were found in microinvasive cancer. Thirty percent of patients with invasive cancer, characterized by low histologic malignancy, showed a striking mixture of lymphocytes and plasmacytes and a highly significant inability of mononuclear cells to differentiate into mature macrophages. Sixty percent of cases with rapid invasion of cancer showed dispersed aggregation of monocytes and macrophages. The lymphoid elements exhibited an unequal tendency to differentiate.

Heterogeneity of Effector Cells

In addition to difficulties in identifying cells and inherent problems of in vitro methods, there is the problem that different cells may perform the same function. This is exemplified by suppressor cells. Some suppressor systems are specific for one antigen only (37–40) while others exhibit nonspecific activity, suppressing immune response to relevant antigen as well as to irrelevant antigens and mitogens (41). Suppressor cells have been described as macrophages in some systems (41,42), as T cells (39,40,43) or B cells (44) in others, and as null cells (37,45,46) in still others. In some patients with Hodgkin's disease the suppressor cells are described as T cells, whereas in others with the same disease the suppressor cells are described as macrophages (47). The efficiency of suppressor

cells varies with different tumor host systems (37,45). The physical properties of suppressor cells in various tumor host systems also vary. Some
supressor cells are sensitive to x-irradiation (48) while others are resistant to it (49). Some are sensitive to hydrocortisone (50) or cyclophosphamide (51) while others are resistant (52). Mitomycin C inactivates
some suppressor cells (53) but not others (54). The velocity of suppressor
cells in the bovine serum albumin (BSA) gradient is different from one
system to another (55,56). In some cases the tumors themselves or the
viruses infecting them stimulate immunosuppression (57–59).

Lang et al (60) reported interaction between two different mechanisms
of macrophage-mediated cytotoxicity—the lymphokine-induced and antibody-dependent cytotoxicity. Compared with normal hosts, tumor-bearing mice were more susceptible (tenfold more) to the immunosuppressive
effect of tumor cells; this increase in susceptibility was mediated by a
population of splenic adherent cells (61). The presence of different subpopulations of macrophages in the lymph node and spleen may also be of
importance. According to some data, spleen macrophages of the S-type
exhibit suppressive activity in their interaction with T_1 lymphocytes. Both
the spleen and the lymph nodes contain L-type macrophages capable of
stimulating T_2 lymphocytes (62). Tumor cells may switch on the host's
own suppressor mechanism (63,64). The tumor-cell-triggered suppressor
mechanism has been shown to require collaboration of at least two populations of macrophages, splenic and peritoneal, in a specific sequence
(splenic must precede peritoneal macrophages) (62).

The variability in the tumor-host system is also reported in studies on
natural killer (NK) cells, which effect spontaneous cell-mediated cytotoxicity. NK cells have been shown to be important in the surveillance mechanism operative in nude mice. Animals deficient in NK cells, such as
beige mutant mice, have been shown to be prone to metastatic spread and
to have low resistance to transplantable syngeneic leukemias (65). There
is one report of NK cells infiltrating solid tumors induced by methylcholanthrene (66). But there is still no definite knowledge about the in vivo
relevance of NK cell activity measured in vitro using peripheral blood
lymphocytes of patients. Draining lymph node cells exhibit the same degree of NK activity as control lymphocytes from normal lymph nodes
(67,68). Both activities are significantly lower on a cell-to-cell basis than
are blood lymphocytes (68). In patients with localized tumors, NK cell
activity has not been found to be significantly different from that of
healthy controls (68,69). Only patients with disseminated disease show
decreased NK cell activity (70,71). NK cell activity may be reflective of
the functional state of the hematopoietic system (72). Most conditions
associated with impairment of bone marrow function, such as leukemias,
preleukemias, osteomyelofibrosis, polycythemia vera, and myeloma have
been found to be associated with a more or less pronounced depression of
NK cell activity (73). It has been suggested that the NK cell activity of

human peripheral blood lymphocytes against tumor targets may reflect, in some way, the functional integrity of the hematopoietic system, rather than indicating a degree of antitumor immunity (73).

Lymphokines in Tumor-Bearing Hosts

Lymphokines are important mediators of immune function but have received little systematic investigative attention, except for studies on the detection of lymphokine activity in the sera of certain cancer patients. Lymphokine assays such as the leukocyte-migration inhibition test, and direct LIF assay utilizing peripheral blood lymphocytes as a lymphokine source, have been used primarily as indicators of sensitization of the host to tumor antigen. It is important to realize that a negative result in such tests could mean any of the following three things: (a) the host's lymphocytes are not sensitized to tumor antigen, (b) sensitization may be present and lymphokine production may be affected, or (c) sensitization and lymphokine production may be there, but the indicator cells may lack the ability to respond to the lymphokines.

The importance of macrophages in direct tumor killing and in tumor regression has been well documented (74–78) and lymphokine-containing supernatants capable of activating monocytes have been shown to be of therapeutic benefit in regression of local tumor lesions (79,80). Snyderman and his co-workers found that chemotaxis of macrophages is abnormal in melanoma patients (81), breast cancer patients (82), and patients bearing other solid tumors (83–85). Surgical removal of tumor-normalized chemotaxis suggests that the tumor itself was the cause of the defect in monocyte function.

Heterogeneity of Tumor Cells

In addition to the variability in the effector systems already mentioned, heterogeneity of the tumor also plays a crucial role in determining the nature of immune response to it. It is generally believed that tumors induced by chemical carcinogens have tumor-associated transplantation antigens (TATAs) that do not show cross-reactivity; it is believed also that TATA of virally induced tumors are common to all tumors induced by the same virus (86). This concept of tumor immunology has been questioned recently; some authors described cross-immunity among chemically induced tumors (87–93).

Martin and Imamura (94) suggest that altered expression of histocompatibility antigens may be a common, although not invariable, feature of tumor cells. These alterations may benefit the host by providing new tumor antigens, but they may also impede host immunity by restricting the host's capacity to develop and utilize cytotoxic T-cell-mediated immunity. Differences in expression of H-2 antigens on the cell surface of a localized T-10 tumor and its metastatic descendant MT-10 were shown.

LT-10 differed qualitatively and quantitatively from MT-10 in expression H-2 antigens (95). Using a highly metastatic tumor variant of a chemically induced DBA/2 lymphoma, Basslet and Schirrmacher (96) showed that tumor cells isolated from liver and bone marrow were TATA-positive, whereas those isolated from spleen were TATA-negative. Tumor variants isolated from spleens of nude mice remained TATA-positive. Loss of TATA expression thus depended on the presence of T cells and may represent an immune escape mechanism produced within clones of tumor cells. The importance of heterogeneity of tumors in eliciting the immune response and of its role in metastases has been reviewed recently (3,64).

Evaluation of the Immune Status of Cancer Patients

The battery of tests now employed to assess the immune status of the patient has given varied prognostic results; some tests correlate with the prognosis (97–99), but others show no correlation (100,101). Therefore, we need to develop comprehensive tests that delineate the defect more precisely. We also need to develop "scales" of antitumor reaction that help to achieve perspective regarding immune status vis-à-vis tumors (102). Any one test may fail to represent responses to those antigens that make for resistance (103). Tests similar to the skin-window technique (83, 104), which would identify responses in the intact host and take into account all attendant variables, are needed as in vitro tests may not truly represent the in vivo situation.

Before resorting to use of cytotoxic agents such as chemotherapeutic drugs or radiation, it is essential to understand that the immune status of the tumor-bearing host; cytotoxic agents do compromise the immune status of the host. Proper evaluation of the immunologic profile of a patient allows the advantage of choosing an appropriate modality of treatment and helps us to avoid the deleterious effects of chemotherapeutic agents through proper circumvention. This consideration is all the more important when we are resorting to circumvention by immunotherapeutic means, because we cannot assume that the understanding we have gained about these procedures from normal recipients would be properly comparable to a host bearing an autochthonous neoplasm (105–109).

Radiotherapy

Radiotherapy (RT) is employed when a tumor is localized. Whole body irradiation (WBI) is also used to control metastasis and lymphoid tumors. Unlike chemotherapy (CT) and immunotherapy, RT is limited by the extension of the tumor. However, tumor size is not a limiting factor in RT, as it is in CT and IT.

RT-Induced Changes in Antitumor Immunity

Effects of radiation on the immune response have been studied in detail during the last 20 years (110,111). Lymphoid tissues and small lymphocytes are extremely radiosensitive and suffer interphase death after irradiation. RT of a tumor not only irradiates the tumor mass, but it also irradiates the lymphoid system, blood, and bone marrow in the vicinity of the tumor. The effect of RT on antitumor response is essentially the same as for any other specific immune response directed against a foreign antigen. Radiation, like CT, kills tumor cells by first-order kinetics. There is doubt about whether the antitumor immune response, which acts by zero-order kinetics in eliminating the remaining viable tumor cells after RT, is kept intact or is abrogated by RT. To reach an understanding we need to know the relationship between RT, the tumor, and the host's immune system.

Radiosensitivity of Elements of Specific Immune Systems

If elements of the immune system happen to be in the radiation field, there will be an alteration in the function of the immune system. Modern cellular immunology helps to delineate the nature of the radiation response to various compartments of the immune system and to the nonlymphoid cells involved in the expression of the immune response. It has been reported that there are two types of specific cytotoxic lymphocytes with reference to the radiosensitivity—one retains cytotoxicity after doses of 2,000 rads and forms the major fraction, the other is markedly inhibited after doses of approximately 500 rads (112). It has been shown that murine cytotoxic lymphocytes activated seven days previously demonstrated cytotoxic activity even after exposure to 20,000 rads in vitro. But, when sensitization was done 21 days previous to irradiation, even doses less than 500 rads were inhibitory (112). This is an important observation because it may be that in the tumor-bearing host the sensitivity of tumor-specific lymphocytes to irradiation depends on their extent of stimulation by tumor antigen. Immunosuppression by WBI does not abrogate concomitant tumor immunity in mice; also, lymphocytes from irradiated tumor-sensitized animals still transfer antitumor immunity adoptively (63,113). Both T and B small lymphocytes die in interphase soon after irradiation, but B cells die more rapidly than T cells. Of the two, antigen-activated T cells appear to be more resistant (114). However, mature B cells, ie, plasma cells, are extremely radiation-resistant (115,116). Moroson and Schechter (117) observed an enhanced cytotoxic reactivity of rat splenic cells after lethal or sublethal irradiation. This could be because x-rays enrich a subpopulation of nonspecific killer cells by preferentially depleting the general pool of a splenic cell population (117). The T-cell subset involved in the suppression of immune response was found to be quite sensitive to radiation (118,119). These observations may have relevance in subjects bearing lymphoid tumors. In addition, they help to explain the augmentation of immune response in certain cases followed by RT. Selective elimination of suppressor cells may be useful in augmenting the generalized immune response, including the antitumor immune response in a tumor-bearing host.

Radiosensitivity of Elements of the Nonspecific Immune Response

In general, the cells involved in nonspecific immune response are relatively radioresistant. NK cells and ADCC in mice were not affected appreciably by 350-rad WBI. Only at a higher dose of 800 rads was there a decrease of 70% in NK cell and ADCC activity (120). In rats substantial loss of NK cell activity was observed with 500-rad WBI, and there was complete elimination of NK cells at 900 rads (121).

Macrophages, especially mature and activated macrophages, are relatively radiation-resistant (122–124). Doses lower than 1,000 rads do not alter the macrophage function. Immune response of macrophages to sheep red blood cells (SRBC) remains unaltered following irradiation (122,123). The above observations suggest that specifically activated components of the lymphoid system, and nonspecific effector cells such as NK cells and macrophages, offer resistance to the immunosuppressive effects of radiation. It is logical to presume that RT, which interacts with the immune system at the effector phase of antitumor immunity, may not alter the antitumor status appreciably, at least in tumors of demonstrable immunogenicity. Summarizing all the above findings, we have a variety of interrelated but separable immunological interactions that differ greatly with respect to their response to radiation damage. This understanding may help to eliminate the negative influences of RT on antitumor immunity. It means that the destructive effect of radiation of the immune system can be put to use in accelerating tumor rejection. At this juncture it is relevant to mention Feldman's observation, wherein he finds accelerated destruction of renal grafts by WBI of recipient rats (125). The possibility of retaining and sometimes increasing host immunity following RT exists, but it depends on a detailed understanding of radiation effects on the immune system.

Recovery of the Immune System Following RT

An important aspect of RT is the opportunity for recovery of immune status following immunosuppression. In mice sensitized against growing tumors, recovery of the spleen following immunosuppression is rapid and proportional to the extent of host sensitization to the tumor. It is also found that tumor-sensitized animals are resistant to the immunodepressive effect of radiation (126). Recovery of the spleen explains the prevention of metastasis in animals irradiated after sensitization with the tumor. There was also retention of Winn-assay demonstrable antitumor immunity in mice immunosuppressed after tumor sensitization. This suggests that specific antitumor immunity is capable of resisting immunosuppression caused by radiation (63).

Lymphoid recovery after RT for breast cancer parallels the recovery of general immune competence to PPD (127). It is often observed that recovery of immune competence depends on the clinical status of the cancer patients. After RT, mitogen response of lymphocytes from patients with recurrent disease continues to decrease, but mitogen response of patients receiving RT, who do not have evidence of disease, increases rapidly. In fact, the post-treatment response exceeds the pretreatment response within 1 to 3 weeks (128). Thus, the recovery pattern after RT may have prognostic value. It has been observed that regeneration of lymph nodes, after WBI, proceeds at a slightly slower pace than does regeneration of the spleen. Regeneration of lymph nodes after local irradiation is extremely rapid, probably owing to the influx of normal immunocompetent cells from nonirradiated lymphoid tissues and the circulating pool of small lymphocytes (129). But a large dose of 3,000 rads result in vascular damage, destruction of stroma, and extreme atrophy (130). Repeated irradiation of local draining nodes prevents both local and distant development of antibody-forming cells (131). These studies help to interpret the results of local RT of solid tumors, eg, breast cancers that involve irradiation of regional lymph nodes.

Immune Status of Patients Receiving RT

The concept of immune surveillance, proposed by Thomas (132), rests on the assumption that potential antitumor immunity works against the development of cancer and that irradiation depresses the antitumor responses. But RT, like CT, deals with established antitumor immunity. In the clinical situation, the criterion used to monitor immune status following RT, in the majority of cases, is the general immune competence, which is thought to reflect antitumor immunity following RT. Effects of RT on the immune response are equivocal. In patients with lung cancer, in vivo response to antigens and also lymphocyte transformations in vitro were impaired; this is in contrast to responses in age- and sex-matched controls. Further impairment of cellular immunity was seen after x-ray therapy (133). Peripheral blood analysis of cancer patients given regional irradiation showed long-term aberration of T and B lymphocytes. Even after 3 years of therapy, many patients had decreased lymphocyte counts. Phytohemagglutinin (PHA) response was also altered for a considerable length of time. Mixed leukocyte reaction (MLR) recovery took from 4 to 5 years (134). In lung cancer patients, E and EAC rosette-forming cells (RFC) plus response to mitogens decreased immediately after RT and continued to decrease for several months (135). In breast cancer the mixed lymphocyte culture (MLC) response of peripheral blood lympho-

cytes was found to decrease after RT. Lymphoid cells collected after RT
inhibited the response and stimulatory capacity of the patient's cryopreserved lymphoid cells that had been obtained before treatment (25). Blomgren observed the appearance of nonspecific suppressor cells in the blood
of breast cancer patients after local radiation therapy (136). RT also resulted in lymphopenia and decreased response to PPD in vitro (136).
Stjernsward reviewed the immunologic alteration after RT for mammary
carcinoma. He suggests a possible relation between radiation-induced
change in the immune system and distant metastases (137). He also found
decreased lymphocyte response to PHA and reduced T-RFC (rosette-
forming T cells) and increased B-RFC (rosette-forming B cells) (138).
Marked and prolonged lymphopenia after local RT is usually observed
(138,139). Byfield et al reported similar findings (35). Usually the T lymphopenia following RT persists for a long time. Postoperative RT for
cancer of the breast resulted in the fall of both B and T lymphocytes. But
the B lymphocyte number reverted to a normal level by the 10th month,
whereas T lymphopenia persisted from 2 to 4 years.

Potentiation of Antitumor Immune Response During RT of Cancer Patients

In contrast to what has been discussed above, many reports indicate an
improvement or recovery of immune response in the host following RT.
For example, Rafla et al reported improvment in PHA and RFC responses
following RT (140). It has been suggested that there is a relationship
between tumor load and immune status. The latter returns to normal
when the tumor load is reduced by RT. This improvement indicates that
immunosuppressive effects, brought about by the growing tumor, are
eliminated by the RT-induced reduction of tumor mass. McCredie found
an increase in the proliferative response of lymphocytes to PHA in patients with carcinoma of the breast or of the uterine cervix (141). It was
also observed that RT did not adversely affect immune response to either
microbial recall antigens or dinitro-chlorobenzene (DNCB) in cancer patients (142). Ovarian cancer patients undergoing RT showed a reduction
of T cells. Cell-mediated immunity was depressed significantly by RT
seven days after treatment; it remained low when measured on the 14th
day, but recovered despite continuation of RT. In osteosarcoma patients
receiving high-dose RT, immunologic reactions were found to be operative. The group treated with RT fared significantly better than the group
undergoing amputation. This was thought to be due to antitumor immunity following RT. Using the spleen-cell migration test for specific antitumor immunity in an experimental model, the same authors observed that
antitumor immunity was eliminated by amputation. This study reveals
that RT is involved in the development of antitumor immunity (143).
Cytotoxicity of lymphocytes against allogeneic target cells in broncho-

genic squamous-cell carcinoma was increased after RT (144). Thus we find that RT can bring about varied changes in antitumor response—from immunodepression to immunostimulation. Our limited knowledge of radiation immunology (145) precludes trying to explain the above findings. Future investigations will bring more definitive information about these matters.

Potentiation of Antitumor Immune Response by RT in Experimental Models

Many significant findings regarding antitumor immunity following RT come from animal studies. It has been shown, in a murine fibrosarcoma system, that injection of radiation-killed tumor cells potentiated cure of the autologous host when in vivo irradiation of the tumor occurred. The tumor cells left remaining after RT may have been eliminated by the immune response, which was initiated by the irradiated autologous tumor cells. This synergy between RT and immunologic effector mechanisms has been studied by several investigators.

Suit et al increased the radiosensitivity of C3H fibrosarcoma by *C. parvum* treatment (146). Another bacterial immunopotentiator, PS-K, was shown to increase significantly the number of uterine and cervical carcinoma patients who showed increased sensitivity to RT (147). Radiation-killed autologous tumor cells eliminate the tumorigenicity but retain the immunogenicity (148,149). It has also been observed that radiation-killed tumor cells offer a certain degree of antitumor immunity when injected into the host prior to challenge with viable tumor cells (148). Lymphoid cells retain their immunogenicity in MLC reactions after irradiation with 1,200 rads (150). Contrary reports are also available (151) to this effect. Maruyama found a significant increase in immunogenicity of irradiated isologous tumor cells (152).

It appears that irradiation of tumor cells may expose hidden antigenic sites on the tumor cell-surface or might enrich the tumor population for the more antigenic cells by selectively destroying the less antigenic tumor cells. Thus, it is possible that during RT a major fraction of the tumor is killed by the ionizing radiation, and these killed cells, or immunogenic cell membrane fragments, sensitize the host specifically against the tumor. Some studies have shown, in fact, that tumor cells exposed to doses of 2,000 rads release an immunogenic component into the tissue culture medium that is capable of potentiating an antitumor response (153,154). Local x-irradiation (4,000 rads) of syngeneic carcinoma or fibrosarcoma in rats resulted in an increased lymphocytotoxicity against both syngeneic and allogeneic tumor cells. This effect vanished after 1 week of RT (155). This result has been explained as a reduction in the release of tumor-specific antigen which can act to inhibit cell-mediated cytotoxicity (CMC) or deplete suppressor lymphocytes. In mice given varied doses of local x-rays to solid sarcomas, metastasis was less frequent in those whose tumor had received the most irradiation. This could have occurred because of the tumor immunity that developed subsequent to tumor sterilization by RT (156). But, a reverse phenomenon was observed also, ie, there was increased metastasis with increased local tumor irradiation, in a very weakly immunogenic murine lymphosarcoma (157). These experiments suggest that RT may induce tumor immunity only in immunogenic tumors. The elements of antitumor immune response may be relatively radiation-resistant, and radiation may interfere with suppressive influences of the immune system; or, radiation may increase the immunogenicity of the tumor and thus increase the immunologic response of the host against the tumor, thereby giving a better therapeutic index.

Immunologic Component in RT-Induced Tumor Cure

Evidence supporting the concept that RT-induced tumor cures have an immunologic component is also provided by the studies performed by Suit and Kastelan (158). They showed that the x-ray dose required for cure in 50% of the mice was about 4,300 rads if the host was immunosuppressed, 3,500 rads in normal mice, and 2,700 rads in actively immunized mice. Crile and Deodhar (159) showed that local irradiation of tumor was able to sustain concomitant antitumor immunity to allogeneic and syngeneic tumors for a much longer period than it could be sustained following surgical excision of tumors. Mice cured of a fibrosarcoma by local irradiation were found to retain the antitumor immunity for a long time because they become refractory to fresh challenge by viable syngeneic tumor cells. The lymphoid cells from cured mice could adoptively transfer the antitumor immunity, as assessed by Winn's assay (160).

RT-Induced Immunosuppression

There are many observations of RT having suppressed the antitumor response. In mice-bearing tumors, T-dependent antigen-specific cytolytic lymphocytes (CTL) could be detected. RT abrogated this specific CTL. It has been observed that scattering of a 1,600-rad single dose for treatment of a tumor was sufficient to provoke this effect (161). Vaage et al (162) investigated the effect of local RT on tumor growth and studied specific tumor immunity in mice actively sensitized to syngeneic sarcoma. RT was found to be therapeutic for tumor growth within the radiation field. Extensive-field radiation could facilitate tumor growth in nonirradiated parts. Metastasis was extensive when radiation was given soon after tumor implantation. This is in accordance with the observation that host sensitization to a tumor prevents metastasis induced by WBI only at the early phase of tumor implantation (63). The above observations suggest the need to prevent damage that might occur to the normal lymphoid tissues adjacent to the tumor because of scattered radiation during the course of RT. Another important observation relevant to these findings is involvement of regional lymph nodes in antitumor immunity; these, too, can be along with primary tumors significantly reduced the immunity of the host to subsequent implant of tumor cells in a contralateral site. Irradiation of the node by 1,000 rads five to seven days after tumor transplantation also abrogated the antitumor immunity, as evidenced by the incidence and extent of pulmonary metastasis (163). If one finds abrogation of antitumor immunity, the sensitization of the host to the growing tumor may be weak or localized. This leads us to an important and controversial issue, that of using RT as an adjuvant to surgical resection of tumor. A collaborative study to find the efficacy of preoperative irradiation of cancer of the lung had disappointing results (164). It may be that the immunosuppressive effects of RT cancel the potential benefits of this treatment. This seems plausible, as immune response against lung cancer is well known (165). The removal or elimination of regional lymph nodes (RLN) in radical mastectomy for breast cancer has received wide attention. Reports are available indicating that postoperative RT for breast cancer increases the chance of distant metastases (137,166). Earlier studies have suggested decreased survival in breast cancer patients who had regional lymph nodes removed. It was suggested that removal of seemingly uninvolved regional lymph nodes along with primary tumor may be detrimental to the immune defense of the host against systemic metastasis. A detailed study by the Cancer Research Campaign Working Group found no significant difference in survival between those with simple mastectomy and those with simple mastectomy followed by RT. In fact, a highly significant risk of local recurrence was found in the simple mastectomy group (167). These authors argue that if RT abrogates tumor immunity by regional lymph node destruction, one should see increased mortality in the group of patients receiving regional RT. But caution must be used in extrapolating from mouse to man the finding that regional lymph nodes are involved in maintaining systemic immunity. The relatively short duration of the presence of a primary tumor in animals cannot be compared with human tumors, which may be present over a protracted period, allowing for the development of systemic immunity (168).

Although lymphopenia persists for a long period following RT in breast cancer patients, it is argued that T-dependent CTL are unaffected in number, or might have actually increased (141). It is further suggested that cellular immune response to breast cancer is unlikely to have been impaired by local RT. Blastogenic response to PHA and RFC in the peripheral blood, which were suppressed, showed a favorable upward trend after RT (140). RT followed by mastectomy for breast cancer showed a prolonged depression of T lymphocytes, but B lymphopenia was short-lived (97).

Relevance of In Vitro Parameters to Clinical Immune Status

The above observations have an important message. The in vitro parameters for general immune competence may not always truly represent the actual clinical status of the patients. Patients with carcinoma of the uterine cervix, when given pelvic RT, had a depressed antibody, neutrophil and lymphocyte count. T and B lymphocytes dropped in number initially, then reverted to the normal level. In vitro tests for cellular immunity remained depressed for 3 to 12 months, but skin response was normal. Thus, a variable response in immune indices has been observed in patients in remission after treatment of localized carcinoma of the cervix. This stresses the importance of assessing several aspects of immune function and implies that persistent depression of certain indices does not adversely affect the host tumor response (169).

The immune function in patients with mammary, pulmonary, head, or neck tumors was investigated after irradiation. The treatment caused an initial lymphopenia and a long-lasting depression in the lymphoid-proliferative response to PHA, concanavalin A (Con A), and PPD. The percentage and ratio of E and EAC-rosette forming cells remained unchanged (170). Serial studies of immunocompetence in head and neck cancer patients undergoing radiation therapy revealed that response to recall antigens did reflect the antitumor immunity. However, DNCB sensitization did not show any statistically significant difference following RT (171). In breast cancer patients postoperatively irradiated, the immune capacity shows varied results with regard to the proliferative response of the lymphocytes to mitogens. Lymphoproliferative response to PHA decreased during the progress of RT, but in some cases the response temporarily increased after irradiation. However, response to Con A was varied during and after RT, indicating a difference in radiosensitivity between lymphocytes stimulated by Con A and PHA. On the other hand, the response to Pokeweed mitogen (PWM) was only slightly affected by RT (172). Therefore, the immunologic test used to monitor immune status should carefully dissect the compartment of immune system affected by RT. The in vitro test has to be made in parallel with the in vivo test, and the assay system has to be carefully chosen so that the test selected truly reflects antitumor immunity.

The foregoing discussion explains the complex interaction of RT with the host immune system. If the host, tumor, and RT interact favorably, there is a good therapeutic index; but if the interaction is not favorable, the outcome of the therapy may be deleterious. In another study, RT was shown to decrease peripheral blood leukocytes (PBL) and total WBC in mammary, esophageal, and lung cancer. When the patient's immune capacity was impaired, the primary and metastatic disease was found to accelerate. Secondary infection also set in (173). Thus, immune status can be used to predict the therapeutic course of cancer patients.

Effect of Whole Body Irradiation on Immune System

WBI is becoming increasingly popular as a modality for controlling neoplasia affecting the lymphoid system. Many studies have shown that the
response rate of WBI is comparable to that of CT, with minimal side
effects during the treatment (174,175). Monitoring the immune system
becomes increasingly important. Usually the peripheral blood picture is
analyzed to get an idea of bone marrow failure and immune status. It was
observed in mice that WBI of 20 to 50 rads twice weekly, with a total dose
of 200 to 500 rads, showed a sustained depression of stem-cell activity,
but the peripheral blood count was normal. This finding indicates that
readily available peripheral blood indices may not truly reflect incipient
marrow failure (176). It may also indicate that peripheral-blood immune
competence does not reflect satisfactorily the antitumor response.

It was found that when only WBI was administered, it induced a transient depression of peripheral blood count. Some authors advance the
hypothesis that WBI and nodal irradiation lead to immunologic and hematopoietic stress, with resultant malignancy. But WBI alone is without
such an outcome. Since WBI usually involves a low dose for a prolonged
period, it may not affect the potential antitumor immunity. WBI in fractional doses administered to patients with non-Hodgkin's lymphoma did
not show any suppressive effect on mitogen-induced lymphoproliferative
response, and it was also noted that an improved mitogen response after
WBI correlates with good clinical progress (177). Hellstrom and Hellstrom attribute the antitumor effect of WBI to the possible elimination of
x-ray-sensitive T-suppressor cells (178). Thus, if one can carefully monitor the immune system while delivering the WBI, the potential antitumor
immunity will not be affected significantly and, therefore, better therapeutic success can be achieved.

Another modality of radiation delivery is extracorporeal irradiation
(ECI). This, too, can be used in leukemia (179). The advantage is that the
lymphoid organs and bone marrow are totally excluded from irradiation.
This method is known to reduce allograft immunity. There are no reports
of alteration in tumor immunity following ECI.

Physical Parameters of Irradiation as They Pertain to Immune Response

Physical parameters also become important in radiation-induced alteration of immune response. There are not many studies that explore the
effects of dose rate, field size, location of the tumor site, or the type of
radiation. Kutzner et al (180) studied the percentage of B and T lymphocytes in peripheral blood monitored before, during, and after RT according to tumor types, tumor localization, field size, and radiation doses.
Most of the patients had a reduced percentage of T cells, which was
sometimes accompanied by a relative increase in the number of B cells.
They could not demonstrate any correlation between the decrease in the

number of T and B cells and field size, location of the tumor, or radiation dose. High-dose radiation administered to an anatomic site that excludes the thymus gland, usually produces suppression of the immune system. It is likely that the suppression results from irradiation of a large volume of blood in the treatment fields (181). This deduction is supported by another observation wherein a remarkable reduction in lymphocytes occurred when large blood vessels were included in the radiation field (182). Wara et al suggested that the contributing factors in immunosuppression were large blood volume in the radiation field, irradiation of the thymus, and malnourishment (98).

Monitoring the scattered-radiation dosage to the lymphoid system, bone marrow, and blood is a useful procedure for determining the extent of immunosuppression. With x-rays and gamma rays the amount of damage to the lymphoid system is directly proportional to the dose (183). With x-rays and gamma rays there is a possibility for sublethal recovery, but with high-energy radiation, such as neutrons and high-energy particles, the potential for recovery from sublethal radiation is minimal (184). Immunosuppression by x-rays and gamma rays depends on the fractional radiation dose, rate, and total dose, whereas neutrons suppress the immune response irrespective of the dosage. Knowledge of these parameters can be made use of during RT for achieving the maximum therapeutic effect while avoiding damage to normal tissue. Currently we have little knowledge about the effects of high-dose radiation on the immune response. Modern radiation therapists should focus on the possible effects of their therapy on the immune response, whichever of the various agents are used in the therapy. Special attention should be paid to the effects of radiosensitizers, molecular oxygen quality of radiation, and the influence of fractionation. Attempts should also be made to determine if lower doses of radiation are effective when given in association with other treatments such as chemotherapy. It should also be attempted if newer radiosensitizing agents can be developed. Better technology should be found as to how to shield the surrounding areas of the tumor so that radiation can be administered only to the target tumor, even though the tumor is located inside an internal organ.

Chemotherapy-Induced Changes in Antitumor Immunity

Cytotoxic chemotherapy is basically a systemic modality of treatment that depends to a great extent on the preferential toxicity of drugs for dividing cells. The drugs circulate throughout the body, except perhaps in certain pharmacologically forbidden zones, such as brain. They can seek out and destroy cancer cells seeded at different locations, or those becoming established as metastatic tumors. Most of the chemotherapeutic drugs lead to toxicity, mainly to the gastrointestinal system, bone marrow, and lymphoid system. Berenbaum (185) found that antitumor agents, even in nontoxic dosage, were often found immunosuppressive; toxic compounds lacking in antitumor properties tended not to be immunosuppressive. This suggests that antitumor properties and immunosuppressive properties go hand in hand. A detailed review of immunosuppression by antineoplastic agents has been published by Gabrielsen and Good (186). Since antitumor immunity has been implicated in control of growth and spread of tumors, it is logical to ask how self-defeating this immunosuppressive property of antineoplastic drugs would be in the treatment of cancer. We shall consider in this section the effect of chemotherapeutic drugs on antitumor immunity.

Types of Chemotherapeutic Agents

Antineoplastic drugs can be conveniently classified as (a) adrenal steroid hormones and their derivatives, (b) alkylating agents, (c) antimetabolites, (d) antibiotics, (e) plant alkaloids, (f) synthetic chemicals, and (g) enzymes. Most of them have been shown to be immunosuppressive (186). Certain drugs are highly immunosuppressive whereas others are nonimmunosuppressive or only mildly so (187). The more immunosuppressive drugs include thiopurines, folic acid antagonists, alkylating agents, doxorubicin hydrochloride (formerly known as adriamycin) nitrosoureas, and corticosteroids. Less immunosuppressive drugs include imidazole carboxamide, bleomycin, vincristine, 5-fluorouracil (5-FU), and cytarabine (formerly known as cytosine arabinoside) (188,189). Uracil mustard is not immunosuppressive at therapeutic doses, but the rest of the mustards suppress both primary and secondary immune response, as tested by DTH and skin graft experiments (190). There are instances wherein host tumor immunity is actually increased after chemotherapy. This has been observed with many antineoplastic drugs, such as cyclophosphamide (CY), doxorubicin, cytarabine, and 5-FU in experimental tumor models.

Antineoplastic Agents Having Immunosuppressive Effects

The immune response, which is perhaps of primary importance in spontaneous cure of cancer, appears to play a significant role as an adjunct to chemotherapy in treatment of cancer (191–197). A survey of the literature reveals a wide range of observations, from highly immunosuppressive effects of drugs to drug-induced antitumor response. It is unfortunate that this latter mechanism if often overlooked or not understood by those who offer chemotherapy to cancer patients. The effectiveness of chemotherapeutic treatment may be altered either in a favorable or in an unfavorable direction by the modification of the host's immunologic responses. In animal models the many variables encountered are

(a) species of experimental animals
(b) type of antigenic material

(c) quality of antigen
(d) the number of injections of antigen
(e) dose and route of inoculation of antineoplastic drugs
(f) type and combination of drugs
(g) the time of administration of the drug in relation to antigenic stimulation
(h) immunogenicity of the tumor
(i) immunosuppressive property of the tumor
(j) tumor load on the animal at the time of treatment
(k) the parameters of immunosuppression
(l) the time of scoring the immune parameters in relation to antigen and drug injection

Some drugs cause a more persistent inhibition of cell-mediated immunity and humoral antibody production than CY when given before antigen presentation (198). Doxorubicin significantly inhibits the titer of hemolytic and hemagglutination antibodies in mice immunized with SRBC. The greatest immunosuppressive effect was observed when doxorubicin was administered after antigen injection, indicating that the drug does not act on the very early stages of the immune response (199,200). Corticosteroids and busulfan (Myleran) produce maximal suppression of immune response in mice when given some one to two days before antigen. Many alkylating agents (e.g., nitrogen mustard), CY, and antimetabolites such as 8-azaguanine, 6-mercaptopurine, and thioguanine, show maximal suppression if given one to four days after the antigen (185). If the immune response was already established, treatment with anticancer drugs had little effect (185,201). Berenbaum (202) studied the time dependence and selectivity of immunosuppressive agents and classified the drug into two classes. Class I inhibits the response if administered either before or one to two days after antigen presentation; class II inhibits only if given one to two days after antigen. These findings may have relevance in chemotherapy, as antineoplastic drugs are administered at a stage when the host is probably sensitized to the growing tumor. Antineoplastic agents may not suppress antitumor immunity if it is already established. Therefore, if one observes a strong antitumor immunity, the chemotherapeutic drugs may possibly be given more safely than otherwise. Unfortunately, such considerations are seldom given adequate attention during chemotherapy of cancer.

Effects of Chemotherapeutic Agents on Antitumor Immune Response

To delineate the complex interaction of chemotherapeutic drugs with the host immune system, it is necessary to understand the effect of the drugs on the various components of the immune response. It has been observed that CY causes a reduction of greater than 70% of NK cell activity one to three days after treatment (121). CY therapy of MCA-induced murine tumor shows an initial increase of macarophages within the tumor, followed by accumulation of granulocytes. After seven to ten days, granulocytic cells replace neoplastic cells, but bone marrow and peripheral WBC decrease rapidly after CY therapy. Differential counts indicate that lymphocyte recovery takes 21 days (203). Single or repeated administration of CY or AZA resulted in dose-dependent inhibition of NK activity two days later and a reduction of spleen cell number. By seven days NK cell activity in treated animals recovered to a normal level. Recovery of NK cell activity may be a good parameter regarding scheduling of chemotherapy. Essentially, the chemotherapeutic index can be increased by amplifying the difference in susceptibility of the immune system and the tumor to chemotherapy. Doxorubicin did not substantially impair NK cytotoxicity per unit number of lymphoid cells, although it did reduce the lymphoid cell number (204). Thus the effect of doxorubicin on NK activity is similar to that of irradiation. Five consequent daily injections of CY caused a decrease in percentage of B cells and an increase of T cells in murine spleen and lymph nodes. HCA had the same effect on spleen. Mitomycin C, FT 207, and AZA had no significant effect on the proportion of B and T cells in spleen. CY had more marked effects on activated spleen cells than on normal spleen cells. CY treatment also caused marked suppression of antibody production to SRBC and LPS whereas treatment with AZA, HCA, mitomycin C, or FT 207 caused only moderate suppression of LPS-induced plaque-forming cells. Treatment with CY or AZA increased blastogenic response to PHA, whereas treatment with CY or mitomycin C decreased response to LPS and mitomycin C, also decreasing the response to PHA (205). These results indicate that CY depletes lymphoid cells and also has a preferential toxicity for NK cells and B cells; however, NK cells are relatively resistant to doxorubicin. AZA selectively inhibits K-cell activity without affecting T- and B-cell responses (206). It has been observed that mice immunized with antigen develop augmented DTH response if they are pretreated with CY (207). The potentiation appears to be through CY-mediated depletion or else inactivation of T-suppressor cells (208). Doxorubicin is not found to impair ADCC responses in terms of specific cytotoxicity (209). Doxorubicin induced a decrease in AFC after primary stimulation with SRBC, whereas daunorubicin was suppressive in secondary immune response. Primary reactivity of T-independent antigen S III was decreased by doxorubicin whereas daunorubicin was ineffective even at higher doses. Daunorubicin was found to be immunosuppressive in tumor allografts (210). This observation suggests that doxorubicin affects the humoral limb of the immune response preferentially and daunorubicin the cellular limb. The above observations are important in explaining why drugs such as doxorubicin suppress host tumor immune responses, whereas drugs such as daunorubicin suppress host tumor immunity. (This is based on the fact that humoral limb usually inhibits antitumor immune response.)

*Effects of Chemotherapeutic Agents on Various Elements of
Immune Response*

Chemotherapeutic agents that inhibit the antibody response may correct
depression of tumor immunity. To retain antitumor immunity, the drug or
drug combination might be selected in a manner that assures that the
effector mechanisms are not subjected to severe suppression. Wide variation in the effects of chemotherapeutic drugs on the immunologic system
may help to explain both chemotherapy-induced suppression of tumor
immunity and chemotherapy-induced activation of tumor immunity.

Ray and Raychaudhuri (51) recently observed that preinjection of inbred male C3H/Hej mice with a low dose of CY (500 μg/animal) either
delayed or inhibited tumor appearance, following the inoculation of transplantable 3-methylcholanthrene-induced fibrosarcomas. This dose of CY
potentiated (a) the foot-pad swelling reaction to *Staphylococcus aureus*
antigen, (b) the blastogenic response to phytohemagglutinin-M and bacterial lipopolysaccharides. Augmentation of immune reactivity has been
attributed to the depletion of suppressor cells. These authors (Ray and
Raychaudhuri, *unpublished observation*) have also noted an increase in
ADCC and killer cell response in CY-treated tumor-bearing animals.

Thus, drug selectivity may become an important factor in determining
the course of chemotherapy because it is becoming increasingly evident
that anticancer drugs exhibit both immunosuppressive and immunoaug-
menting effects through their selective action on specific cells at different
stages of development of immune response.

Immune Competence in Patients Following Chemotherapy

In clinical practice, most commonly the general immune competence is
the parameter assessed following chemotherapy. The effect of chemotherapeutic drugs on the immune response in normal subjects cannot be
directly extrapolated to cancer patients, since progressive growth of the
tumor itself induces alteration in the host immunity, notably immunosuppression, and also changes in drug metabolizing rates.

It was observed in malignant melanoma patients following monthly
cycles of vincristine that B-, T-, non-B-, and non-T-cell numbers tended
to fall early in the cycle, as did PHA-induced cytotoxicity to CRBC. PHA
transformation and cytotoxicity returned to normal by day 29. B- and T-
cell numbers remained subnormal (211). In another group of patients
treated with lomustine (CCNU) and vincristine for various types of malignancies associated with metastasis, suppression of blastogenic response
to PHA and streptolysin O (SLO) was observed. Recovery occurred with
significant overshoot above pretreatment level for PHA and SLO in those
patients whose tumors regressed and whose survival was prolonged (212).
This observation suggests that chemotherapy-induced tumor regression is
probably accompanied by antitumor immunity and that tests for general
immune competence have a positive prognostic value. It also suggests

that general immune competence may parallel antitumor immunity. However, the immunosuppressive response to chemotherapy may also have a differential effect on tumor immunity and general immunity. MLR responses of lymphocytes from dogs with lymphosarcoma given multiple cycles of combination chemotherapy were depressed for tumor cells, but were intact for allogeneic cells (213). This suggests a differential immunosuppressive effect of chemotherapeutic drugs on the capacity of lymphocytes from lymphosarcoma dogs to respond to MLR. It also highlights the importance of monitoring both specific and nonspecific antitumor immunity. In another clinical trial, the effects of chemoimmunotherapy on immune status were explored in patients with stage II-B breast cancer. On the parameters examined, only the percentage of RFC was markedly depressed during CY, methotrexate (MTX) and 5-FU therapy (214). This does not necessarily reflect antitumor response. The immune status of patients with Hodgkin's disease was tested after intensive chemotherapy. In patients achieving remission, overall cellular immunity, after deteriorating with cytotoxic chemotherapy, returned to the pretreatment level. Serum IgG and IgM levels decreased during intensive chemotherapy in splenectomized patients. IgA and IgM levels were lower (irrespective of splenectomy and therapy status) in remission than at presentation or after treatment. Relapse or nonresponse was usually associated with deteriorating cellular immunity (215). This study brings out the relationship between the level of immune status and chemotherapy. In patients with defective cellular immunity, infection sets in. All of the above considerations stress the need to maintain an effective host immunity. In sarcoma patients given adjuvant chemotherapy with doxorubicin and high-dose MTX with citrovorum rescue, in vitro lymphocyte function for the HDM therapy group was significantly depressed 24 hours following treatment, but it returned to pretreatment level by 48 hours. Long-term administration of doxorubicin and HDM does not appear to alter in vivo and in vitro cell-mediated immunity, although transient depression was observed (216). The preservation of intact cell-mediated immunity may account, in part, for the effectiveness of these agents as surgical adjuvants. Patients with acute myelogenous leukemia in remission had pronounced deficiency in ADCC and mitogen-induced cellular cytotoxicity. Cytotoxic functions were further suppressed by the administration of monthly cycles of combination chemotherapy. Following each chemotherapy cycle, progressive recovery of cytotoxic functions occurred during the third and fourth week, with occasional increase above the baseline in patients for whom chemotherapy was withheld for more than 5 weeks. Single doses of intravenous (IV) daunorubicin had no effect on cytotoxic function (217). Thus, effector cells involved in ADCC and in mitogen-induced cytotoxicity take a longer time for recovery. Split-dosage chemotherapy should give enough time for the recovery of all effector mechanisms, and this could help to keep the antitumor immunity intact. Ideally, recovery of the immune capacity should be monitored, as it depends on the extent of sensitization and stimulation of the host prior to immunosuppressive treatment (126). Multidrug chemotherapy is much more immunosuppressive, whereas single-drug chemotherapeutic schedules may bring about transient depression (218). In canine lymphosarcoma, MLR response to autochthonous tumor antigen is significantly depressed by multiple cycles of combination chemotherapy (213). This finding indicates that polychemotherapy suppresses tumor immunity, so judicial selection of drugs or drug combinations along with constant monitoring of the immune status of cancer patients following therapy may be rewarding.

Chemotherapy-Induced Nonspecific Stimulation of Immune Response

Chemotherapy-induced antitumor immunity has been well-documented in experimental tumors. There is evidence indicating that host defense mechanisms contribute to the antitumor immunity of cancer chemotherapeutic drugs, such as doxorubicin, CY, cytarabine, and 5-FU. It has been described that immunosuppression can impair the antitumor efficacy of drugs (193–195,219–222). Despite these findings on the effect of antineoplastic agents on different lymphoid populations, understanding of the role played by different lymphoid cells in antitumoral activity of cancer chemotherapeutic drugs is still far from complete.

In mice a single intraperitoneal administration of doxorubicin resulted in the rapid increase of cytolytic activity caused by PEC. The effector cells were identified as NK cells. In contrast to the stimulatory effect on NK activity of PEC, doxorubicin caused a transient dose-dependent depression of NK activity in the spleen, with a peak reduction at day 3 and recovery within a few days. The depressed activity could be reversed by removal of adherent cells. Moreover, doxorubicin induced cytostatic activity against tumor cells by macrophages. This suggests that activated macrophages may be responsible for the suppression of splenic NK cells. The idea of possible modulation of NK activity by doxorubicin-induced macrophages was supported by experiments in which plastic adherent spleen cells from doxorubicin-treated mice, but not from normal mice, inhibited NK activity of normal spleen cells (223). This experiment demonstrates the effect of doxorubicin on two different effector mechanisms. It has been suggested that macrophages are one of the candidates for giving doxorubicin a better chemotherapeutic index (224). Doxorubicin-induced antitumor response is abrogated by antimacrophage agents such as carrageenan or silica (194).

Effect of Structural Alteration of Chemotherapeutic Drugs on Antitumor Response

Interaction of antineoplastic drugs with the immune system can be modulated by altering the structure of the drug. Many workers have shown the superiority of doxorubicin as an antineoplastic agent over its structural analog daunorubicin (224). Doxorubicin given to C_3H mice 24 hours before allogenic L1210 inoculation significantly increased survival of these mice over survival of mice given the daunorubicin analog. The doxorubicin pretreated mice had higher cell-mediated cytotoxicity in the peritoneal cavity (at the site of tumor growth) (209). It was observed that immunosuppression of DBA/2 mice bearing lymphocytic leukemia abrogates the antitumor effect of doxorubicin, whereas immunosuppression has no effect on the antineoplastic agent daunorubicin (195). It has also been shown that daunorubicin is at least four times more toxic than doxorubicin to macrophage monolayers in vitro. Even in vivo daunorubicin is more suppressive than doxorubicin in abrogating C parvum-induced splenic macrophage cytotoxicity (225).

Doxorubicin and daunorubicin were tested on L1210 leukemia variants of different immunogenicity. It was found that the higher the immunogenicity of the tumor, the greater the therapeutic efficacy of doxorubicin. Immunosuppression of the host mice markedly impaired efficacy of the drug for immunogenic tumors. Further, it was observed that mice that remained immunosuppressed for more than nine days after the completion of therapy succumbed to the tumor, whereas mice that were immunocompetent achieved tumor cures. On the other hand, the antitumor property of daunorubicin was not significantly affected by tumor immunogenicity and host immune status (193). These observations suggest that doxorubicin has a relatively sparing effect on the immune system compared with the analog daunorubicin; this property gives doxorubicin superiority as an antineoplastic drug, particularly in cases where there is existing antitumor immunity. The above studies also bring out the difference in interactions between drugs and the host immune system, even when the drugs are close structural analogs. The possibility of drug interaction with different limbs of the immune system, as an explanation for the observed difference between doxorubicin and daunorubicin, has been discussed in the literature (34). Synergistic antitumor activity was observed in vivo when doxorubicin was combined with C parvum, a well-known macrophage activator, whereas combination of daunorubicin with C parvum did not show any significant therapeutic advantage (224,225). Observations such as these have proved very useful in designing chemoimmunotherapy.

Specific Antitumor Immunity Following Chemotherapy

Animal models have given valuable information regarding specific antitumor immunity following chemotherapy. In the mouse syngeneic plasmacytoma model, using 5-FU, good correlation among the efficacies of various therapies (222,226) was found. The most effective antineoplastic drug not only yielded a higher proportion of cures, it rendered the mice comparatively more refractory to challenge from syngeneic tumor cells. Immunity of cured mice was found to be highly specific. The immunity decreased with time but was still evident as late as 12 months post-therapy. Balb/c mice cured of their palpable plasmacytoma MOPC 1046 by a single dose of CY remained tumor-immune for at least 4 months post-therapy. Mice given CY either 4, 11, or 20 days after tumor transplantation rejected either 6, 60, or 400 times as many tumor cells, respectively, as did controls (227). This finding indicates that exposure to greater amounts of tumor antigen results in increased amount of residual tumor immunity following cure. The results suggest the involvement of two factors in the induction of tumor immunity: effectiveness of the drug in killing the tumor cells and ability of host immune-mechanisms to function so that tumor immunity is induced and immunity becomes functional despite any immunodepressive effects of the drug or of the tumor. Another report indicates the necessity of intact antitumor response for the eradication of established tumors by CY therapy (228). In addition to the pathways mentioned so far, the drug may render residual tumor cells more susceptible to immune lysis (229) or potentiate cytotoxic immunity by eliminating suppressor elements that interfere with an effective antitumor immune response (194,230). It has been suggested that drug-induced immunosuppression is minimal when the drug is bringing about tumor reduction (222). One can, of course, speculate that the chemotherapeutic drug is diverted toward the tumor mass, thus relieving its effect on the host immune system. Relevant to this point is the observation that intestinal mucosal cells, from mice bearing progressively growing L1210 tumors, were not subjected to the toxic effects of therapy until the tumor load was significantly reduced by drug administration (231). Again, these observations should help to program chemotherapy for inducing remission. Since an intact antitumor response is essential to the efficacy of some drugs, one expects a corollary observation of low effectiveness for the same drugs in immunosuppressed animals, but these observations are not available in the literature. Irradiation and antilymphocyte serum (ALS) treatment of hosts decrease the antineoplastic effect of CY and melphalan on mammary carcinoma (232). CY response to murine sarcoma is poor in immunosuppressed animals and is potentiated in specifically immune animals (220). The success of ı-asparaginase therapy of mouse lymphoma is found to depend on the host's immune response (233). CY treatment of tumor bearers that are immunosuppressed by antithymocyte serum (232,234), x-irradiation (232,235), or high doses of drugs (236) has been reported to be less effective than similar treatment of immunocompetent tumor bearers.

Screening Chemotherapeutic Agents for Immunosuppressed Activity

It will be very convenient when one can design in vitro experiments to screen the suppressive effect of chemotherapeutic drugs on antitumor immunity. Twelve anticancer agents have been tested for their effect on the development of primary cell-mediated immunity by spleen cells from C57BL/6J against irradiated allogenic P815 in culture (237). The test is quite sensitive and is able to differentiate the sensitivity of the immune response to closely related drug analogs. With this sensitive system it was possible to measure drug effect on the developing immune response. Similarly, drugs can be classified according to their bone marrow toxicity, as detected by CFU-S and CFU-C. Such tests are very useful in selecting drugs or drug combinations, so that deleterious effects on tumor immunity are kept to a minimum.

Drug-Induced Alteration in Tumor-Cell Immunogenicity

Another important aspect of chemotherapy is drug-induced alteration of the tumor target. It has been observed in vivo that DTIC treatment induced increased immunogenicity of the tumor-cell population in a virus-induced leukemia system (238–240). The drug-induced change in immunogenicity may be attributable to mutation, since it can be prevented by antimutagenic compounds such as quinacrine (241) CY has also induced the appearance of "new" markers in normal murine cells; these markers stimulate self-reactive lymphocytes (242–244). The authors suggest that similar events may affect cancer cells and stimulate cancer-reactive lymphocytes. It has been suggested, too, that altered immunogenic tumor cells may initiate an immune response directed against previously tolerant tumor cells. Therefore, a single dose or short course of CY would have the advantage of allowing activated cytotoxic lymphocytes to follow the changes in tumor antigenicity, whereas a long course of CY might eliminate the cytotoxic effector cells required for protective response. Selected sulfhydryl inhibitors such as iodoacetate, carbasone, or thiomurin could induce tumor immunity in mice, unlike other commonly used antitumor agents (245). These sulfhydryl inhibitors have been shown to modify the surface texture of cancer cells. This has wide implications, since these drug-induced immunogenic tumor cells perhaps can be controlled by host tumor immunity if drug-induced immunosuppression is regulated.

Circumvention of Immunosuppression Induced by Chemotherapy and Radiotherapy

Introduction

Although the aim of RT and CT is elimination of tumors without damaging normal tissue, in practice this goal is not attainable. Both treatments are notoriously blunt weapons, despite having been in use for some time. In the process of cancer therapy, normal tissues also suffer damage from both modalities. The gastrointestinal system, bone marrow, and lymphoid tissues are the most vulnerable sites. The primary concern in retaining the host's immunity against infection and immune surveillance of tumors should be to protect the lymphoid organs, both primary and secondary. In what follows, methods should be explored to circumvent CT- and RT-induced immunosuppression, so that the host's immunity against the residual tumor cells is kept intact.

Circumvention can be effected by means of both the target, ie, the tumor-bearing host, and the effector, ie, the modality of treatment. Development of compounds of low leukocytotoxicity is an essential requirement for achieving further success in the area of cancer chemotherapy. Various methods employed to eliminate the myelosuppression and immunosuppression include (a) chemical modification of neoplastic agents to decrease the immunosuppression and increase the selectivity against tumor cells, (b) combination chemotherapy to achieve additive or synergistic antitumor effect without increasing immunosuppression, (c) proper drug scheduling, (d) administration of metabolite intermediates to counteract the effect of the agent on the host's immune system, (e) drug delivery to the target organs, and (f) dose of drug to be used.

For RT the development has to be aimed at (a) the source of radiation, (b) the mode of delivery of radiation, and (c) search for techniques to give radiation only to the tumor target.

Circumvention at the Effector Level of Chemotherapy

Structural Alteration of Chemotherapeutic Drugs

In the current repertoire of chemotherapeutic agents, bleomycin is least immunosuppressive in both man and animals. We discussed earlier in this chapter how doxorubicin spares the host's immune system while its structural analog, daunorubicin, suppresses the antitumor response (193,195,210,224,225). CY and ifosfamide exert a more pronounced immunosuppression than trofosfamide, which has a relatively slight immunosuppressive effect (246). To develop a new drug with low immunosuppressive effect, one needs to know the relation between the chemical structure of the antineoplastic drug and its interaction with the immune system. Currently, we are far from having this understanding. The chemotherapeutic index of 5'dFU was shown to be greater than that of 5-FU; however, the former did not show any detectable immunosuppression (247). Chlorozotocin is a nitrosourea derivative that has curative activity against L1210 leukemia, but produces little or no bone marrow toxicity. Chlorozotocin has twice the in vitro alkylating activity of its structural analog, carmustine (BCNU), at equimolar concentration (248). Drugs with low immunosuppressive capacity, but which have potent cancerotoxicity, are the drugs of choice for maintenance therapy.

There have been attempts to study the metabolic pool in tumor cells.

The metabolic pool can be expected to affect activation of certain anti-metabolic drugs by competing for a common enzyme site. Antimetabolic drugs are more useful if the metabolic pool in the tumor cells is comparatively lower than that in normal tissues (204). This offers the possibility of increasing drug selectivity and, at the same time, sparing other sensitive tissues. The enzyme L-asparaginase (L-asnase) has been found to vary with respect to its immunosuppressive capacity, depending on the source of the enzyme. L-Asnase from *Escherichia coli* is immunosuppressive in both man and mice (249,250). L-Asnase from *Vibrio succinogenes* is not suppressive, although both derivatives show potent antilymphoma activity (249). It has been suggested that the immunosuppressive effect *E coli* enzyme is due to the presence of glutaminase. Asparaginase, which is not immunosuppressive, may be more beneficial therapeutically than *E coli* enzyme; it reduces the primary tumor, but induces development of metastasis, which is shown to be due to its immunosuppressive activity (251).

Combination Chemotherapy

Another approach to decreasing immunosuppressive and myelosuppressive effects while increasing the chemotherapeutic index is to use combination chemotherapy. Since differential killing of the lymphoid cells of the immunoregulatory circuit by CT drugs can produce either an enhanced or depressed response to an antigen, drugs must be carefully selected so that potential bone marrow and lymphoid toxicity is kept at a minimum. It has been observed that a combination of doxorubicin and MTX is synergistic in killing L1210 cells; however, cytotoxicity to normal hematopoietic stem cells is less than additive. The extent of synergy depends on the dose of doxorubicin only (197). Knowledge of the relative immunosuppression and myelosuppression caused by each drug helps to achieve a maximum chemotherapeutic index and also to maximally spare lymphoid and marrow tissue (252,253). The class of drugs with minimal bone marrow toxicity can be supplemented with other drugs. The experimental work of Goldin et al (254), Skipper et al (255), and Bruce et al (256) laid the conceptual framework for combination chemotherapy. The drugs employed in these early combinations were selected on the basis of their demonstrated efficacy against leukemias and because their toxic manifestations on normal tissues were within tolerable limits. Chlorozotocin is active against metastatic melanoma to the same degree as other chloroethyl nitrosoureas in clinical use, but the fact that chlorozotocin does not cause bone marrow toxicity has made them the choice for use in combination chemotherapy (252). Platinum complexes, which are found to have little toxicity on hematopoietic precursor cells (257), possibly can be used in combination with CT. A nonmyelotoxic combination of CT interspersed with a myelotoxic combination of CT gave a very good response in oat cell carcinoma patients. This combination showed neither drug cross-resistance with myelotoxic combination nor significant bone marrow toxicity (258).

Drug Presentation

Presentation of chemotherapeutic drugs has differential effects on host tissues. Drug synergism between CY and doxorubicin was observed in L1210 only when the two drugs are given together; this regimen was found to have relatively little toxicity to bone marrow (259). Intermittent drug therapy is to be preferred to continuous daily therapy for preventing immunosuppression of the host (188). Split dose therapy may aid recovery of immune function following chemotherapy. Recovered immune status has been correlated with better response to therapy (212), but even intermittent therapy becomes immunosuppressive if maintained for long periods, especially for B-cell function (260).

Rescue from Chemotherapeutic Toxicity

Rescue from chemotherapeutic toxicity, especially from antimetabolite chemotherapy, is becoming common. Of particular interest is the citrovoram factor (CF) in rescuing patients from MTX toxicity. Combination of vincristine, MTX, and CF, if appropriately monitored, is nonmyelosuppressive. It should be possible to include doxorubicin with these combinations. Such combination has proved to be of value in treating hematologic malignancies (261). Some observers find myelosuppression, but not hematopoietic toxicity, with high doses of MTX and CF (18). The remarkably mild toxicity of high-dose MTX-CF reported in clinical studies was substantiated by studying their effect on erythropoiesis and granulopoiesis. Bone marrow granulocyte reserves were marginally depressed, however. The decrease of peripheral blood CFU-c pool size, and of the relative number of bone marrow CFU-c, is moderate; recovery to pretreatment value occurs within 7 to 14 days (262). High-dose MTX-CF reduced the bone marrow CFU-c only moderately, compared with the severe myelosuppressive effect of CY (263).

Drug Delivery

Another novel approach to chemotherapy lies in the mode of drug delivery. Methods have been developed that allow the antitumor drug or radioactive isotopes to be carried selectively to tumor tissue, thus sparing other sensitive tissues. A potentially attractive approach is to employ specific antibodies as carriers of cytotoxic drugs or radioactive isotopes. Globulin combined with the nitrogen mustard, chlorambucil, has been used in a mouse lymphoma model; the result was improved survival (264). ^{131}I-labeled antibody when used against CEA has been shown by several investigators to localize with appropriate selectivity in metastatic tumors of the large bowel and colon (265–267). This suggests the possibility of using implantation RT in conjunction with specific tumor-directed antibody. One can also replace antineoplastic drugs for ^{131}I to achieve selective localization of the drugs. One of the problems with using immunoglobulins is that of isolating a specific antibody directed against the tumor. Now, with the advent of monoclonal antibody, one can hope to raise large amounts of specific antibody against human tumor-associated antigen which will have a high degree of selectivity against the tumor in question (268,269). For an effective outcome, antibodies that localize on the plasma membrane of tumor cells should be degraded after their attachment. Destruction, or release in an inactive form, of antibody bound to the tumor cell may be through pinocytosis or through an enzymatic mechanism. To achieve a more selective accumulation of chemotherapeutic drugs, the drug conjugated to the antibody should be biologically inert until activated at the tumor cell surface (270). Monoclonal antibodies can be used to carry selectively the chemical radiosensitizer to the tumor mass, so that radiation dose to the tumor can be reduced, with a concomitant decrease in the immunosuppressive effect of RT. Liposomes delivered more than four times MTX to murine tumors heated to 42 °C. Most of the accumulated drug was intracellular and bound to dihydrofolate reductase, the enzyme blocked by MTX (271,272). Microwave radiation was found to augment the cellular uptake of MTX, besides inhibiting DNA synthesis (273). This approach was found to increase the survival of L1210-bearing mice. Another experimental approach is complexing of the drug with DNA. It has been proposed that complexing of doxorubicin or daunorubicin with DNA confers lysosomotropic properties on the drug and enables higher incorporation into neoplastic cells. Experimental tumor studies in Belgium and at the National Cancer Institute in Bethesda, Maryland, have indicated potentially less toxicity and increased efficacy when DNA complexes are formed (274,275). Another study indicated that insulin enhanced the rate of absorption of mannosulfan from the peritoneal cavity and prolonged its elimination from the body. Insulin probably enhances not only passage of mannosulfan from the peritoneal cavity to blood, but also from blood to tissues. Since increased antitumor effectiveness of mannosulfan was accompanied by decreased toxicity, it may be concluded that insulin causes selective accumulation of cytostatics only in certain tissues, among others in the tumor (276). Selective concentration of antineoplastic drug can be achieved also by manipulating the route of administration of the drug. Protracted intra-arterial infusion chemotherapy, besides eliminating systemic toxicity, improves local drug concentration (277). Prolonged, slow infusion of 5-FU to cancer patients eliminates myelosuppression, and this may be related to the resultant lower levels of 5-FU in bone marrow (278). Thus, route-dependent pharmacokinetics can be important to eliminating drug toxicity in sensitive normal tissues. Experimental observations suggest that damage to the hemopoietic system is also reduced by means of priming the host. The method involves administering a preliminary small dose of a cytotoxic agent at a specific interval before subsequent injection of a large dose of the same or of a different cytotoxic agent, or before RT. This reduces the dosage to normal tissues (136,234).

Circumvention by Varying the Radiotherapy Mode and Schedule

In the field of RT the technique of using megavoltage has been found to have minimal complications. Technicalities such as delineation of treatment fields and dosimetry beam-alignment procedures have helped a great deal in minimizing harmful effects of radiation on normal tissues. There are two different methods of improving RT. One is to concentrate more of the dose on the tumor itself, thereby reducing the dose to the other parts of the body. The other treatment involves the treatment schedule and radiation qualities that are more destructive to tumor cells than normal cells. Vital normal tissues can be protected selectively by adopting a fractionation regime. Split-dose irradiation of mice has been shown to help recovery of bone marrow and the lymphoid system (279,280). A fractionation regimen consists of a number of variables such as the dose per fraction, the number of fractions, and the time interval between individual fractions. One can profitably vary the individual components in a clinically established fractionation regimen, so that damage to normal tissues, including the lymphoid organs, is minimized. Much less radiobiologic work has been done on normal tissues than on tumors. Therefore, our inability to account satisfactorily for the changes in the immune system following radiation makes it difficult, if not impossible, to have an RT program with minimal effects on the immune system (145). More damage can be done to hypoxic tumor cells by fast neutrons than by x-rays for a given degree of injury to well-oxygenated normal tissues. Since absorption of neutron energy is proportional to hydrogen content of the tissue, bone receives a relatively small dose, thus decreasing bone marrow injury (281). This may be one of the reasons for the lower relative biologic efficiency (RBE) of 15 MeV neutrons for bone marrow than for some animal tumor cells (282) whereas 300 KeV x-ray reduced the recovery of bone marrow CFU. In general, the variation in radiosensitivity between various cell populations, due to either external or internal factors, tends to be smaller for neutrons than for x-rays, possibly owing to smaller amounts of sublethal damage by neutrons as compared with x-rays (184). Neutron irradiation suppresses the antibody formation independent of the dose rate. Immunosuppression by x-ray depends on both radiation rate and total dose (283). X-ray dose rate has been found to have a differential immunosuppression effect. For a given total radiation dose, high dose rates significantly suppressed the xenograft immunity and humoral immunity in mice more than did lower dosages (284,285). This suggests that low x-ray dose rate may have a sparing effect on host immunity. X-rays, if used judicially, besides having economic feasibility, may be more efficient than neutron therapy in certain tumors. Electron therapy of tumors offers the advantage that the depth dose-curves can be accommodated to the needs of therapy by changing the primary energy of the electrons. Thus, doses administered to the tumor can be reduced, and this offers an opportunity to reduce radiation damage to the lymphoid system and bone marrow if they are situated adjacent to the tumor. Electron therapy is more sparing to normal tissue than is RT; also electron therapy produces significantly less leukopenia in cancer patients than does RT (286,287).

Host Protection Against Radiotherapy-Induced Immunosuppression

Circumvention at the level of the host involves preferential protection of the lymphoid system. Physical protection can be achieved in the case of RT by shielding whatever lymphoid tissue is close to the tumor and is uninvolved in the tumor spread. In mice and rats, recovery of hematopoietic organs is more rapid when the spleen is protected from the radiation field (288). Methods have been suggested for selective accumulation—in the bone-marrow, spleen, and other lymphoid organs—of protective substances combined with corpuscular or macromolecular carriers. Svet-Moldavsky et al (289) have used the principle of differential distribution of large molecules and particles in the body. They used folic acid attached to corpuscular or macromolecular carriers to protect the bone marrow, spleen, and liver without reducing the effect of chemotherapeutic agents on the tumor (289). Similarly, injection of corpuscular particles conjugated with well-known radiation protectors such as cystamine has been found to be of value in preventing radiation damage to bone marrow (290). The scheme becomes very active if nontoxic radioprotectors are available. Interferoninducers protected the host against acute and prolonged x- and gamma irradiation, as assessed by a test of survival and by examination of spleen colony formation (291). Compound WR 2721 selectively protects against alkylating agent injury without affecting antitumor properties in a murine tumor (292). Injection of WR 2721 before radiation exposure significantly increases radiation resistance of skin and bone marrow of mice without altering radiation sensitization of solid tumors (293). Such differential protection has been found to be due to the ability of this compound to preferentially concentrate in sensitive tissues such as bone marrow (294). Drugs that selectively radiosensitize hypoxic tumor cells might be exploited in RT to decrease the dose required to sterilize the resistant hypoxic cells (295). A combination of lymphoid-cell sensitizer and normal-tissue radioprotector may produce a more favorable therapeutic dose than can be achieved with either type of drug used independently (296). A new method of radioprotection of mammalian systems, by means of a gas hypoxic mixture containing 10% oxygen and 90% nitrogen, has been worked out by Russian scientists. They report the protective effect of this method on normal human tissues, including the lymphoid system. They recommend this method for oncologic practice, for the purpose of selective protection of patients' healthy tissue during radiotherapy (297). The concept of synergism between therapeutic modalities can be made use of in circumventing CT- and RT-induced alteration of the immune system. Suit et al reported that the dose of radiation to treat a murine fibrosarcoma, which usually requires a toxic, high dose of local RT, could be reduced if used in combination with *C parvum* (298). Similarly, chemotherapeutic dosage of CY could be reduced in experimental tumor systems if the animal was specifically sensitized (220).

Immunologic Reconstitution

The above methods, in principle, cannot protect the elements of antitumor immunity inside the tumor. Haskill et al have shown the importance of in situ lymphocytes in the destruction of tumor cells (29). Modern cellular and molecular immunology has contributed to the development of several novel approaches of modulating, restoring, and enhancing the potential antitumor response. One can engineer the immune response to tumors in several ways so that any depression of antitumor immune response brought about by CT and RT can be reversed and possibly transcended. The various possible ways to circumvent immunosuppression are (a) replacement of inadequate immune functions by various elements of the immune system, (b) nonspecific active immunotherapy, (c) specific active immunotherapy, and (d) specific adoptive immunotherapy. Potential applicability of each of these methods for overcoming host immunosuppression will be considered separately.

Reconstitution of Elements of the Immune System

Thoracic-duct lymphocytic-transfer to seven cancer patients resulted in complete regression of one patient's tumor and partial regression in two other patients. Skin reaction to normal recall antigens was restored in five of the patients (299,300). Administration of 10^9 autochthonous lymphocytes, activated with mitogen PHA, resulted in the regression of pulmonary nodules, although hepatic metastases continued to grow. Lack of response in the liver may be the result of a tumor mass beyond the size that immunotherapy can handle. Also, the outcome may depend on the anatomical site of the tumor (301). This method has the limitation of requiring a large number of lymphocytes to achieve a favorable response; negative results have been attributed to insufficient number of lymphocytes being available. Recently, there are elegant in vitro methods to cultivate a large number of lymphocytes, which may help to overcome the above limitation (302). Intensive CT or WBI in the management of lymphoid tumors often results in bone marrow failure and severe immunosuppression. It has been known for quite some time that animals can be saved from lethal doses of drugs or radiation by the transplantation of their own or genetically identical bone marrow cells.

Immunologic engineering has recently become a new discipline concerned with the restoration of the deprived immune system. In fact, severe impairment of the immune system has become a blessing in disguise in the sense that the "take" of transplanted marrow in the host becomes more likely in the immunosuppressed host. Patients with myeloblastic leukemia give a positive response after intensive CT followed by WBI. This has been attributed to the antitumor effect of high-dose CT and WBI and also to the antitumor-effect by immune competent grafts (303). In a murine experimental model, normal bone marrow has been found to have a unique capacity for inhibiting tumor growth in the presence of tumor-sensitized splenocytes (304). The major complication encountered during immunocompetent cell transplantation is the graft v host (GVH) reaction. An increasing understanding of the pathophysiologic aspects of GVH disease and of the mechanism of graft rejection has helped to overcome this problem. Significant progress has been made in donor selection. Total lymphoid-system irradiation appears to be a promising approach for inducing transplantation tolerance without GVH reaction in histoincompatible bone marrow grafts (305). Other major limiting factors are toxicity of RT and CT to other sensitive tissues, especially the gastrointestinal tract. In a study by Fefer and Thomas, using identical twin bone marrow, long-term survivors were not subject to frequent infections and showed adequate recovery of humoral and cellular immune responses (306). Recovery of immune function in patients with bone marrow transplants has been studied and reviewed by Van Bekkum (307). In general, it appears that the larger the degree of histoincompatability between the recipient and the donor, the longer it takes for the full immunologic reconstitution to be attained.

Nonspecific Immunotherapeutic Intervention in RT

The evidence available today from both animal and clinical studies strongly suggests that nonspecific immunotherapeutic intervention is most likely to be of benefit when it is given along with conventional treatment (87). There are various modalities of restoring the immunodeficient patient to normal status. Levamisole has been tested widely to correct therapy-induced immunosuppression in the host. Significant life prolongation, and even cure, of murine tumors was observed when levamisole was employed in a combined chemoimmunotherapeutic approach (308). It has been suggested that levamisole enhances bone marrow recovery after cytostatic treatment (309). This observation may permit shortening of the interval usually observed between successive courses of antineoplastic treatment, thereby allowing a more aggressive and perhaps more effective anticancer therapy with reduced effect on host immunity.

Many pharmacologic immune-restorations in cancer patients have been reported. Indomethacin appears to restore the immune status, and monocytes seem to play an important role in this (310). The immunopotentiator OK 432, when given along with the cytostatic drug 5-FU to patients with gastrointestinal cancer, markedly augmented the lymphocyte response to PHA; but the cytotoxic activity of lymphocytes was not elevated (311). Combined use of OK 432 in multidrug CT of carcinoma was effective in reducing the duration of hematologic disorders (312). Lithium carbonate was found to increase the circulating polymorphonuclear neutrophils (PMN) and perhaps granulopoiesis in patients with advanced malignancies (313). Lithium may be most useful when used in combination with cytotoxic drugs for treating malignant diseases. Lithium given along with CT shortens the median duration of granulocytopenia in patients undergoing remission induction for acute myeloid leukemia and also reduces the degree of leukopenia (314). It also reduces infection and leukopenia associated with systemic CT of small cell carcinoma (315). Nandrolone decanoate was found to increase the immune status of patients receiving RT for head and neck cancer (316). Cepharanthine is found to increase the number of peripheral lymphocytes, especially T lymphocytes, in some patients when administered continuously during and after RT (173). PS-K administered during and after RT slightly aided recovery of lymphocyte and T-cell count, as well as lymphocyte response to PHA (172). Retinoic acid derivatives were observed to restore the immune status of cancer patients with advanced solid tumors who were receiving CT (317). It has been reported that retinoic acid suppresses tumor growth as a result of stimulation of thymus-dependent effector cells (318). Levan, an immunomodulating polysaccharide, in combination with CY, increases the antitumor effect and decreases the damage caused by CY to the immune system (319). Enhancement of the immune system of CT-treated patients was observed during simultaneous treatment with thymic extract (320). Treatment of rats with pyridoxine after irradiation brings an earlier and rapid restitution of leukocytes, lymphocytes, and granulocytes of peripheral blood (321). If the blood cell picture is any indication of immune recovery, it is worth considering such pharmacologic immune restoration.

Nonspecific Intervention in Chemotherapy

Chemoimmunotherapy with BCG and *C parvum* are well documented. It was found that BCG given five days after CY in L 1210 leukemic cells increases the effect of a less than optimal dosage and reduces the toxicity of higher doses. This possibly reflects the recovery of immune status following immunotherapy. Here the sequencing of the agents is very important. It is seen that BCG, given 15 days before the optimum dose of CY required for tumor cure, decreased the effect of optimum dose (16). Another observation of a similar nature is the increased sensitivity of C parvum-treated mice to ionizing WBI. It was observed that CFU from spleen of mice treated with C parvum was more sensitive to irradiation than CFU from normal spleen (322).

Chemoimmunotherapy also gave encouraging results in a pilot study of active immunotherapy (IT) of acute lymphoid leukemia (323). BCG-CWS enhanced the recovery of PBL of lung cancer patients receiving RT, and the PHA and PWM response recovered rapidly. This suggests that BCG-CWS injection to patients receiving RT is effective for recovery of T-cell response (135). BCG-CWS also restored the immune competence of late-stage bronchogenic carcinoma and prolonged the survival of the patients (324). MER of tubercle bacilli prevented the immunosuppression induced by chemotherapeutic agents. MER could successfully restore both contact hypersensitivity and antibody response in CY-treated mice (325,326). It could also prevent the suppression of contact hypersensitivity in guinea pigs and mice treated with 5-FU and MTX.

Patients with advanced lung cancer who had received CT-RT showed a stonger cutaneous reactivity to recall antigens and increased lymphocyte stimulation following treatment with MER. Although MER treatment did not significantly increase the survival period, it did prevent distant metastasis (327). Patients with stage II breast cancer receiving C parvum IT along with CT did not show a depressed immune status, but those receiving only CT did show a depression in the immune status (214). Lung cancer patients receiving RT and CT showed impairment in cellular immunity. IT with BCG and levamisole caused an increase in skin reaction and lymphocyte response to PPD (133).

Another novel approach to increasing the antitumor immunity during conventional therapy is to control the host immunosuppressive arc by means of immunoadsorption (IA) of plasma-blocking factors, using Protein A bearing Staphylococcus aureus (328–332). It was observed that when IA was coupled with low-dose CY therapy, the therapeutic response, as assessed by the growth inhibition of rat primary mammary adenocarcinoma, improved (328). It is essential to understand the interaction of immunostimulants with one another and with other modalities of treatment, particularly with chemotherapeutic protocols. It has been shown that some of these agents can affect the drug-metabolizing enzymes of the liver (333,334). Immunomodulation in neoplasia is an attempt to alter, in a predictable direction, exceedingly delicate relationships among cell types: host immunocytes and other accessory cells on the one hand, and tumor cells on the other. Immunologic activation, in addition to its capability to induce immune recovery, can also complement CT in destroying tumor cells that may be drug-resistant. Negative effects can also result from multifactorial treatment. It has been observed that the immunomodulator BCG can at times accentuate rather than prevent the immunosuppressive influence of chemotherapeutic drugs (335).

Specific Immunotherapy

Efforts toward specific IT of cancer patients have been made since the beginning of experimental and clinical oncology. Supplementation of specific IT with CT has yielded some promising results. Immunochemotherapy of lung cancer with MTX and soluble antigens, from histologically matched allogeneic tumors, in Freund's complete adjuvant, resulted in the enhancement of patient response to recall antigens. Late testing with tumor antigens, 12 to 30 months following surgery, showed moderate to very strong reactions in the immunochemotherapy group, weak to moderate reactions in the IT group, and anergy in half of the patients tested after administration of CT alone.

MTX was found to counter MLC-blocking factors induced in patients who received IT. This observation promises active specific IT to be an important addition to the chemotherapeutic treatment (336). It also suggests that even CT circumvents the immunosuppressive factors induced by IT (337). This is an important feature in chemoimmunotherapy protocols. In a canine lymphosarcoma model, combination chemotherapy gave a favorable response, but dogs that also received autogenous vaccine with chemically altered tumor-cell extracts survived significantly longer (338). The encouraging results in this group suggest a complementary role of IT in CT. Enzyme-modified tumor cells have been shown to be more immunogenic than the untreated cells. Neuraminidase has been successfully used in developing a specific vaccine in animal tumor models (339). Mice bearing L 1210 leukemia show prolongation of survival following MTX treatment, but no cures. However, by adding a single inoculation of neuraminidase-treated L 1210 cells, much greater extension of survival occurred, and some 40% of the mice were cured (340). It was suggested that with a better experimental drug, capable of producing 20% cures by itself, perhaps 80% to 90% of animals could be cured following a timed inoculation of neuraminidase-treated tumor cells. Patients with acute myelocytic leukemia have shown an increased remission rate when neuraminidase-treated allogeneic myeloblasts were given along with CT (341).

Passive and Adoptive Immunologic Intervention

To circumvent circumstances that suppress the host immune system, attempts at passive and adoptive immunologic intervention in cancer are still in their initial stage, but are promising. This approach has definite advantages, especially with regard to generation of cytotoxic effector cells and antibodies in tissue culture (342). The attempt at passive adoptive IT in vitro with sensitized cells is based on a sound understanding of cellular immunobiology and helps to avoid at least some of the problems associated with active immunotherapy. This, together with the capability to store responder lymphoid cells and tumor-stimulator cells by cryopreservation for prolonged periods without significant loss of reactivity (343, 344), makes the approach a very promising one. Cryopreservation has been successful in both human and murine systems. But it has been observed that some techniques of cryopreservation, storage, and thawing have a negative influence on cell characteristics that are of immunologic significance (345,346). A numberof investigators have demonstrated the feasibility of in vitro sensitization of lymphoid cells to specific cytotoxic reactivity against neoplastic cells (347–353). Sensitization can be achieved even against neoplastic cells that evoke little or no response in the host (343,354).

In man peripheral white blood cells obtained from a high proportion of patients with solid tumors, and from leukemia patients in remission, can be sensitized effectively against autochthonous tumors (349,353). In vitro sensitization to autochthonous tumors can be potentiated by addition to allogeneic stimulator cells to autochthonous neoplastic stimulators (353,355,356). Chemically and enzymatically altered neoplastic cells often effect increased sensitization of responding lymphoid cells (357). Enzymatic treatment of responder cells before and after sensitization also amplifies the cytotoxic potential (358). The presence of microgram quantities of MER in the culture medium also augments the specific cytotoxic response (342,359). The attractive feature of the potentiation of sensitization is the possibility of close correlation, in some systems, between the in vitro and in vivo activities of murine effector cells sensitized in culture, thus permitting an increased therapeutic response (351,352). The responding cells that are generated can adoptively transfer the antitumor immunity, as assessed by Winn assay (343,360,361,362). Such effector lymphoid cell transferred in animals bearing syngeneic tumors have yielded encouraging results. Cell transfer also controlled metastasis (342,351,352,360,363). Autochthonous effector cells are preferable, because their immunologic compatibility with the host to be treated favor their retention for a very long time, thus maintaining the antitumor immunity for an extended period. This procedure also minimizes the complications of GVH reactions. If an adequate quantity of autochthonous cells is not available, it may be possible to enlarge the relevant T-cell population by enrichment of sensitized peripheral white blood cells cultured with factor(s) released by lymphoid cells upon mitogenic stimulation (302,364).

When effector cells were employed therapeutically in mice bearing syngeneic leukemia or lymphoma, without CT only a small percentage of cures were observed, although survival of the mice is significantly prolonged (351,352,360,365). In contrast, when chemotherapy was used in addition to adoptive IT, permanent cures were observed in more than 90% of the animals. CT alone was curative in less than half of the mice

(347,351,360). Even allogeneic effector cells were effective in a chemoimmunotherapy protocol, with minimal GVH (351). In leukemia a combination therapy, which included CT, RT, and adoptive IT with allogeneic lymphoid cells, yielded prolonged survival with only moderate and transient GVH reaction (366). The above studies clearly focus on the need to increase host tumor-immunity in conjunction with RT and CT to get greater tumor control and cure. The accomplishments attained using inbred mice bearing laboratory-induced tumors give a firm foundation for clinical exploration. Although some attempts in the direction of specific adoptive immunotherapy in man have been made, so far clinical trials have not yielded beneficial results (342).

The Lawrence transfer factor, which is a dialyzable factor from leukocyte extract from a sensitized donor, possess the property of immunologic reconstitution of cell-mediated immunity (367). Immune RNA (I-RNA) from lymphoid cells of sheep sensitized against rat sarcoma was shown to be inhibitory to tumor growth (368). Unlike adoptive lymphocyte transfer, this transfer factor and I-RNA do not cause homograft rejection or GVH reaction. Therefore, these factors are worth considering when attempting to restore the immune systems of patients after CT- and RT-induced immunosuppression and to provide better therapeutic benefit to the patients.

Immunologic intervention to restore or increase antitumor immunity in CT or RT is an exceedingly complex bioengineering task, requiring an understanding of the various elements of immune response and of the interaction between the tumor and host, which are still not very clear. The timing of IT with reference to other modalities of treatment, frequency, quality, course of IT, type of IT, and tumor-host relationships all contribute to the success or failure of increasing antitumor immunity.

Antitumor Immune Reactions Following Surgical Resection of Tumor

Introduction

It is becoming increasingly evident that all three major modalities of cancer treatment, although they may be immunosuppressive at times, have the ability to potentiate the immune reactivities of the host to fight back against cancer under appropriate conditions. These benefits are obtained as an unexpected "extra," rather than being a goal. If adequate attention was focused on these areas, where various parameters of these treatments are known, it might be possible to obtain much better therapeutic successes in cancer management.

Of course, surgery is related to immune functions of the cancer patient. For a long time it has been speculated that (a) removal of tumors, (b) decreasing the size of the tumor by CT or RT, or (c) decrease in tumor volume by autogenous regression are all associated with the potentiation of immunologic functions of the host, but not much attention has been paid in this area to exploit its benefit therapeutically. On the contrary, it has been observed that increase in the load of tumors is usually associated with immunosuppression (58,59). Tumor-specific immune responses, which develop at a very early stage of tumor growth, decline and often disappear entirely (58,59,369–371). A number of studies have indicated that generalized immune responses such as delayed hypersensitivity reactions to recall antigens and in vitro lymphocyte stimulation by mitogens and antigens are usually depressed in cancer patients (372,373) and in tumor-bearing mice (374,375).

Immunologic phenomena related to growth of tumors, which are believed to be induced by the tumors, are termed as "blocking phenomena." Several types of humoral factors are found to have the ability to block the immune reactivities of the host (58,59,376,377). They include antigens, antibodies, and antigen-antibody complexes (58,59,376,377). Cellular blocking components, such as suppressor cells, are also described (58,59,378,379) in tumor-bearing hosts. Apart from the specific immunosuppressive factors, humoral and cellular, there are a number of nonspecific immunosuppressive components that can exert immunosuppressive activity in a tumor host. This aspect has been discussed by Yamagishi and colleagues (in this volume).

Surgery as an Immunosuppressant

Although surgery is perhaps the best single modality of cancer therapy, at least for solid tissue tumors, several studies indicate that either surgical intervention by itself, or with associated procedures, may be immunosuppressive.

Lundy and colleagues (380) reported that the anesthesia used for surgery was itself immunosuppressive. They reported that major surgery itself may also be immunosuppressive. It causes a decrease in cell-mediated cytotoxicity and an increase in the number of pulmonary metastases. Using a methylcholanthrene-induced sarcoma model, they inoculated tumor cells on day 0. On day 14 the animals were subjected to halothane anesthesia and the hind limb amputated. The control animals, of course, had no injections of tumor cells. These investigators observed that the major surgery of limb amputation resulted in impaired cell-mediated cytotoxicity postoperatively and also in an increase in the number of pulmonary metastases. The mechanism of immunosuppression was not clear. Mechanical dissemination of tumor cells appeared to be ruled out, because the limb of the animal was cross clamped prior to amputation, hence obviating the possibility of tumor dissemination due to surgical manipulation. It is not clear whether the primary tumor had an inhibitory

influence on possible metastasis, so that its elimination removed the inhibition and thereby facilitated metastatic spread (380).

Simpson-Herren and colleagues (381) demonstrated that surgery may
effect cell genetics, ie, incomplete removal of tumors appears to cause
increased growth of the residual tumor. Using a Lewis lung-tumor model,
they were able to quantify an increase in cellular uptake, as measured by
thymidine index. The uptake increased up to 14 days after surgery. They
suggest that surgery stimulated the growth of lung nodules, resulting in a
slightly decreased median life span. There was a decrease in median life
span after noncurative lung surgery, as well as after sham surgery. They
concluded that mice with widely metastatic lung cancer may have a decreased life expectancy after surgical manipulation, because the residual
tumor tissue is stimulated and grows more rapidly. But altered cell kinetics
may be favorable to chemotherapeutic intervention, so this finding may be
therapeutically useful. In a series of studies Saba et al (382,383) demonstrated that surgery resulted in the host having decreased resistance to
tumor cell growth. They suggested that this depression resulted in a compromise of the host's reticuloendothelial system. Saba et al (382) investigated the influence of surgical stress on the resistance of tumor challenge
with Walker-256 tumor cells in rats. After the experimental animals were
challenged with tumor cells, there was decreased phagocytic activity,
decreased immune clearance, and decreased opsonin levels. The activity
of the reticuloendothelial system was decreased for 60 minutes post-
surgery. The surgery performed was a celiotomy plus jeujunostomy.
Thus, it appeared that tumor surgery resulted in both decreased humoral
and cell-mediated immunity. Decreased phagocytosis was the most pro-
nouncd effect owing to impaired Kupfer cells of the liver, which are a
component of the reticuloendothelial system.

Surgical Manipulation. Does It Result in Increased
Tumor Dissemination?

Several studies have demonstrated that surgical manipulation may release
tumor cells into the circulation. The question has always been whether or
not these tumor cells always result in clinically significant metastases.
Roberts et al (384) demonstrated the isolation of cancer cells from the
bloodstream of patients undergoing uterine curretage. It has been shown
that surgery in tumor-bearing hosts results in an increased number of
viable tumor cells in the blood and in an increased incidence of pulmonary
metastasis.

What then is the implication of these tumor emboli in the circulation?
Several experimental studies have shown that the majority of tumor emboli failed to become established as metastatic tumors. Schatton et al
(385) summarized the status of tumor emboli in their report (386–388).

There has been no demonstrable correlation between the presence of tumor cells in the blood and subsequent development of distant metastases. It appears that tumor cells enter the bloodstream continually. In some patients with carcinomas the tumor emboli survive and grow only when proper conditions exist. What are these proper conditions? It is tempting to speculate that some aspects in the preoperative period may tip the tumor-host relationship in favor of the tumor. In the study by Schatten et al (385) utilizing transplanted myeloma S91 tumors in DBA animals, they demonstrated that there was an increase in the number and size of pulmonary metastases after amputation of a tumor-bearing limb. However, they noticed that there was no increase in metastases when major surgery was performed on the contralateral leg. They concluded that "there was no effect of surgery, anesthesia, or cortisone on the number of artificial pulmonary metastases." This point was disputed in another report by Vose and Moudgil (389). These investigators observed a significant depression of cell-mediated cytotoxicity in breast cancer patients for at least 1 week postoperatively. After the operation under general anesthesia, there appeared to be a transient fall or else diminished activity of peripheral-blood lymphocyte-mediated cytotoxicity lasting from 2 hours to 1 week postoperatively. Other investigators have corroborated this transient fall of response secondary to surgery; notably, Riddle and Berembaum (390) also demonstrated postoperative depression of lymphocyte response to PHA.

Immunorestorative Capacity of Surgery

Le Francois and colleagues (391) reported that peritoneal cells from mice at the beginning of tumor growth had a moderate immunologic activity that disappeared entirely when the tumors reached 7 mm or more in diameter. After surgical removal of the tumors, this activity reappeared, after nearly 20 days.

Mikulska et al (392) showed that lymphoid cells from rats carrying chemically induced sarcomas, when mixed in vitro with corresponding tumor cells, showed no depressive action on their growth when reintroduced in vivo; however, lymphoid cells showed full functional activity when taken from rats 3 weeks after surgical removal of the tumor.

Heppner (393) and Baldwin et al (191) showed that tumor excision effects an increase or return of cell-mediated immunity, with a decline in serum-blocking factor. Alexander et al (394) demonstrated the presence of immunoblast cells in the thoracic-duct lymph after tumor removal.

Bray and Keast (395) studied the changes in cell-mediated and humoral immunity following excision of a transplantable melanoma growing in the foot-pad of its syngeneic host. Spleen-cell cytotoxicity did not change significantly. Cells from the regional lymph nodes stimulated tumor growth before tumor excision. Three days following tumor excision this stimulatory effect was undetectable. Loss of serum factors capable of blocking the cytotoxicity of spleen cells occurred 24 hours after tumor excision. Serum cytotoxicity increased after tumor excision, reaching its maximum on the third day. Thus, following tumor excision, the rise in serum cytotoxicity and loss of regional lymph node tumor stimulation were concomitant with the loss of blocking activity.

From the above discussion, it appears logical that the observed changes in host immunity are directly related to removal of the source of tumor antigen, leading to loss of serum blocking and to a rise in serum cytotoxicity. With the loss of blocking factor locally, stimulation of tumor growth by regional lymph node also disappears. If these in vitro findings are directly applicable to the in vivo situation, it suggests that excision of tumors confers a number of beneficial effects on the host. These benefits are immunologic by nature and may contribute to the inhibition of tumor growth.

A number of studies have reported that after a tumor attains a certain size, tumor-specific immunity of the host becomes nonfunctional. In these cases, surgical resection of the tumor helps to regain the immunologically responsive state in the host (391,393). Other workers have shown that nonspecifically depressed cell-mediated immunity in tumor-bearing hosts could be restored to normal levels after surgical resection of the tumor (374). Snyderman and colleagues (81) found that chemotaxis of macrophages is abnormal in melanoma patients (81), breast cancer patients (82), and patients bearing other solid tumors (83–85). Surgical removal of tumor normalized chemotaxis, suggesting that the tumor itself was the cause of the defect in monocyte function.

In a recent study Shafer et al (396) observed that in postoperative colon and rectal cancer patients, reduced IgG and IgM values returned gradually to normal levels.

Greco et al (397) examined an earlier suggestion that electrocoagulation of carcinoma of the rectum was an acceptable alternative to abdominoperineal resection and that electrocoagulation acted as an immunostimulant. The authors reported that electrocoagulation was less of an immunosuppressant than was abdominoperineal resection. In a separate study (398) the same authors did leukocyte migration inhibition assays in patients with carcinoma of the colon and rectum treated by electrocoagulation, abdominoperineal resection, or low anterior resection. No statistically significant differences in cell-mediated immunity, measured by leukocyte migration inhibition, were noticed between those in the electrocoagulated group and those undergoing resection. However, electrocoagulation cured some carcinomas of the rectum and afforded a superior quality of survival.

Cryosurgery has been found to effect disappearance of metastates from the lung in human cancer patients. In mice, significantly increased humoral and cellular immune response was observed following cryosurgery. Cryosurgery has been shown capable of eradicating a local tumor sometimes, but the contributions of the systemic immune response to local and metastatic tumor control, and the conditions necessary to maximize this response, have not been fully evaluated as yet. Future trials should attempt to determine the optimal methods for delivering cryosurgery to control local tumors and utilize the augmented immune response of the host to treat the metastatic lesions.

Conclusion

From the foregoing it appears that every conventional modality of cancer treatment modifies the immune response of the host. Given suitable subjects and proper planning, immune response can be made to favor the host; that is, the immune response can be augmented subsequent to the use of conventional modalities of treatment, either to arrest or inhibit tumor growth and/or metastases. Achieving a favorable state of immune balance may even be designed to achieve minimal residual tumor mass after conventional treatment modalities.

Exactly how an immune balance can be achieved, which favors the host, is not currently well understood. However, it is known that RT and CT can kill tumor cells, and one can speculate that if killed tumor cells act as a source of autogenous vaccination, then antitumor immunity may develop, which in turn may control progressive tumor growth or destroy the residual tumor mass. We can speculate that surgical resection of a tumor may also alter the immunologic balance in favor of the host by conferring the ability to counteract the residual tumor growth or even a new growth. Long-term disease-free survivals, or else cures, are probably related directly to the development of antitumor immunity subsequent to RT, CT, or surgery, but one cannot be more definitive at this point as to how this can be achieved until more information is available.

Exhaustive research in this area is urgently needed to understand how to achieve shifts in the immune balance that favor the host's immunity against the tumor in the first place during and/or subsequent to conventional cancer therapy.

References

1. Fidler IJ: Tumor heterogenity and the biology of cancer invasion and metastasis. *Cancer Res* 38:2651–2658, 1978.
2. Fidler IJ, Gersten DM, Hart IR: The biology of cancer invasion and metastases. *Adv Cancer Res* 28:149–165, 1978.
3. Fidler IJ, Kripke ML: Tumor cell antigencity, host immunity and cancer metastases. *Cancer Immunol Immunother* 7:201, 1980.
4. Nossal GJV: The case history of Mr. Tumor Immunology. Terminal patient or still curable? *Immunol Today* 1:5–12, 1980.

5. Catalona WJ, Sample WF, Chretient PB: Lymphocyte reactivity in cancer patients: Correlation with tumor histology and clinical stage. *Cancer* 31:65–79, 1973.
6. Ducos J, Migueres J, Colombies P, Kessous A, Pougoulet N: Lymphocyte response to PHA in patients with lung cancer. *Lancet* i:1111–1113, 1970.
7. Garrioch DB, Good RA, Tatti RA: Lymphocyte response to PHA in patients with nonlymphoid tumors. *Lancet* i:618–627, 1970.
8. Gerosa MA, Amadori G, Semenzato P, Gasparotto G, Carteri A: Immunobiology of primary CNS tumor in infancy and childhood: Bone marrow derived, thymus dervied, cell dependent immunity and cytotoxicity and cell kinetics evaluation. *Child's Brain* 6:92–105, 1980.
9. Han T, Takita H: Immunological impairment in bronchogenic carcinoma: A study of lymphocyte response to PHA. *Cancer* 30:616–624, 1972.
10. Herberman RB: Assessment of cellular immune response to cancer of the breast. *Ann Clin Lab Sci* 9:467–474, 1979.
11. Klippel KF, Hutschenreiter G, Jacobi G, Graff J: Urological primary multiple neoplasias: Diminished immunocompetence. *Onkologie* 2:12–26, 1979.
12. Lander I, Bone G: Lymphocyte transformation in large bowel cancer. *Br J Cancer* 27:409–421, 1973.
13. Leb L, Merritt JA: Decreased monocytic function in patients with Hodgkin's disease. *Cancer* 41:1794–1812, 1978.
14. Menconi E, Barzi A, Greco M, Caprino MC, de Vecchis L, Muggia F: Immunologic profile of breast cancer patients in early or advanced disease. *Experientia* 35:820–825, 1979.
15. Menconi E, Barzi A, Grew M: Immunological reactivity in patients bearing solid tumors. *Tumori* 66:311–317, 1980.
16. Solowey AC, Rapaport FT: Immunologic responses in cancer patients. *Surg Gynecol Obstet* 121:756–764, 1965.
17. Umeda T, Yokoyama H, Kobayashi K, Akaza H, Nijime T: Subsets of thymus derived lymphocytes of patients with maligancies of urogenital tract. *Cell Mol Biol* 25:95–104, 1979.
18. Pitman SW, Parker LM, Tattersall MHN, Jaffe N, Frei E, III: Clinical trial of high dose Methotrexate with Citrovorum factor-toxicologic and therapeutic observations. *Cancer Chemotherap Rep Part 3* 6:43–51, 1975.
19. Whittaker MG, Rees K: Reduced-lymphocyte transformation in breast cancer. *Lancet* i:892–894, 1971.
20. Yanagawa E, Yasumoto K, Manabe H, et al: Cytostatic activity of peripheral blood monocyte against bronchogenic carcinoma cells in patients with lung cancer. *Gann* 70:533–542, 1979.
21. Gross RL, Steel CM, Levin AG, Singh S, Brubaker G: In vitro immunological studies on East African cancer patients. III. Spontaneous rosette formation by cells from Burkitt lymphoma biopsies. *Int J Cancer* 15:139–148, 1975.
22. Haskill JS, Yamamura Y, Radov L: Host responses within solid tumors: non-thymus derived specific cytotoxic cells within a murine mammary adenocarcinoma. *Int J Cancer* 16:798–807, 1975.
23. Haskill JS, Proctor JW, Yamamura Y: Host responses within solid tumors. I. Monocytic effector cells within rat sarcomas. *J Natl Cancer Inst* 54:387–394, 1975.

24. Jondal M, Klein G: Classification of lymphocytes in nasopharyngeal carcinoma biopsies. *Biomedicine* 23:163–172, 1975.
25. Juhlin I, Blomgren H, Wasserman J: Evidence for the appearance of nonspecific inhibitory cells in the blood after radiation therapy for breast carcinoma. *Cancer Lett* 3:311–316, 1977.
26. Klein E, Becker S, Svedmyr E, Jondal M, Vanky F: Tumor-infiltrating lymphocytes. *Ann NY Acad Sci* 276:207–212, 1976.
27. Underwood JCE: Lymphoreticular infiltration in human tumors: Prognostic and biological implication. A review. *Br J Cancer* 30:538–543, 1974.
28. Yata J, Desgranges C, The G De, et al: Nasopharyngeal carcinoma. VII. B and T lymphocytes in the circulating blood and in tumor tissue. *Biomedicine* 21:244–254, 1975.
29. Haskill JS, Yamamura Y, Radov L, Parthenasis E: Are peripheral and in situ tumor immunity related? *Ann NY Acad Sci* 276:373–385, 1976.
30. Holden HT, Haskill JS, Kirchner H, Herberman RB: Two functionally distinct antitumor effector cells isolated from primary murine sarcoma virus induced tumors. *J Immunol* 117:440–449, 1976.
31. Iochim HL: The stromal reaction of tumors: an expression of immune surveillance. *J Natl Cancer Inst* 57:465–472, 1976.
32. Vanky F, Klein E, Stjernsward J, Rodriguez L, Peterffy A, Steiner L, Nilsonne U: Human tumor lymphocyte interaction in vitro. III. T lymphocyte in autologous tumor stimulation. *Int J Cancer* 22:679–688, 1978.
33. Vose BN, Vanky F, Fopp M, Klein E: In vitro generation of cytotoxicity against autologous human tumor biopsy cells. *Int J Cancer* 21:588–594, 1978.
34. Pelouze GA, Pelletier G: Lack of in situ cell mediated cytotoxicity in human lung cancer. *Abstr No 10.3.30,* 4th International Congress of Immunology, 1980.
35. Byfield PE, Stratton JA, Small R: Lymphocyte response after radiotherapy. *Lancet* 1:309–310, 1974.
36. Kozlowski H, Hrabowske M: Types of cell mediated immune response in invasive zones of carcinoma of uterine cervix. *Arch Geschwulstforch* 49:240–245, 1979.
37. Deutsch O, Devens B, Naor D: Immune responses to weakly immunogenic murine leukemia virus induced tumors. VIII. Characterization of suppressor cells. *Isr J Med Sci* 16:538–547, 1980.
38. Devens B, Galili N, Deutsch O, Naor D, Klein E: Immune responses to weakly immunogenic virally induced tumors. II. Suppressive effects of the in vivo carried tumor YAC. *Eur J Immunol* 8:575–584, 1978.
39. Fujimoto S, Greene MI, Sehon AH: Regulation of the immune response to tumor antigens. I. Immunosuppressor cells in tumor bearing hosts. *J Immunol* 116:791–799, 1976.
40. Takei F, Levy JG, Kilburn DG: Characterization of suppressor cells in mice bearing syngeneic mastocytoma. *J Immunol* 118:412–421, 1977.
41. Kirchner JH, Chusadm TM, Herberman RB, Holden HT, Larvin DH: Evidence of suppressor cell activity in spleens of mice bearing primary tumors induced by Moloney Sarcoma virus. *J Exp Med* 139:1473–1482, 1974.
42. Kold JP, Arrian S, Zolla-Pazner S: Suppression of tumor immune response

by plasmacytomas: mediation by adherent mononuclear cells. *J Immunol* 118:702–714, 1977.

43. Treves AJ, Cohen IR, Feldman M: Suppressor factor secreted by T lymphocytes from tumor bearing mice. *J Natl Cancer Inst* 57:409–417, 1976.
44. Gorczynski RM: Immunity to murine sarcoma virus induced tumors. II. Suppression of T cell mediated immunity by cell from progressor animals. *J Immunol* 112:1826–1834, 1974.
45. Cerny J, Stiller RA: Immunosuppression by spleen cells from Moloney leukemia. Comparison of the suppressive effect on antibody response and on mitogen induced response. *J Immunol* 115:943–955, 1975.
46. Stiller RA, Cerny J: Immunosuppression by spleen cells from Moloney leukemia. II. Studies on the mechanism of suppression and failure to detect an extracellular suppressive product. *J Immunol* 117:889–894, 1976.
47. Hillinger SM, Herzig GP: Increased suppressor cell activity in Hodgkin's disease. *Proc Am Assoc Cancer Res* 18:152, 1977.
48. Broder S, Poplack D, Whang-Peng J, Drum M, Goldman C, Maul L, Waldman TA: Characterization of a suppressor cell leukemia. Evidence for the requirement of two T cells in development of a tumor suppressor effector cell. *N Engl J Med* 298:66–72, 1978.
49. Kumar V, Bennet M: H-2 compatibility requirements for T suppressor cell function induced by Friend leukemia virus. *Nature* 265:345–346, 1977.
50. Schechter B, Feldman M: Hydrocortisone affects tumor growth by eliminating precursors of suppressor cells. *J Immunol* 119:1563–1573, 1977.
51. Ray PK, Raychaudhuri S: Low dose cyclophosphamide inhibition of transplantable fibrosarcoma growth by augmentation of the host immune responses. *J Natl Cancer Inst* 67(6):1341–1352, 1981.
52. Fujimoto S, Greene MI, Sehon AH: Regulation of the immune response to tumor antigens. II. The nature of immunosuppressor cells in tumor bearing host. *J Immunol* 116:800–810, 1976.
53. Stelzer GT, Wallace JH: Suppressor cells in mice bearing B-16 melanoma. *Proc Am Assoc Cancer Res* 18:68–72, 1977.
54. Rudczynski AB, Mortensen RF: Suppressor cells in mice with murine mammary tumor virus induced mammary tumors. I. Inhibition of mitogen induced lymphocyte stimulation. *J Natl Cancer Inst* 60:205–212, 1978.
55. Schaaf-Lafontaine N: Separation of lymphoid cells with a suppressor effect on the activity of cytotoxic cells in vitro during the growth of a syngeneic mouse tumor *Int J Cancer* 21:329–334, 1978.
56. Small M, Trainin N: Separation of population of sensitized lymphoid cells into fractions inhibiting and fractions enhancing syngeneic tumor growth in vivo. *J Immunol* 117:292–302, 1976.
57. Kamo I, Friedman H: Immunosuppression and the role of suppressive factors in cancer. *Adv Cancer Res* 25:271–284, 1977.
58. Raychaudhuri S, Ray PK, Bassett JG, et al: Changing pattern of blocking and effector immune mechanisms during the growth of methylocholanthrene fibrosarcomas. *Fed Proc* 39(3):696, 1980.
59. Saha S, Ray PK: Tumor antigen mediated induction of humoral and cellular tumor growth enhancing factors. *Fed Proc* 41(3):411, 1982.
60. Lang H, Domzig W, Lohmann-Mathes ML: Cooperative effects between

lymphokine-induced and antibody-dependent macrophage-mediated cytotoxicity in C_{57} BL/10 and C_3 H/HeJ mice. *Immunobiol* 157:109–114, 1980.

61. Ting CC, Rodrigues D: Increased susceptibility to tumor cell immunosuppressive effect in tumor bearing mice. *J Natl Cancer Inst* 65:205–212, 1980.
62. Ting CC, Rodrigues D: Subversion by tumor cells of the host immune surveillance via macrophages. *4th Int Cong Immunol Abstr* 10.3.42, 1980.
63. Seshadri M, Poduval TB, Sundaram K: Studies on Metastasis. I. Role of sensitisation and immunosuppression. *J Natl Cancer Inst* 1205–1214, 1979.
64. Seshadri M, Poduval TB: Immunity stimulation and Metastasis. *Cancer Immunol Immunother* 9:213–218, 1980.
65. Karre K, Klein G, Kiessling R, Klein G, Roder J: Low resistance against transplantable syngeneic leukemias in natural killer deficient C_{57} BL Biege mutant mice. *4th Int Cong Immunol Abstr* 10.2.17, 1980.
66. Flannery GR, Robins RA, Baldwin RW: Natural killer cell infiltrates solid tumors. *4th Int Cong Immunol Abstr* 10.2.08, 1980.
67. Eremin O, Ashby J, Stephens JP: Human natural cytotoxicity in the blood and lymphoid organ of healthy donors and patients with malignant disease. *Int J Cancer* 21:35–44, 1978.
68. Heindenreich W, Jagla K, Schussler J, Borner P, Dehnhard F, Kalden JR, Liebold W, Peter H-H, Deicher H: Spontaneous cell mediated cytotoxicity and antibody dependent cellular cytotoxicity in peripheral blood and draining lymph nodes of patients with mammary carcinoma. *Cancer Immunol Immunother* 7:65–74, 1979.
69. Peter HH, Eife RF, Kalden JR: Spontaneous cytotoxicity (SCMC) of normal human lymphocyte against a human melanoma cell line: A phenomenon due to a lymphokine-like mediator. *J Immunol* 116:342–354, 1976.
70. Peter HH, Pavite-Fischer J, Fridman WH, Aubert C, Cessarini JP, Rouhin R. Kourilsky FM: Cell-mediated cytotoxicity in vitro of human lymphocytes against a tissue culture melanoma cell line (IGR 3). *J Immunol* 115:539–546, 1975.
71. Takasugi M, Ramsemeyer A, Takasugi J: Decline of natural nonselective cell-mediated cytotoxicity in patients with tumor progression. *Cancer Res* 413:419, 1977.
72. Peter HH, Heidenrich W: Spontaneous cell-mediated cytotoxicity. *Cancer Immunol Immunother* 8:79–88, 1980.
73. Peter HH, Lange B, Serbin A, Euler S, Stangl W, Avenarius HJ, Deicher H: Natural killing in hemopoietic disorders and immunodeficiency syndromes. Evidence for the bone marrow dependency of human NK effector cells. *Immunobiology* 156:206–210, 1979.
74. Hanna MG, Zbar B, Rapp HJ: Histopathology of tumor regression after intralesional injection of Mycobacterium bovis. I. Tumor growth and metastasis. *J Natl Cancer Inst* 48:1441–1452, 1972.
75. Lala PK: Dynamics of leukocyte migration into the mouse ascites tumor. *Cell Tissue Kinet* 7:239–304, 1974.
76. Levy MH, Wheelock EF: The role of macrophage in defence against neoplastic disease. *Adv Cancer Res* 20:131–152, 1974.
77. Nelson DS (ed): *Immunobiology of the Macrophage.* New York, Academic Press, 1976.

78. Shin HS, Hayden M, Langley S, Kaliss N, Smith MR: Antibody-mediated suppression of grafted lymphoma. III. Evaluation of the role of the thymic function, non thymus derived lymphocytes, macrophages, platelets, and polymorphonuclear leukocytes in syngeneic and allogeneic hosts. *J Immunol* 114:1255–1264, 1975.

79. Klein E: Immunotherapy of cutaneous and mucosal neoplasms. *NY State J Med* 68: 900–910, 1968.

80. Papermaster BW, Holterman OA, Rosner D, Klein E, Dao T, Kjerassi, I: Regressions produced in breast cancer lesions by a lymphokine fraction from a human lymphoid cell line. *Res Commun Chem Pathol Pharmacol* 8:413–424, 1974.

81. Snyderman R, Seigler HF, Meadows L: Abnormalities of monocyte chemotaxis in patients with melanoma: Effects of immunotherapy and tumor removal. *J Natl Cancer Inst* 58:37–46, 1977.

82. Snyderman R, Maedows L, Well SA, Jr, Hoder W: Abnormal monocyte chemotaxis in patients with breast cancer: evidence for a tumor-mediated effect. *J Natl Cancer Inst* 60:737–743, 1978.

83. Black MM: Human breast cancer. A model for cancer immunology, *in* Weiss DW(ed): Immunological parameter of host-tumor relationship. New York, Academic Press, 1973, pp 80–105.

84. Hausman MS, Brosman S, Snyderman R: Defective monocyte function in patients with genitourinary carcinoma. *J Natl Cancer Inst* 55:1047–1054, 1975.

85. Fink MA (ed): *The Macrophage in Neoplasia.* New York, Academic Press, 1976.

86. Klein G, Sjogren HO, Klein E, Hellstrom KE: Demonstration of resistance against Methylcholantherene induced sarcomas in the primary autochthonous. *Cancer Res* 20:1561–1574, 1960.

87. Cohen D, Yron I, Grover NB, Weiss DW: Chemoimmunotherapy of Syngeneic mouse mammary carcinomas employing methanol extraction residue. *Ann NY Acad Sci* 277:195–204, 1976.

88. Hellstrom KE, Hellstrom I, Brown JP: Unique and common tumor specific transplantation antigens of chemically induced mouse sarcomas. *Int J Cancer* 21:317–326, 1978.

89. Kudo H, Waga T, Sato T, Ogasawara M, Ito I, Usubuchi I: Cross immunity between syngeneic tumors in mice immunized with gamma irradiated ascites tumors. *Tohoku J Exp Med* 131:285–292, 1980.

90. Leffel MS, Coggin JH, Jr: Common transplantation antigen on Methylcholanthrene-induced mouse sarcomas detected by three assays of tumor rejection. *Cancer Res* 37:4112–4121, 1977.

91. Parmiani G, Invernizzi G: Alien histocompatability determinants on the cell surface of sarcomas induced by MCA. 1. *in vivo* studies. *Int J Cancer* 16:756–762, 1975.

92. Usubuchi I, Sobajima Y, Kudo H, Sugawara M: Cross immunity among syngeneic tumors of mice. *Tohoku J Exp Med* 108:79–89, 1972

93. Usubuchi I, Nishimura S, Kudo H, Ito I, Sobajima Y: Further studies on cross immunity among syngeneic tumors of mice. *Tohoku J Exp Med* 116:373–384, 1975.

94. Martin WJ, Imamura M: Variable expression of histocompatibility antigens on tumor cells. *Cancer Immunol Immunother* 8:219–224, 1980.

95. De Baetselier P, Katzav S, Feldman M, Segal S: H-2 antigenic differences between a primary tumor and its descendant pulmonary metastasis. *4th Int Cong Immunol* 10.3.09, 1980.

96. Basslet K, Schirrmacher V: Escape of spleen metastasising tumor cell variant from T cell immunity. *4th Int Cont Immunol* 10.3.04, 1980.

97. Anderson JM, Campbell JB, Wood SE, Boyd JE, Kelly F: Lymphocyte subpopulations in mammary cancer after radiotherapy. *Clin Oncol* 1:201–213, 1975.

98. Wara WM, Phillips TL, Wara DW, Ammann AJ, Smith V: Immunosuppression following radiation therapy for carcinoma of the nasopharynx. *Am J Roentgenol* 123:482–492, 1975.

99. Weber W, Missmahl HP, Mazloumi B: Tuberculin and dinitrochlorobenzene tests in cancer patients before and after cytostatic drug therapy. *Klin Wochenschr* 56:905–909, 1978.

100. Golub SH, Rangel DM, Morton DL: In vitro assessment of immune competence in patients with malignant melanoma. *Int J Cancer* 20:873–886, 1977.

101. Teasdale C, Hillyard JW, Webster DJT, Bolton PM, Hughes LE: Pretreatment general immune competence and prognosis in breast cancer. A prospective 2 year follow up. *Eur J Cancer* 15:975–982, 1979.

102. Schullenberger CC: Chemoimmunotherapy of 3 categories of solid tumors (sarcoma, melanoma and lymphoma), in Crispen RG (ed): *The Problem of Immunoresistant Tumors*. Chicago, ITR Press, 1973, pp 193–225.

103. Herberman RB: Cell mediated immunity to tumor cells. *Adv Cancer Res* 19:207–218, 1974.

104. Black MM: Cellular and biological manifestation of immunogenicity in precancerous mastopathy. *Natl Cancer Inst Monograph* 35:73–82, 1972.

105. Alexander P: Back to the drawing board: The need for more realistic model systems for immunotherapy. *Cancer* 40:467–479, 1977.

106. Baldwin RW: Relevant animal models for tumor immunotherapy. *Cancer Immunol Immunother* 1:197–204, 1976.

107. Bartlett GL, Kreider JW, Purnell DM: Immunotherapy of cancer in animals: Models or muddles? *J National Cancer Inst.* 56:207–215, 1976.

108. Fidler IJ: Experimental Basis of Immunotherapy of Metastatic Disease, in The Univ Texas System Cancer Center: *Immunotherapy of Human Cancer*. New York, Raven Press, 1971, pp 63–85.

109. Fidler IJ, Hart IR: Host Immunity in Experimental Metastasis, in Castro JE (ed): *Immunological Aspects of Cancer*. Lancaster, England, MTP Press, 1978, pp 193–192.

110. Anderson RE, Warner NL: Ionizing radiation and the immune response. *Adv Immunol* 24:215–221, 1976.

111. Taliaferro WH, Taliaferro LG, Joroslow BN: *Radiation and Immune Mechanisms*. New York, Academic Press, 1964.

112. Denham S, Grant CK, Hall JG, Alexander P: Occurrence of two types of cytotoxic lymphoid cells in mice immunized with allogeneic tumor cells. *Transplantation* 9:366–373, 1970.

113. Poduval TB, Seshadri M, Sundaram K: Studies on development of concomi-

tant immunity in a murine fibrosarcoma. *Aspects Allergy Appl Immunol* 11:240–251, 1978.

114. Anderson RR, Sprent J, Miller JFAP: Radiosensitivity of T and B lymphocytes. I. Effect of irradiation on cell migration. *Eur J Immunol* 4:199–207, 1974.

115. Makinodan T, Nettesheim P, Morita T, Chadwick CJ: Synthesis of antibody by spleen cells after exposure to kiloroentgen doses of ionizing radiation. *J Cell Physiol* 69:355–362, 1967.

116. Miller JJ III, Cole LJ: The radiation resistance of long-lived lymphocytes and plasma cells in mouse and rat lymph nodes. *J Immunol* 93:982–991, 1967.

117. Moroson H, Schechter M: Enhanced cytotoxic reactivity of rat splenic cells after lethal or sublethal whole body X-irradiation. *Int J Radiat Biol* 33:595–602, 1978.

118. Dutton RW: Inhibitory and stimulatory effects of Concanavalin A on the response of mouse spleen cell suspension to antigen: I. Characterization of the inhibitory cell activity. *J Exp Med* 136:1445–1457, 1972.

119. McCullagh P: Radiosensitivity of suppressor cells in newborn rats. *Aust J Exp Biol Med Sci* 53:399–412, 1975.

120. Herberman RB, Holden HT: Natural cell mediated immunity. *Adv Cancer Res* 27:305–315, 1978.

121. Shellam GR: Gross virus induced lymphoma in the rat. V. Natural cytotoxic cells are non T cells. *Int J Cancer* 19:225–234, 1977.

122. Ellis ST, Govans JL, Howard JC: Cellular events during the formation of antibody. *Cold Spring Harbor Symp Quant Biol* 32:395–400, 1967.

123. Gershon H, Feldman M: Studies on the immune reconstitution of sublethally irradiated mice by peritoneal macrophages. *Immunology* 15:827–834, 1968.

124. Kornfeld L, Greenman V: Effects of total body X-irradiation on peritoneal cells of mice. *Radiat Res* 29:433–442, 1966.

125. Feldman JD, Pick E, Lee S, Silvers WK, Wilson DB: Renal homotransplantation in rats. III. Tolerant recipients. *Am J Pathol* 52:687–692, 1968.

126. Poduval TB, Seshadri M, Ray PK, Thakur VS, Sundaram K: Effect of host sensitization to tumor on splenic depletion and recovery following severe immunosuppressive treatment. *Ind J Exp Biol* 17:1064–1074, 1979.

127. Baral E, Blomgren H, Petrini B, Wasserman J: Blood lymphocytes in breast cancer patients following radiotherapy and surgery. *Int J Radiat Oncol Biol Phys* 2:289–293, 1977.

128. Stratton JA, Fast PE, Weintraub I: Enhanced or repressed mitogen responses of peripheral blood mononuclear cells after radiation therapy and prognosis in cancer. *4th Int Cong Immunol* 10.7.29, 1980.

129. Benninghoff DL, Tyler RW, Everett NB: Repopulation of irradiated lymph node by recirculating lymphocytes. *Radiat Res* 37:381–392, 1969.

130. Engeset A: Irradiation of lymph nodes and vessels. Experiments in rats, with reference to cancer therapy. *Acta Radiol* (Suppl) 229:1–7, 1964.

131. Weissman IL, Peacock M, Eltringham JR: Regional lymph node irradiation: Effect of local and distant generation of antibody forming cells. *J Immunol* 110:1300–1315, 1973.

132. Thomas L: Discussion, in Lawrence HS (ed): *Cellular and Humoral Aspects of the Hypersensitive States*. London, Cassell, 1959, 529–539.

133. Grapp C, Havemann K: Cellular immune reactions in patients with bronchogenic carcinoma before and after radio-chemo-and immunotherapy. *Z Immunitaetsforsch* 153:236–242, 1977.
134. Hoppe Richard T, Freks ZY, Strober S, Kaplan HS: The long term effects of radiation on the T and B lymphocyte in the peripheral blood after regional irradiation. *Cancer* 40:2071–2076, 1977.
135. Nishikawa H, Yasaki S, Yoshimoto T, Sakatani M, Itoh M: Effect of BCG cell-well skeleton immunotherapy on the peripheral blood lymphocytes in patients with lung cancer after radiotherapy. *Jpn J Cancer Res* 69:819–826, 1978.
136. Blomgren H, Wasserman J, Baral E, Petrini B: Evidence for the appearance of nonspecific suppressor cells in the blood after local radiation therapy. *Int J Radiat Oncol Biol Phy* 4:249–254, 1978.
137. Stjernsward J: Immunological changes after radiotherapy for mammary carcinoma. *Ann Inst Pasteur* 122:833–891, 1972.
138. Stjernsward J, Jondal M, Vanky F, Wigzell H, Sealy R: Lymphopenia and changes in distribution of human B and T lymphocytes in peripheral blood induced by irradiation for mammary carcinoma. *Lancet* i:1352–1353, 1972.
139. Meyer KK: Radiation-induced lymphocyte-immune deficiency. *AMA Arch Surg* 101:114–118, 1970.
140. Rafla S, Yang SJ, Maleka F: Changes in cell-mediated immunity in patients undergoing radiotherapy. *Cancer* 41:1076–1084, 1978.
141. McCredie JA, Inch WR, Sutherland RM: Effect of postoperative radiotherapy on peripheral blood lymphocytes in patients with carcinoma of the breast. *Cancer* 29:349–354, 1972.
142. Clement JA, Kramer S: Immunocompetence in patients with solid tumors undergoing Cobalt-60 irradiation. *Cancer* 34:193–202, 1974.
143. Fukushima H: Immunological studies concerned with high dose radiotherapy for osteosarcoma. *Nippon Seikei Geka Gakkai Zasshi* 53:1607–1614, 1979.
144. Manabe H, Yasumoto K, Ohta M, Toyahira K, Nomoto K: Effect of anticancer therapy on lymphocytic cytotoxicity in lung cancer patients. *Gann* 68:477–482, 1977.
145. Doria G: Immunological effects of irradiation: Waiting for a model. *Int J Rad Oncol Biol Phys* 5:1111–1118, 1979.
146. Suit HD, Sedlacek R, Wagner M, Orsi L, Silobric V, Rothman KJ: Effect of *Corynebacterium parvum* on the response to irradiation of a C_3H fibrosarcoma. *Cancer Res* 36:1305–1311, 1976.
147. Tsukahara Y, Shiozawa I, Shoji I, Tohoru F: Effect of protein binding polysaccharide PS-K on radiotherapy of uterine cervical carcinoma. *Gan No Rinsho* 25:783–786, 1979.
148. Ray PK, Thakur VS, Sundaram K: Antitumor immunity. I. Differential response of neuraminidase-treated and X-irradiated tumor vaccine. *Eur J Cancer* 11:1–11, 1975.
149. Ray PK, Thakur VS, Sundaram K: Antitumor immunity II. Viability, tumorigenicity and immunogenicity of neuraminidase-treated tumor cells: Effective immunization of animals with a tumor vaccine. *J Natl Cancer Inst* 56:83–94, 1976.

150. Elves MW: Comparison of Mitomycin C and X-rays for the production of one way stimulation of mixed Leucocyte cultures. *Nature* 223:90–92, 1969.
151. McKhann CF: The effect of X-ray on the antigenicity of donor cells in transplantation immunity. *J Immunol* 92:811–816, 1964.
152. Maruyama Y: Contribution of host resistance to radiosensitivity of an isologous murine lymphoma *in vivo*. *Int J Radiat Biol* 12:277–282, 1967.
153. Nio Y: Studies on the cells producing an antitumor agent (Japanese). *Nippon Acta Radiol* 30:481–487, 1970.
154. Sato I, Nio Y, Abe M: In vitro production of an antitumor agent by Reticuloendothelial cells. *Gann* 59:273–279, 1968.
155. Moroson H, Nowakowski J, Schechter M: Enhanced lymphocyte-mediated killing of tumor irradiation *in vivo*. *Int J Radiat Biol* 33:473–481, 1978.
156. Sheldon PW: The effect of irradiating a transplanted solid sarcoma on the subsequent development of metastasis. *Br J Cancer* 30:416–424, 1974.
157. Sheldon PW, Fowler JF: The effect of irradiating a transplanted murine lymphosarcoma on the subsequent development of metastases. *Br J Cancer* 28:508–515, 1973.
158. Suit HD, Kastelan A: Immunological status of host and immune response of a MCA-induced sarcoma to local X-irradiation. *Cancer* 26:232–242, 1970.
159. Crile G Jr, Deodhar SD: Role of preoperative irradiation in prolonging concomitant immunity and preventing metastasis. *Cancer* 27:629–634, 1971.
160. Seshadri M, Poduval TB, Ray PK, Sundaram K: Involvement of immune surveillance in radiotherapy. *Aspect Allergy Appl Immunol* 11:256–262, 1978.
161. Gerber M, Budois JB, Gauci L, Serrou B: The effect of local irradiation on the immune response in mice. II. Alteration due to low dose scattering. *Ann Immunol* (Paris) 130:735–742, 1979.
162. Vaage J, Doroshow JH, DuBois TT: Radiation-induced changes in established tumor immunity. *Cancer Res* 34:129–134, 1974.
163. Crile G Jr: The effect of metastasis of removing or irradiating regional nodes of mice. *Surg Gynecol Obstet* 126:1270–1278, 1968.
164. Warram J: Preoperative irradiation of the cancer of the lung: Final report of a therapeutic trial: A collaborative study. *Cancer* 36:914–923. 1975.
165. Stewart THM, Hollinshead AC, Herberman RB: Soluble Membrane antigens of human malignant lung cells, in Maltoni C (ed): *Advances in Tumor Prevention, Detection and Characterization*. Vol 2, New York, American Publ. Co, Inc, 1974, pp 638–674.
166. Fisher B, Slack NH, Cavanaugh PH, Gardner B, Ravdin RG: Postoperative radiotherapy in the treatment of breast cancer. *Ann Surg* 172:711–721, 1971.
167. CRC Working party: Cancer Research campaign King's Cambridge troa; for early breast cancer. A detailed update at the tenth year. *Lancet* ii:55–65, 1980.
168. Fisher B, Fisher ER: Studies concerning the regional lymph node in cancer. II. Maintenance of immunity. *Cancer* 29:1496–1507, 1972.
169. Hancock BW, Bruce L, Heath J, Sugden P, Ward AM: The effects of radiotherapy on immunity in patients with localised carcinoma of the cervix uteri. *Cancer* 43:118–124, 1979.
170. Nordman E, Toivanen A: Effects of irradiation on the immune function in patients with mammary, pulmonary or head and neck carcinoma. *Acta Radiol Oncol Radiat Biol* 17:3–14, 1978.

171. Stefani S, Krman R, Abbate J: Serial studies of immunocompetence in head and neck cancer patients undergoing radiation therapy. *Am J Roentgenol* 126:880–892, 1976.
172. Sciichi K: *Immunocompetence in Human Cancer Patients.* Nippon Geka Hokan 120:504–512, 1979.
173. Makidono R, Madidono A, Matsura K: Leukopenia and lymphopenia during the radiotherapy and their recovery by anti-leukopenia drugs. *Nippon Igaku Hoshasen Gakkai Zasshi* 37:1153–1161, 1977.
174. del Regato JA: Total body irradiation in the treatment of chronic lymphogenous leukemia. *Amer J Roentgenol* 120:504–512, 1974.
175. Johnson RE: Total body irradiation as primary therapy for advanced lymphosarcoma. *Cancer* 35:242–253, 1975.
176. Melamed JS, Michael GC, Brown JW, Katagiri CA: Acute hematological tolerance to multiple fraction, whole body low dose irradiation in an experimental murine system. *Radiology* 134:503–514, 1980.
177. Yonkosky DM, Feldman MI, Cathcart ES, Kim S: Improvement of *in vitro* mitogen proliferative responses in non Hodgkin's lymphoma patients exposed to fractionated total body irradiation. *Cancer* 42:1204–1215, 1978.
178. Hellstrom I, Hellstrom KE: Antitumor effect of whole body X-irradiation: Possible role of an X-ray sensitive T suppressor cell population. *Transplant Proc* 11:1073, 1979.
179. Chanana AD, Cronkite EP, Joel DD, Stevens JB: Prolonged renal allograft survival: extracorporeal irradiation of the blood. *Transplant Proc* 3:838–844, 1971.
180. Kutzner J, Goldhofer R, Kreienberg R, Lemmel EM: Examinations carried out in order to determine the effects of radiotherapy on the immunity stimulation in tumor patients. *Strahlentherapie* 155:341–349, 1979.
181. Wara WM: Immunosuppression associated with radiation therapy. *Int J Radiat Oncol Biol Phys* 2:593–597, 1977.
182. Chee CA, Ilbery PLT, Rickinson AB: Depression of lymphocyte replicating activity in radiotherapy patients. *Brit J Radiol* 3:562–567, 1969.
183. Ruhl H, Vogt W, Ruhl U: Effect of hydrocortisone treatment and whole body irradiation on mouse lymphocyte stimulation in vitro. *Immunology* 25:753–759, 1973.
184. Barendsen GW: Responses of cultured cells, tumors and normal tissues to radiations of different linear energy transfer in Ebert M, Howard A (ed): *Current Topics in Radiation Research,* Vol. IV, Amsterdam, North Holland Biological Company, 1968, pp. 332-346.
185. Berenbaum MC: The effect of cytotoxic agents on the production of antibody to TAB vaccine in the mouse. *Biochem Pharma* 11:29–34, 1962.
186. Gabrielsen AE, Good RA: Chemical suppression of adoptive immunity. *Adv Immunol* 6:91–99, 1967.
187. Hersh EM, Friereich EJ: Host defence mechanism and their modification by cancer chemotherapy. *Methods in Cancer Res* IV:355–382, 1968.
188. Hersh EM, Gutterman JU, Mavligit GM, et al: Host defence, chemical immunosuppression and transplant recipient, relative effect of intermittent versus continuous immunosuppressive therapy with reference to objective of treatment. *Transplant Proc* 5:1191–1205, 1973.
189. Yamaki H, Tanaka N, Umezawa H: Effects of several tumor inhibitory antibiotics on immunological responses. *J Antibiot* 22:315–322, 1969.

190. Schwartz RS: Are immunosuppressive anticancer drugs self defeating? *Cancer Res* 28:1452–1462, 1968.
191. Baldwin RW, Embleton MJ: Assessment of cell mediated immunity to human tumor associated antigens. *Int Rev Exp Pathol* 17:49–54, 1977.
192. Cerottini JC, Brunner KT: Cell mediated cytotoxicity, allograft rejection with tumor immunity. *Adv Immunol* 19:67–84, 1974.
193. Mantovani A, Potentarutti N, Luine W, Peri G, Spreafico F: Role of host defence mechanism in the antitumor activity of adriamycin and Daunomycin in mice. *J Natl Cancer Inst* 63:61–72, 1979.
194. Riccardi C, Puccetti P, Santoni A, Herberman RB, Bonmassar E: Adriamycin-induced antitumor response in lethally irradiated mice. *Immunopharmacology* 1:211–224, 1979.
195. Schwartz HS, Grindey GB: Andriamycin and Daunorubicin: Comparison of antitumor activities and tissue uptake in mice following immunosuppression. *Cancer Res* 33:1837–1845, 1973.
196. Segerling M, Ohanian SH, Borsos T: Enhancing effect by metabolic inhibitors on the killing of tumor cells by antibody and complement. *Cancer Res* 35:3195–3211, 1975.
197. Valeriote F, Vietti T, Coulter D: Cytotoxicity of Adriamyoin combined with Methotrexate against L 1210 leukemia in mice. *J Natl Cancer Inst* 64:801–810, 1980.
198. Vecchi A, Fioretti MC, Mantovani A, Barzi A, Spreafico F: The immunodepressive and hematotoxic activity of imidazole 4-carboxamide, 5-(3,3-dimethyl-1-triazeno)K in mice. *Transplantation* 22:619–624, 1976.
199. DellaBurna C, Sanfillippo A: Immunodepressive activity of Adriamycin in experimental infection of the mouse with *Nippostrongylus brasiliensis*. *Experientia* 27:841–852, 1971.
200. Isetta AM, Intini C, Soldatai M: On the immunodepressive action of Adriamycin. *Experientia* 27:202–214, 1971.
201. Berenbaum MC, Brown IN: Dose response relationships for agents inhibiting the immune response. *Immunology* 7:65–74, 1964.
202. Berenbaum MC: Time dependence and selectivity of immunosuppressive agents. *Immunology* 36:355–362, 1979.
203. Evans R, Madison LD, Eidler DM: Cyclophosphamide induced changes in the cell compartment of Methylcholantherene induced tumor and their relation to bone marrow and blood leucocyte levels. *Cancer Res* 40:395–408, 1980.
204. Mihich E: New leads towards antitumor selectivity in therapeutics. *Chemotherapy* 7:51–62, 1976.
205. Wanebo HJ, Jun MY, Strong EW, Oettgen H: T cell deficiency in patients with squamous cell cancer of the head and neck. *Am J Surg* 130:445–452, 1975.
206. Parves EC, Barenbaum MC: Selective suppression of murine antibody-dependent cell-mediated cytotoxicity by azathioprine. *Transplantation* 19:274–281, 1975.
207. Mitsuoka A, Baba M, Morikawa S: Enhancement of delayed hypersensitivity by depletion of suppressor T cells with Cyclophosphamide in mice. *Nature* 262:77–79, 1976.
208. Askenase PW, Hayden BJ, Gershon RK: Augmentation of delayed type

hypersensitivity by doses of Cyclophosphamide which do not effect antibody responses. *J Exp Med* 141:697–704, 1975.

209. Mantovani A, Vecchi A, Tagliabue A, Spreafico F: The effects of Adriamycin and Daunomycin on antitumoral immune effector mechanisms in an allogeneic system. *Eur J Cancer* 12:371–379, 1976.

210. Vecchi A, Mantovani A, Tagliabue A, Spreafico F: A characterization of the immunosuppressive activity of Adriamycin and Daunomycin on humoral antibody production and tumor allograft rejection. *Cancer Res* 36:1222–1300, 1976.

211. Reynolds PM, Dawkins RL, Byrme MJ: Immunological effects of cancer chemotherapy in malignant melanoma: Differential effects on function of lymphocyte subpopulations. *Cancer Immunol Immunother* 4:185–191, 1978.

212. Cheems AR, Hersh EM: Patient survival after chemotherapy and its relationship to in vitro lymphocyte blastogenesis. *Cancer* 28:851–859, 1971.

213. Bowles CA, Lucas D, Norton L, Graw RG, Jr.: Immunological studies of canine lymphosarcoma: Mixed leucocyte reactivity following chemotherapy. *Clin Immunol Immunopathol* 9:211–214, 1978.

214. Weese JL, Oldham RK, Torney DC et al: Immunologic monitoring of carcinoma of breast. *Surg Gynecol Obstet* 145:209–214, 1977.

215. Hancock BW, Bruce L, Dunsmore IR, Ward MA, Richmond J: Follow up studies on the immune status of patients with Hodgkin's disease after splenectomy and treatment, in relapse and in remission. *Br J Cancer* 36:347–352, 1977.

216. Roth JA, Eilber FR, Morton DL: Effect of Adriamycin and high dose Methotrexate chemotherapy on in vivo and in vitro cell mediated immunity in cancer patients. *Cancer* 41:814–821, 1978.

217. Zighelboim J: Deficiency of antibody-dependent cell-mediated cytoxicity and mitogen-induced cellular cytotoxicity effector cell function in patients with acute myelogenous leukemia in remission. *Cancer* 39:3357–3362, 1979.

218. Krienberg R, Melchert F, Lemmel EM: Monitoring of the immunological status of breast cancer patients treated with adjuvant chemotherapy and polychemotherapy. *Onkologie* 2:181–186, 1979.

219. Mihich E: Combined effects of chemotherapy and immunity against leukemia L_{1210} in DBA/2 mice. *Cancer Res* 29:848–851, 1969.

220. Moore M, Williams DE: Contribution of host immunity to cyclophosphamide therapy of a chemically induced murine sarcoma. *Int J Cancer* 11:358–362, 1973.

221. Steele G, Pierce GE: Effects of cyclophosphamide on immunity against chemically induced syngeneic murine sarcoma. *Int J Cancer* 13:572–581, 1974.

222. Teller MN, Faanes RB: Association of host immunity with 5-Flurouracil initiated cure of plasmacytoma LPC-1 in BALB/c mice. *Cancer Res* 40:2790–2799, 1980.

223. Santoni A, Riccardi C, Sorci V, Herberman RB: Effects of Adriamycin on activity of mouse natural killer cells. *J Immunol* 124:2329–2334, 1980.

224. Mantovani A, Tagliabaue A, Luini W, Facchinetti T, Spreafico F: The Role of Macrophages in the Antitumoral Activity of Adriamycin or in Combination with *C. parvum,* in James K, McBride B, Stuart A (ed): *The Proc*

EURES Symp on 'The Macrophage and Cancer'. Edinburgh, Ecoprint, 1977, pp 203–225.

225. Mantovani A: *In vitro* and *in vivo* cytotoxicity of Adriamycin and Daunomycin on murine macrophages. *Cancer Res* 37:815–824, 1977.

226. Teller MN, Bowie M, Mountain IM, Stock CC: Combination chemotherapy of advanced murine myeloma and subsequent resistance to tumor challenge. *J Natl Cancer Inst* 52:667–672, 1974.

227. Lubet RA, Carlson DE: Immunity against MOPC 104E plasmacytoma: Effects of tumor size and time post therapy on *in vivo* tumor immunity. *J Natl Cancer Inst* 60:1107–1114, 1978.

228. Hengst JCD, Mokyr MB, Dray S: Importance of timing in cyclophosphamide therapy of MOPC315 tumor bearing mice. *Cancer Res* 40:2135–2142, 1980.

229. Borsos T, Bast RC Jr, Ohanian SH, Segerling M, Zbar B, Rapp H: Induction of tumor immunity by anti-tumoral chemotherapy. *Ann NY Acad Sci* 276:565–574, 1976.

230. Glaser M: Regulation of specific cell mediated cytotoxic response against SV40 induced tumor associated antigen by depletion of suppressor T cells with cyclophosphamide in mice. *J Exp Med* 149:774–782, 1979.

231. Philips FS, Chou TC, Hutchinson DJ, Schmid F, Sternberg SS: Selective Toxicity and Chemotherapeutic Efficacy, in *Pharmacological Basis of Cancer Chemotherapy,* MD Anderson Hospital and Tumor Institute, Williams and Wilkins Co., Baltimore, MD. 1975, pp 469–492.

232. Radov LA, Haskill JS, Korn JH: Host immune potentiation of drug responses to a murine mammary adenocarcinoma. *Int J Cancer* 17:773–781, 1976.

233. Carter RL, Connors RA, Weston BJ, Davies AJS: Treatment of a mouse lymphoma by L-asparaginase: Success depends on the host's immune response. *Int J Cancer* 11:345–352, 1973.

234. Gregory SA, Fried W, Knopse WH, Trobaugh FE: Accelerated regeneration of transplanted hemopoietic stem cells in irradiated mice pretreated with cyclophosphamide. *Blood* 37:196–208, 1971.

235. Lubet RA, Carlson DE: Therapy of the murine plasmacytoma MOPC 104E: role of the immune response. *J Natl Cancer Inst* 61:896–904, 1978.

236. Mathe G, Halle-Pannenko I, Bourut C: Effectiveness of murine leukemia chemotherapy according to the immune state. *Cancer Immunol Immunother* 2:139–146, 1977.

237. Orsini F, Eppolito C, Ehrke MJ, Mihich E: Inhibition by selected anticancer agent of the development of primary cell-mediated immunity against allogeneic tumor cells in culture. *Cancer Treat Rep* 64:211–219, 1980.

238. Bonmassar E, Bonmassar A, Vadlamudi S, Goldin A: Immunological alteration of leukemic cells in vivo after treatment with anti-tumor drug. *Proc Natl Acad Sci* (USA) 66:1089–1097, 1970.

239. Houchene DP, Bonmassar E, Gershon MR, Kende M, Goldin A: Drug mediated immunogenic changes of virus induced leukemia in vivo. *Cancer Res* 36:1347–1354, 1976.

240. Mihich E: Modification of tumor regression by immunological means. *Cancer Res* 29:2345–2351, 1969.

241. Giampietri A, Fioretti MC, Goldin A, Bonmassar E: Drug induced antigenic

changes in murine leukemic cells: Antagonistic effects of quinacrine, and antimutagenic compound. *J Natl Cancer Inst* 64:297–304, 1980.

242. Dye ES, North RJ: Macrophage accumulation in murine ascites tumors. I. Cytoxan induced dominance of macrophage over tumor cells and the antitumor effects of endotoxin. *J Immunol* 125:1650–1657, 1980.

243. L'age-Stehr J, Diamantstein T: Studies on induction and control of cell mediated autoimmunity. I. Induction of "autoreactive" T lymphocytes in mice by cyclophosphamide. *Eur J Immunol* 8:620–627, 1978.

244. Wander RH, Hilgard HR: Does cyclophosphamide alter tumor cell antigenicity? *Lancet* ii:1077–1078, 1980.

245. Knock F, Galt R, Oester Y, Sylvester R, Rebechini-Zasadny H: Selected Sulfhydryl inhibitors capable of inducing immunity against cancer in mice. *Oncology* 36:197–208, 1979.

246. Brock N: Experimental basis of cancer chemotherapy. *Chemotherapy* 7:19–26, 1976.

247. Ohto Y, Sucki K, Kitta K, Takcmoto K, Ishitsuka H, Yagi Y: Comparative studies on the immunosuppressive effect among 5'-Deoxy-5Fluorouridine, *Ftorafu* and 5FU. *Gann* 71:190–199, 1980.

248. Anderson T, McManamin M, Schein P: Chlorozotocin 2-(3-(2-chlorothyl))-3-nitosourea, an antitumor agent with modified bone marrow toxicity. *Cancer Res* 35:761–768, 1975.

249. Durden DL, Distasio JA: Comparison of the immunosuppressive effects of Asparaginase from *E. coli* and *Vibrio succinogenes*. *Cancer Res* 40:1125–1132, 1980.

250. Schwartz RS: Immunosuppression by L-asparaginase. *Nature* 224:275–281, 1969.

251. Deodhar SD: Enhancement of metastases by L-asparaginase in a mouse tumor system. *J Reticuloendothelial Soc* 10:212–219, 1971.

252. Hoth DF, Schein PS, Winokur S et al: A phase II study Chlorozotocin in metastatic malignant melanoma. *Cancer* 46:1544–1552, 1980.

253. Millar JL, Hudspith BN, Blackett NM: Reduced lethality in mice receiving a combined dose of Cyclophosphamide and busulfan. *Cancer* 32:193–201, 1975.

254. Goldin A, Venditti JM, Hymphreys SR, Mantel N: Quantitative evaluation of chemotherapeutic agents against advanced leukemia in mice. *J Natl Cancer Inst* 21:495–505, 1958.

255. Skipper HE, Schabel FM Jr, Wilcox WS: Experimental evaluation of potential anticancer agents. XIII. On the criteria and kinetics associated with curability of experimental leukemia. *Cancer Chemother Rep* 35:3–11, 1964.

256. Bruce WR, Mechker RE, Powers WE, Valeriote FA: Comparison of the dose and time survival curves for normal hematopoietic and lymphoma colony forming cells exposed to Vinblastine, Arabinosyl cytosine and Amethopterin. *J Natl Cancer Inst* 42:1015–1022, 1969.

257. Wierda D, Pazdernik TL: Toxicity of platinum complexes on hemopoietic precursor cells. J Pharmacol Exp Ther 211:531–537, 1979.

258. Israel L, Dapierre A, Choffel C, Milleron B, Edelstein R: Immunochemotherapy in 34 cases of oat cell carcinoma of lung with 19 complete responses. *Cancer Treatment Rep* 61:343–349, 1977.

259. Mulder JH, Van Putten LM: Adriamycin—Cyclophosphamide combination

chemotherapy: the importance of drug scheduling. *Eur J Cancer* 15:1503–1508, 1979.

260. Sen L, Borell L: Expression of cell surface markers and T and B lymphocyte after long term chemotherapy of acute leukemia. *Cell Immunol* 9:84–91, 1973.

261. Frie E. III: Methotrexate revisited. *Med Pediat Oncol* 2:227–234, 1976.

262. Schreml W, Lohrmann HP: Effect of high dose Methotrexate with ci-trovorum factor on human granulopoiesis. *Cancer Res* 39:4195–4204, 1979.

263. Lohrmann HP, Schreml W, Lang M, Betzler M, Fliedner TM, Heimpel H: Changes of granulopoiesis during and after adjuvant chemotherapy of breast cancer. *Br J Haematol* 40:369–374, 1976.

264. Ghose T, Rapth MRC, Nigam SP: Antibody as carrier of chlorambucil. *Cancer* 29:1398–1402, 1972.

265. Goldernberg MD, DeLand F, Klin E, Bennet S, Primus JF, Van Nagel JR, Estes N, DeSimone P, Rayburn P: Use of radiolabelled antibody to carci-noembryonic antigen for detection and localization of diverse cancers by external photoscanning. *N Engl J Med* 298:1384–1395, 1978.

266. March JP, Carrel S, Merenda C, Sordat B, Cerrotoni JC: *In vivo* localization of radiolabelled antibody to carcinoembryonic antigen in human colon carci-noma grafted into nude mice. *Nature* 248:704–715, 1974.

267. Order SE, Klein JL, Sgagias M, Ettinger E, Trump D: Isotopic immuno-globulin therapy: A phase I-II trial. *Proc Am Assoc Cancer Res* 20:366–372, 1979.

268. Kohler G, Milstein C: Continuous cultures of fused cells secreting antibody of predefined specificity. *Nature* 256:495–504, 1975

269. Woodbury RG, Brown JP, Yeh MY, Hellstrom I, Hellstrom KE: Identifica-tion of a cell surface protein, p 97, in human melanomas and certain other neoplasms. *Proc Natl Acad Sci* (USA) 787:2183–2192, 1980.

270. Bale WF, Contreras MA, Grady ED: Factors influencing localisation of labelled antibodies in tumors. *Cancer Res* 40:2965–2974, 1980.

271. Weinstein JN, Magin RL, Yatvin RL, Zaharko DS: *Science* 204:188–195, 1979.

272. Weinstein JN, Magin RL, Cysyk RL, Zaharko DS: Treatment of solid L 1210 murine tumors with local hyperthermia and temperature sensitive lipo-somes containing methotrexate. *Cancer Res* 40:1388–1397, 1980.

273. Chang BK, Huang AT, Joines WT: Inhibition of DNA synthesis and en-hancement of the uptake and action of Methotrexate by low power density microwave radiation in L 1210 leukemia cells. *Cancer Res* 40:1002–1013, 1980.

274. DeDuve C, Trouet A: Lysosomes and lysosomotropic drugs in host-parasite relationship, in Braun W, Ungar J (ed): *Nonspecific Factors Influencing Host Resistance* Basel, Karger, 1973, pp 153–164.

275. Trouet A, Compeneere DD, DeDuve C: Chemotherapy through lysosomes with a DNA-daunorubicine complex. *Nature* (New Biol) 239:110–118, 1972.

276. Damusz A, Wutkiewicz M, Wierzbe K: Influence of insulin on pharmaco-kinetics of mannosulfan in rats. *Arch Immunol Ther Exp* 27:376–382, 1979.

277. Obefield RA, Cady B, Booth JC: Regional arterial chemotherapy for ad-vanced cancer of the head and neck. *Cancer* 32:82–94, 1973.

278. Fraile RJ, Baker LH, Buroker TR, Horbvitz J, Vaitkevicius VK: Pharmacokinetics of 5-FU administered orally by rapid intravenous and by slow infusion. *Cancer Res* 40:2223–2232, 1980.
279. Till JE, McCulloch EA: Early repair processes in marrow cells irradiated and proliferating *in vivo*. *Radiat Res* 18:96–105, 1963.
280. Vos O: Survival of lymphatic cells after X-irradiation in mice. Effects of ionizing radiations on the hematopoietic tissues. *IAFA,* Vienna, 1967, pp 134–149.
281. Bewley DK: Fast neutron beams for tumor therapy, in Ebert M, Howard A (ed): *Current Topics in Radiation Research,* Vol VI, Amsterdam, North Holland Biological Company, 1970, pp. 249–262.
282. Broerse JJ, Barendsen GW, Freriks G, Van Putten LM: RBE values of 15 MeV neutrons for effects on normal tissue. *Eur J Cancer* 7:171–182, 1971.
283. Gottlieb CF, Gengozian N: The humoral immune response in mice after neutron or X-irradiation at different dose rates. *J Immunol* 109:711–721, 1972.
284. Carlson DE, Gengozian N: The effect of acute radiation exposure rates on formation of hemagglutinating antibody in mice. *J Immunol* 106:1535–1544, 1971.
285. Gengozian N: Transplantation of rat bone marrow in irradiated mice: effect of exposure rate. *Science* 146:663–672, 1964.
286. Vaeth JM (editor): Electron beam therapy. (*Proc 2nd Ann San Francisco Cancer Symp,* 1966) Kargar, Basel, 1968.
287. Zuppinger A, Poretti G (editors): *Proc Symp High Energy Electrons.* Springer, Berlin, 1965.
288. Jacobson LO, Simmons EL, Marks EK, Eldredge Jr: Recovery from radiation injury. *Science* 113:510–514, 1951.
289. Svet-Moldavsky GJ, Pavlotsky AI, Ravkina LI: The principle of selective defence at chemotherapy of malignant tumors. *Vestn Acad Med Sci U.S.S.R.* 5:42–51, 1967.
290. Svet-Moldavsky GJ, Pavlotsky AI: Particular carriage of radio-resistance. *Lancet* ii:779–781, 1967.
291. Talas M, Batkai L: Study of interferon inducers as radioprotective agents. *6th Int Cong Radiat Res Abstr* E-6-1, 1979.
292. Yuhas JM: Active versus passive absorption kinetics as the basis for selective protection of normal tissues by 5-2-(30-aminopropylamino) ethylphosphorothioic acid. *Cancer Res* 40:1519–1524, 1980.
293. Yuhas JM, Storer JB: Differential chemoprotection of normal and malignant tissues. *J Natl Cancer Inst* 42:332–339, 1969.
294. Utley JF, Marlowe C, Waddell WJ: Distribution of ^{35}S-labelled WR-2721 in normal and malignant tissues of mouse. *Radiat Res* 68:264–271, 1976.
295. Denekamp J, Michael BD: Preferential sensitisation of hypoxic cells to radiation in vivo. *Nature* (New Biol) 239:21–23, 1972.
296. Chapman JD, Urtasum RC: The application in radiation therapy substances which modify cellular radiation response. *Cancer* 40 (Suppl):484–491, 1977.
297. Chizhov AY, Strelkov RB: On practical use of a gas hypoxic mixture GHM-10 as a radioprotectant. *6th Int Cong Rad Res Abstr* E-6-5, 1979.
298. Suit HD, Sedlacek R, Wagner M, Orsi L: Radiation response of C_3H fibro-

sarcoma enhanced in mice stimulated by *Corynebacterium parvum. Nature* 255:493–495, 1975.

299. Yonemoto RH, Terasaki PI: Cancer immunotherapy with HLA compatible thoracic duct lymphocyte transplantation. Cancer 30:1438–1441, 1972.

300. Yonemoto RH: Adoptive immunotherapy utilizing thoracic duct lymphocytes. *Ann NY Acad Sci* 277:7–15, 1976.

301. Frenster JH, Rogoway WM: Immunotherapy of human neoplasms with autologous lymphocytes activated in *vitro*, in Harris JE (ed): *Proc Fifth Leucocyte Culture Conf*, New York, Academic Press, 1982, pp 359–378.

302. Gillis S, Smith KA: Long term culture of tumor specific cytotoxic T cells. *Nature* 268:154–156, 1977.

303. Thomas ED, Buckner CD, Banaji M: One hundred patients with acute leukemia treated by chemotherapy, total body irradiation, and allogeneic marrow transplantation. *Blood* 49:511–519, 1977.

304. Scuderi P, Rosse C: Unsensitised bone marrow uniquely interacts with sensitised splenocytes in inhibiting tumor growth. *4th Int Cong Immunol Abstr* 10.2.40, 1980.

305. Kaplan HJS, Strober S, Gottlieb M, et al: Induction transplantation tolerance without graft versus host disease by total lymphoid irradiation. *6th Int Cong Rad Res Abstr* C-23-9, 1979.

306. Fefer A, Thomas ED: Marrow transplants in aplastic anemia and leukemias. *Sem Hematol* 11:353–362, 1974.

307. Van Bekkum DW: Perspectives of immunological reconstitution. *Proc 9th Int Cong Allergology,* Excerpta Medica, Amsterdam, 1977.

308. Amery WK, Spreafico F, Rojas AF, Denissen E, Chirigos MA: Adjuvant treatment with levamisole in cancer. A review of experimental and clinical data. *Cancer Treatment Rev* 4:167–174, 1977.

309. Senn JS, Lai CC, Price GB: Levamisole: Evidence for activity on human progenitor cells. *Br J Cancer* 41:40, 1980.

310. Mavligit GM, Raphael LS, Calvo DB, Wong WL: Indomethacin-induced monocyte-dependent restoration of local graft versus host reaction among cells from cancer patients. *J National Cancer Inst* 65:317–324, 1980.

311. Mashiba H, Yoshinaga H, Matsunaga K, et al: Effect of immunochemotherapy on lymphocyte response of patients with gastrointestinal cancer. *J Surg Oncol* 12:275–282, 1979.

312. Kurukowa T, Nakao I, Furukawa K, Kanko T, Yokoyama T, Obashi Y: Multidrug combination in cancer chemotherapy: Mitomycin C with 5-FU. *Tohoku J Exp Med* 129:337–346, 1979.

313. Grecom FA, Breseton HD: Effect of lithium carbonate on the neutropenia caused by chemotherapy: A preliminary clinical trial. *Oncology* (Basel) 34:153–157, 1977.

314. Stein RS, Flexner JM, Graber SE: Lithium and granulocytopenia during induction therapy of acute myelogenous leukemia. *Blood* 54:636–647, 1979.

315. Lyman GH, Williams CC, Preston D: The use of lithium carbonate to reduce infection and leukopenia during systemic chemotherapy. *N Engl J Med* 302:257–268, 1980.

316. Huys JV, Plum JR: Effect of nandrolone decanoate on thymus derived lymphocyte during radiotherapy. *Clin Ther* 2:352–364, 1979.

317. Cupissol D, Serrou B: Evaluation of the immunorestorative properties of

retinoic acid derivative in patients with advanced solid tumors. *4th Int Cong Immunol Abstr* 10.5.13, 1980.

318. Patek PO, Collins JL, Yogeeswaran G, Dennert G: Antitumor potential of retinoic acid: Stimulation of immune mediated effectors. *Int J Cancer* 24:624–635, 1979.
319. Leibovici J, Stark Y, Wolman M: Combined effects of levan and cyclophosphamide on the growth of Lewis lung carcinoma in $C_{57}BL$ mice. *4th Int Cong Immunol Abstr* 10.5.46, 1980.
320. Shoham J, Brenner HJ, Chaitchik S: Enhancement of the immune system of chemotherapy treated cancer patients by simultaneous treatment with the thymic extract, TP-1. *4th Int Cong Immunol Abstr* 10.5.63, 1980.
321. Stojanovic DB, Milivojevic KS: Reaction of some radiosensitive physiological systems of irradiation and injury, in *Radiobiological Research and Radiotherapy*, Vol. II. (Proc. Symp. Vienna, 1976), IAEA, Vienna 1977, pp 247–272.
322. Basic I, Kastelan, Milas L: Increased sensitivity of *Corynebacterium parvum* treated mice to ionising whole body irradiation. *6th Int Cong Radiat Res Abst* E-19-2, 1979.
323. Mathe G, Amiel JL, Schwarzenberg L, Schneider M, Cattan A, Schulumberger JR, Hayat M, de vassal F: Active immunotherapy for acute lymphoid leukemia. *Lancet* 1:697–699, 1969.
324. Yasumoto K, Manabe H, Ueno M, et al: Immunotherapy of human lung cancer with BCG cell wall skeleton. *Gann* 67:787–794, 1976.
325. Stupp Y, Saltoun R, Weiss DW: Prevention by the methanol extraction residue tubercle bacillus fraction of immunosuppression induced by cancer chemotherapeutic agents. I. Antibody response of mice treated with cyclophosphamide. *Cancer Immunol Immunother* 1:219–224, 1976.
326. Zimber C, Ben-Efraim S, Weiss DW: Prevention by the MER tubercle bacillus fraction of immunosuppression induced by cancer chemotherapeutic agents. II. Contact hypersensitivity in guinea pigs and mice treated with cyclophosphamide. *Cancer Immunol Immunother* 3:35–44, 1977.
327. Robinson E, Cohen BY, Mekori T: Immunotherapy counteracting the immunodepressive effect of radio and chemotherapy, in (Proc. Symp. Vienna, 1976) *Radiobiological Research and Radiotherapy*, Vol II, Vienna, IAEA, 1977, pp 261–274.
328. Ray PK, Mohammed J, Raychaudhuri S, Bassett JG, Cooper DR: Growth inhibition of rat primary mammary adenocarcinomas (MA) by immunoadsorption of blocking immune complexes. *4th Int Cong Immunol Abstr* 10.7.25, 1980.
329. Ray PK, Cooper DR, Bassett JG, Mark R: Antitumor effect of *staphylococcus aureus* organisms. *Fed Proc* 38:1089, 1979.
330. Ray PK, Idiculla A, Rhoads JE Jr, Mark R, Besa E, Thomas H, Bassett JG, Cooper DR: Extracorporeal immunoadsorption of pathologic plasma immunoglobulin G or its complexes. A novel approach for their selective removal from the plasma. *Proceedings of the First Annual Apheresis Symposium: Current Concepts and Future Trends*. Chicago, October 1979, pp 203–215.
331. Ray PK, Idiculla A, Mark R, Rhoads JE Jr, Thomas H, Bassett JG, Cooper DR: Extracorporeal immunoadsorption of plasma from a metastatic colon

carinoma patient by protein A-containing nonviable *Staphylococcus* aureus. Clinical, biochemical, serological, and histological evaluation of the patient's response. *Cancer* 49(9): 1800–1807, 1982.

332. Ray PK, Idiculla A, Mark R, Thomas H, Rhoads JE Jr, Bassett JG, Cooper DR: Immunotherapy of cancer: extracorporeal adsorption of plasma blocking factors using nonviable *Staphylococcus aureus* Cowan I, in Nagel G (ed): *Plasma Exchange Symposium,* 1980, Basel, S Derger, 1981, pp 102–113.

333. Farquhar D, Loo TL, Gutterman JU, Hersh EM, Luna MA: Inhibition of drug metabolising enzymes in rat after Bacillus Calmette-Guerin treatment. *Biochem Pharmacol* 25:1529–1534, 1976.

334. Fisher B, Wolmark N, Robin H: Further observations on the inhibition of tumor growth by *Corynebacterium parvum* with cyclophosphamide. III. Effect of C. parvum on cyclophosphamide metabolism. *J Natl Cancer Inst* 57:225–234, 1976.

335. Sparks FC, Albert NE, Andreone PA, Breeding JH: Effect of Bacillus Calmette-Guerin on immunosuppression from cyclophosphamide, methotrexate, and 5-flurouracil. *Cancer Res* 37:2560–2568, 1977.

336. Stewart THM, Hollinshead AC, Harris JE, S et al: Immunochemotherapy of lung cancer. *Ann NY Acad Sci* 277:436–442, 1976.

337. Jun MH, Johnson RH: Effect of cyclophosphamide on tumor growth and cell mediated immunity in sheep with ovine squamous cell carcinoma. *Res Vet Sci* 27:155–162, 1979.

338. Theilen GH, Worley M, Benjamini E: Chemoimmunotherapy for canine lymphosarcoma. *J Am Vet Med Assoc* 170:607–612, 1977.

339. Ray PK: Bacterial neuraminidase and altered immunological bahaviour of treated mammalian cells. *Adv Appl Microbiol* 21:227–242, 1977.

340. Holland JF: Prospectus from cancer treatment. *Cancer* 36(Suppl):299–306, 1975.

341. Holland JF, Bekesi JG, Cuttner J: Chemoimmunotherapy for acute myelocytic leukemia, in *Immunotherapy of Human Cancer.* The Univ of Texas System Cancer Centre. New York, Raven Press, 1977, pp 237–252.

342. Rosenberg SA, Terry WD: Passive immunotherapy of cancer animals and man. *Adv Cancer Res* 25:323–332, 1977.

343. Kedar E, Schwartzbach M, Raanan Z, Hefetz S: In vitro induction of cell mediated immunity to murine leukemia cells. II. Cytotoxic activity in vitro and tumor neutralizing capacity in vivo of anti-leukemia cytotoxic lymphocytes generated in macrocultures. *J Immunol Methods* 16:39–48, 1977.

344. Kedar E, Raanan Z, Kafka I, Holland JF, Bekesi GJ, Weiss DW: In vitro induction of cytotoxic effector cells against human neoplasms. I. Sensitization conditions and effects of cryopreservation on the induction and expression of cytotoxic responses to allogeneic leukemia cells. *J Immunol Methods* 28:303–312, 1979.

345. Bartlett GL, Katsilas DC, Dreider JW, Purnell DM: Immunogenicity of viable tumor cells after storage in liquid nitrogen. *Cancer Immunol Immunother* 2:127–134, 1977.

346. Golub SH: Cryopreservation of human lymphocytes, in Bloom BR, David JR (ed): *In Vitro Methods in Cell Mediated and Tumor Immunity.* New York Academic Press, 1976, pp 731–756.

347. Fefer A: Adoptive tumor immunotherapy in mice as an adjunct to whole

body X-irradiation and chemotherapy. A review, in Weiss DW (ed): *Immunological Parameter of Host Tumor Relationship.* Vol II, New York, Academic Press, 1973, pp 146–162.

348. Gloderson A: In vitro approach to development of immune reactivity. Current Topics in Microbiol. *Immunol* 75:1–21, 1976.

349. Golub SH, Morton DL: Sensitisation of lymphocytes in vitro against human melanoma associated antigens. *Nature* 251:161–172, 1974.

350. Kall MA, Hellstrom I: Specific stimulatory and cytotoxic effects of lymphocytes sensitised in vitro to either alloantigen or tumor antigen. *J Immunol* 114:1083–1088, 1975.

351. Kedar E, Raanan Z, Schwartzbach M: In vitro induction of cell mediated immunity to murine leukemia cells. VI. Adoptive immunotherapy in combination with chemotherapy of leukemia in mice using lymphocytes sensitised in vitro to leukemia cells. *Cancer Immunol Immunother* 4:161–169, 1978.

352. Kedar E, Schwartzbach M, Raanan Z, Hefetz S: In vitro induction of cell mediated immunity to murine leukemia cells. V. Adoptive immunotherapy of leukemia in mice with lymphocytes sensitised in vitro to leukemia cells. *Cancer Immunol Immunother* 4:151–159, 1978. ·

353. Zarling JM, Raich PC, McKcough M, Bach FH: Generation of cytotoxic lymphocytes in vitro against autologous human leukemic cells. *Nature* 262:691–702, 1976.

354. Kedar E, Unger E, Schwartzbach M: In vitro induction cell mediated immunity to murine leukemia cells. I. Optimization of tissue culture conditions for the generation of cytotoxic lymphocytes. *J Immunol Methods* 13:1–12, 1976.

355. Lee SK, Oliver RTD: Autologous leukemia specific T Cell-mediated lymphocytotoxicity in patients with acute myelogenous leukemia. *J Exp Med* 147:912–921, 1976.

356. Zarling JM, Robins HI, Raich PC, Bach FH, Bach ML: Generation of cytotoxic T lymphocytes to autologous human leukemia cells by sensitization to pooled allogeneic normal cells. *Nature* 274:269–276, 1978.

357. Kedar E, Lupu T: In vitro induction of cell mediated immunity to murine leukemia cells. IV. Amplification of the generation of cytotoxic lymphocytes by enzymatically and chemically modified stimulatory leukemia cells. *J Immunol Methods* 21:35–45, 1978.

358. Kedar E, Lupu T, Schwartzbach M, Avrahan Y: In vitro induction of cell mediated immunity to murine leukemia cells. VIII. Methods for augmenting the induction and expression of the cytotoxic response in vitro to syngenic tumors. *J Immunol Methods* 26:157–162, 1979.

359. Kedar E, Nahas F, Unger E, Weiss DW: In vitro induction of cell mediated immunity to murine leukemia cells. III. Effect of the methanol extraction residue fraction of tubercle bacilli on the generation of anti-leukemia cytotoxic lymphocytes. *J Natl Cancer Inst* 60:1097–1104, 1978.

360. Cheever MA, Kempf RA, Fefer A: Tumor neutralisation immunotherapy and chemoimmunotherapy of a Friend Leukemia with cells secondarily sensitised in vitro. *J Immunol* 119:714–721, 1977.

361. Rollinghoff M, Wagner H: In vitro protection against murine plasma cell tumor growth by in vitro activated syngeneic lymphocytes. *J Natl Cancer Inst* 51:1317–1324, 1973.

362. Rouse BT, Wagner H, Harris AW: In vivo activity of in vitro immunized lymphocytes. I. Tumor allograft rejection mediated by in vitro activated mouse thymocytes. *J Immunol* 108:1353–1362, 1972.

363. Treves AJ, Cohen IR, Feldman M: Immunotherapy of lethal metastases by lymphocytes sensitized against tumor cell in vitro; *J Natl Cancer Inst* 54:777–784, 1975.

364. Rosenberg SA, Schwarz S, Spiess PJ: In vitro growth of murine T cells. II. Growth of in vitro sensitized cells cytotoxic for alloantigens. *J Immunol* 121:1951–1962, 1978.

365. Burton RC, Warner NL: In vitro induction of tumor specific immunity. IV. Specific adoptive immunotherapy with cytotoxic T cells induced in vitro to plasmacytoma antigens. *Cancer Immunol Immunother* 2:91–101, 1977.

366. Bortin MM, Rimm AA, Rodey GE, Giller RH, Saltzstein EC: Prolonged survival in long passage AKR leukemia using chemotherapy, radiotherapy and adoptive immunotherapy. *Cancer Res* 34:1851–1859, 1974.

367. Lawrence HS: in Bach FH, Good RA (ed): *Clinical Immunology*. Vol 2, New York, Academic Press, 1974, pp 115–132.

368. Alexander P, Delorme EJ, Hamilton LDG, Hall JG: Effect of nucleic acids from immune lymphocytes on rat sarcomata. *Nature* (Lond) 213:569–571, 1967.

369. Decker PJ, Davis RC, Parker GA, Mannick J: Effect of tumor size on concomitant tumor immunity. *Cancer Res* 33:33–43, 1973.

370. Whitney RB, Levy JG, Smith AG: Influence of tumor size and surgical resection on cell mediated immunity in mice. *J Natl Cancer Inst* 53:111–116, 1974.

371. Youn JK, Lefrancois D, Barski G: *In vitro* studies on the mechanism of the eclipse of cell-mediated immunity in mice bearing advanced tumors. *J Natl Cancer Inst* 50:921–929, 1973.

372. Golub SH, O'Connell TX, Morton DL: Correlation of *in vivo* and *in vitro* assays of immunocompetence in cancer patients. *Cancer Res* 34:1833–1839, 1974.

373. Krant MJ, Manskopf G, Brandrupp CS, Madoff MA: Immunologic alterations in Bronchogenic cancer. *Cancer* 21:623–631, 1968.

374. Adler WH, Takiguchi T, Smith RT: Phytohemagglutinin unresponsiveness in mouse spleen cells induced by methylcholanthrene sarcomas. *Cancer Res* 31:864–872, 1971.

375. Rowland GF, Edwards AJ, Sumner MR, Hurd CM: Thymic dependency of tumor induced immunosuppression. *J Natl Cancer Inst* 50:1329–1334, 1973.

376. Baldwin RW, Price MR, Robins RA: Inhibition of hepatoma-immune lymph node cell cytotoxicity by tumor-bearer serum and solubilized hepatoma antigen. *Int J Cancer* 11:527–531, 1973.

377. Hellstrom KE, Hellstrom I: Immunological enhancement as studies by cell culture techniques. *Ann Rev Microbiol* 24:373–394, 1970.

378. Waldmann TA, Broder S: Suppressor cells in the regulation of the immune response, in Schwartz RS (ed): *Progress in Clinical Immunology*, Vol 3, New York, Grune and Stratton, 1977, pp. 269–283.

379. Whitney RB, Levy JG: Suppression of mitogen responses by serum from tumor bearing mice. *Eur J Cancer* 10:739–744, 1974.

380. Lundy J, Lovett EJ, Wolinsky SM, Conran P: Immune impairment and

metastatic tumor growth. The need for an immunorestorant drug as an adjunct to surgery. *Cancer Res* 19(19):945–954, 1979.

381. Simpson-Herren I, Sanford AH, Holmquist JP: Effect of surgery on the cell kinetics of residual tumor. Proceedings of Cell Kinetics and Chemotherapy Meeting in Annapolis, Maryland, November 4–6, 1975. *Cancer Treatment Report* 60:1749–1760, 1976.

382. Saba TM, Antikatzides TG: Decrease resistance to intravenous tumor-cell challenge during reticuloendothelial depression following surgery. *Surg Ann* 7:71–76, 1975.

383. Saba TM, Scovill WA: Effect of surgical trauma on host defence. *Surg Ann* 7:71–76, 1975.

384. Roberts S, Long L, Jonassen O, McGrath R, McGraw E, Cole WH: The isolation of cancer cells from the blood stream during uterine curretage. *Surg Gynecol Obstet* 111(1):3–9, 1960.

385. Schatton WE, Kramer WM: An experimental study of postoperative tumor metastases. II. Effects of anesthesia, operation and cortisone administration on growth of pulmonary metastasis. *Cancer Res* 39:501–511, 1961.

386. Warren S, Gates O: Fate of intravenously injected tumor cells. *Ann J Cancer* 27:485–492, 1936.

387. Watanbe S: Metastasizability of tumor cells. *Cancer* 7:215–223, 1954.

388. Zeidman I, McCutcheon M, Coman DR: Factors affecting number of tumor metastases: experience with transplantable mouse tumor. *Cancer Research* 10:357–359, 1950.

389. Vose BM, Moudgil OC: Effect of surgery on tumor-directed leukocyte responses. *Br Medical Journal* 1:56–58, 1975.

390. Riddle PR, Berenbaum MC: Post-operative depression of lymphocyte response to PHA. *Lancet* 1:746–754, 1967.

391. Le Francois DL, Goun Jr, Belehradek J Jr, Barski G: Evaluation of cell-mediated immunity in mice bearing tumors produced by a mammary carcinoma cell line. Influence of tumor growth, surgical removal, and treatment with irradiated tumor cells. *J Natl Cancer Inst* 46:981–988, 1971.

392. Mikulska IB, Smith C, Alexander P: Incidence for an immunological reaction of the host directed against its own actively growing primary tumor. *J Natl Cancer Inst* 36:29–34, 1966.

393. Heppner GH: *In vitro* studies on cell mediated immunity following surgery in mice sensitized to syngenic mammary tumors. *Int J Cancer* 9:119–123, 1972.

394. Alexander P, Bensted J, Delorme EJ, Hall JG, Hodgitt J: The cellular immune response to primary sarcomata in rats. II. Abnormal response of nodes draining the tumor. *Proc Roy Soc Lond B* 174:237–247, 1969.

395. Bray AE, Keast D: Changes in host immunity following excision of a murine melanoma. *Brit J Cancer* 31:170–178, 1975.

396. Safir M, Bekesi JG, Papatestas A, Slatu G, Anfses AH: Preoperative and post-operative immunological evaluation of patients with colorectal cancer. *Cancer* 46:700–708, 1979.

397. Greco RS, Salvati E, Rubin R: Cell mediated immunity in adenocarcinoma of the colo-rectum. *J Surg Res* 24:253–257, 1978.

398. Greco RS, Rubin R, Salvati E: A comparison of cellular immunity in patients undergoing electrocoagulation and resection for adenocarcinoma of the rectum. *Surg Gynec Obst* 151:471–479, 1980.

Chapter 3

Immunologic Methods of Diagnostic and Prognostic Value in Tumor Bearers

KENNETH J. MCCORMICK

Contents

Introduction

Cancer patients, especially those with clinically advanced disease, have demonstrated a variety of immunologic dysfunctions. However, it has not been possible to relate this multiplicity of abnormalities to a primary causal relationship with the host's tumor. Although many reports have linked immune dysfunction to advanced stages of disease, the wealth of conflicting results in studies from various institutions has made it difficult to obtain data that are meaningful to the clinician.

Part of the difficulty in assessing these conflicting reports results from (a) the type of immune assays selected for use, (b) technical differences between laboratories using similar assays, and (c) the statistical analyses used to assess results (1). Nevertheless, clinically relevant data may be obtained in certain instances.

It is important to differentiate between those assays that use immuno-logic techniques or reagents as tools to assess the desired parameter and those assays that assess the status of the patient in regard to a particular immune function. The former assays evaluate host status using the im-mune technique as a sensitive, yet discriminative, tool; the latter methods evaluate the host's immune status, which may be either related to the disease process itself or covariable with it. Clinically relevant assays have either diagnostic or prognostic value and, therefore, aid in the identifica-tion or differentiation of the disease process or provide a probable result in regard to recovery or need for more aggressive therapy.

Current diagnostic assays are usually concerned with either the detec-tion of tumor products (markers) or the detection of products of a host's response to tumor (2). Assays of prognostic significance may evaluate the above parameters, as well as nonspecific or specific immune factors that may correlate with severity of disease.

This chapter reviews immunologic methods that have been utilized in diagnostic and prognostic evaluations of the cancer patient. It describes those immunologic techniques that are used as tools in these assessments and that may provide clinically relevant information about the immune system itself.

General Diagnostic Tests for Cancer

Since the beginning of the 20th century many tests have been proposed to serve as diagnostic tools for malignant diseases in general. These assays and their descent into oblivion were reviewed by Currie (2). More re-cently, two tests, which may or may not be related to immunologic phe-nomena, have been suggested as diagnostic for cancer.

The first, the macrophage electrophoretic mobility test (3), measures the slowing in electrophoretic mobility of guinea pig macrophages or tan-nic-acid-treated sulfosalicylic acid-stabilized sheep erythrocytes (4) in the presence of supernatant fluids from peripheral blood mononuclear cells incubated with antigen (encephalitogenic factor from brain or cancer basic protein from tumor extracts). The assay is technically difficult, and modifi-cations have been made to improve its usefulness (4–7). For those who favor an immunologic hypothesis, it is thought that lymphokines released by specific interaction of antigen with sensitized lymphocytes slow the electrophoretic mobility of the indicator macrophages or erythrocytes by interaction with the cell surface (6). For those who favor a nonimmuno-logic hypothesis, neutralization of the net negative charge on the surface of the indicator cells is thought to result from (a) decreased digestion of protein antigen by lymphocytes from cancer patients, thereby allowing binding to the indicator cell surface (6); or (b) nonspecific release of lymphokines as a result of the aggregation of lymphocytes, which, in cancer patients, is not inhibited by the presence of the antigen (7). What-ever the mechanism, the encouraging initial results (3,4,8) have not been unchallenged. In recent double-blind studies (6,9) the clinical usefulness of the assay has not been confirmed.

The structuredness of cytoplasmic matrix (SCM) test (10) is based on changes in the organization of the cytoplasm of lymphocytes detected by fluorescence polarization following stimulation with cancer basic protein, encephalitogenic factor or phytohemagglutinin (11). The initial work sug-gested that the SCM test could accurately distinguish cancer patients from normal individuals (12,13), but these have been followed by less enthusiastic reports (11,14). The test has been modified extensively (15–17), but its clinical value appears to be uncertain.

In considering diagnostic tests for cancer in general, one should always bear in mind that, even with tests of high sensitivity (>90%) and high specificity (>90%), the predictive value of the assay is related to the prevalence of the disease in an unselected population. For the predictive value to approach the sensitivity and specificity of the assay, the actual prevalence of the disease in an unselected population must approach 50% (18). Therefore, if the prevalence of a particular disease in an unselected population is 0.1% and the false positive rate of a particular test is only 5%, the chance that an individual with a positive test has the disease is less than 2% (19). Bagshawe (20) has discussed the clinical dilemmas that could result from screening the general population with a diagnostic test for cancer that has false positive and false negative rates of only 10%.

Immunologic Techniques as Tools in Diagnosis and Prognosis

These techniques are used as sensitive tools to monitor secreted tumor products or tumor cell constituents in order (a) to assess the host's tumor burden, (b) to localize the distribution of tumor within the host, or (c) to aid in histopathologic diagnosis. This is a relatively new area of cancer research which will continue to expand as the techniques of protein isola-tion, characterization, and monoclonal antibody production are devel-oped further.

Tumor Products

Tumor-associated products are usually nonantigenic within the host and have, at times, been incorrectly designated as tumor "antigens" (21). The humoral biologic markers become useful in assessing tumor burden either as a result of enhanced synthesis of normal cell products by the neoplastic cell or through genetic derepression of oncofetal (onco-developmental) proteins in the neoplastic cell (22). A third category of marker, the eva-nescent "tumor-specific" antigen, may also be considered a tumor product (22). In general, however, the quantitatively elevated levels of normal cell products and the oncofetal proteins are, at this time, the most useful markers in the clinical laboratory.

The monoclonal (M) proteins are markers found in the serum of patients with malignant monoclonal gammopathies (23). They result from the synthesis of a single class and type of normal immunoglobulin (Ig) by an abnormal clone of plasma cells. The monoclonal gammopathies produced by multiple myeloma, Waldenström's macroglobulinemia, and occasionally by malignant lymphoma are detected by serum electrophoresis on cellulose acetate membranes. A homogeneous peak of protein in the γ, γ-β, or β-α_2 regions of the electrophoretic pattern is characteristic of these diseases. If detected, the serum is subjected to immunoelectrophoresis to determine the class of Ig and type of light chain. The patient's serum is added to several wells cut into an agar medium, and the samples are treated with an electric current to separate the various serum proteins. After electrophoresis, troughs are cut into the agar, and each is filled with specific antiserum to one of the Ig classes (G, M, A, D, or E) and one of the light-chain types (κ,λ). The M protein is identified by formation of precipitin arcs in the agar medium. This technique may aid in the differentiation of an isolated plasmacytoma from disseminated disease since successful radiotherapy results in disappearance of the M protein in localized disease (23). Recently, an improved prognostic system for multiple myeloma of the IgA type has been developed utilizing the M protein level in combination with the levels of hemoglobin and calcium (24–26).

The radioimmunoassay (RIA) (27) has been used extensively to detect serum levels of (a) carcinoembryonic antigen (CEA), an oncofetal protein associated with colorectal and other cancers (28); (b) α-fetoprotein (AFP), an oncofetal protein associated with hepatocellular carcinoma (29); (c) prostatic acid phosphatase (PAP), an enzyme synthesized as a normal product by prostatic epithelial cells (30); and (d) calcitonin, a normal peptide product of thyroid C-cells (31). An RIA has also been developed to detect the β subunit of human chorionic gonadotropin (32), which can be used as an indicator of tumor burden in patients with choriocarcinoma (20) or, in conjunction with AFP, in patients with ovarian or testicular teratocarcinomas (33).

Although the details of a particular RIA may vary, the general principle of each assay is similar. Purified radiolabeled antigen is incubated with specific antiserum in the presence of unlabeled standard or unknown. The antiserum added is sufficient to bind approximately 40% to 60% of the labeled antigen in the absence of standard or unknown. During incubation, unlabeled antigen competes with labeled antigen for antibody binding sites. The amount of labeled antigen bound in the presence of unknown is related to the concentration of unlabeled antigen in the standard or unknown. Following incubation, bound and/or free labeled antigen is determined after separation of antigen-antibody complexes by the addition of dextran-charcoal, antiglobulin prepared against the species of the first antiserum, or polyethylene glycol. After assaying bound (or free) radioactivity, the relationship between percent radioactivity bound and the amount of standard added provides a standard curve from which to assess the concentration of antigen in the unknown material. The highly sensitive enzyme-linked immunosorbent assay (34) may replace the RIA for these types of markers in the future.

The RIA for calcitonin may be used for diagnosis of familial medullary carcinoma of the thyroid (35) and that for PAP may diagnose metastatic prostatic carcinoma (30). However, serum PAP cannot be used as a screen to differentiate prostatic cancer from obstructive prostatic hyperplasia (36). The use of these types of markers to screen populations of patients has been disappointing. Nevertheless, the markers can be used as an adjunct in the diagnosis of patients who have symptoms of cancer (37). In addition, assessment of CEA levels may aid in prognosis since elevated preoperative levels are related to more advanced disease (38). Markers may also be used to assess response to therapy (decline in levels) and early recurrence of tumor (sequential evaluations posttherapy with increasing levels of marker) (38). Teichmann et al (39) recently described a quick RIA for insulin that aided the intraoperative localization of benign or malignant insulinomas by assaying insulin in samples obtained by catheterization of the various veins draining the pancreas.

Assays for other tumor-related markers are being developed (40,41) and some of these will undoubtedly make a contribution to the evaluation of the cancer patient. The clinical usefulness of several of these newer tumor markers has recently been reviewed (42).

Radioimmunoimaging

The use of antibodies in the localization of tumors has been shown to be a feasible approach to this clinical problem (43). On injection into human tumor-xenografted nude mice, radiolabeled heterologous antibodies to tumor marker, such as CEA, selectively localize in human tumors producing these proteins (44). CEA circulating in the peripheral blood does not interfere with detection of tumor (45), and antibodies to CEA and AFP have been used to localize tumors in patients (46,47). Computer subtraction technology and the potential usefulness of radiolabeled antibodies (both heterologous and monoclonal) in tumor localization will continue to advance the diagnostic and therapeutic possibilities of nuclear medicine (48,49).

Diagnostic Histopathology

Immunocytochemistry may aid in the pathologic differentiation of certain types of neoplasms. Both immunofluorescence (50) and immunoperoxidase (51) techniques utilize the sensitivity and specificity of the antibody molecule to visualize antigenic markers related to particular tumors. In the former method a fluorescent compound, usually fluorescein isothiocyanate, is conjugated to the antibody-containing globulin fraction of a specific antiserum. In the direct test the fluorochrome-labeled antiserum is used to stain the sectioned specimen. In the indirect test the fluorochrome is conjugated to an antibody prepared against either the species globulin or Ig class in which the first antibody to tumor marker was raised. In this case, sections are treated with either normal serum or serum containing antibodies to tumor marker and, following washing, are treated with the flurochrome-labeled antiglobulin. Using either the direct or indirect method, the preparations are viewed by transmitted (dark-field)- or incident-light microscopy using an ultraviolet light source. A system of exciter and barrier filters permits visualization of antigen to which fluorochrome-tagged antibodies have been bound through the emission of an intense apple-green fluorescence.

In contrast, the immunoperoxidase technique utilizes an enzyme, horseradish peroxidase, which (a) may be conjugated to antibodies and used in direct or indirect staining methods analogous to those described for immunofluorescence, or which (b) may be used in a free form (enzyme bridge technique) or complexed with an antiperoxidase as a final step in sandwich methods employing a primary antitumor antibody and intermediate layers of antiglobulins (52). Visualization of the positive reaction results from incubation with H_2O_2, the substrate for the enzyme, and a chromagen such as diaminobenzidine. A brown granular precipitate is produced at the site of antigen localization. The sections are viewed by light microscopy after counterstaining with hematoxylin.

The immunoperoxidase technique has become widely accepted in the laboratory; as the light microscope may be used to observe the reaction, the histologic detail surpasses that observed in immunofluorescence, and the slide preparations are permanent (51). The procedure may be used on frozen sections or on formalin-fixed paraffin-embedded material. However, frozen sections are necessary in tests of membrane antigenicity, as membrane antigens may be labile to the stress of fixation and embedding.

Immunofluorescence can be used to identify terminal deoxynucleotidyl transferase (53), a DNA polymerase marker for non-T, non-B, and T-cell lymphoblastic leukemias (54), which serves as an adjunct in the classification and management of lymphoid tumors (22). Undifferentiated neoplasms have been categorized as epithelial or mesenchymal tumors on the basis of immunofluorescent staining for prekeratin, an intermediate filament of epithelial cells (55). Immunoperoxidase techniques currently aid in the differentiation of skin (56), prostatic (57), and other urologic (58) cancers, as well as hematopoietic (59,60) and various anaplastic (61,62) tumors. The advent of monoclonal antibodies (63) has provided and will continue to provide valuable reagents for use in diagnostic histopathology (64,65).

The immunologic classification of human lymphoid tumors has progressed rapidly (66). Markers found on normal lymphocyte membranes, ie, receptors for sheep erythrocytes on T lymphocytes and presence of heavy-chain surface immunoglobulin on B lymphocytes as detected by immunofluorescence, were initially used for reliable differentiation of T- or B-cell neoplasms (67). Light-chain typing of B-cell lesions by immunofluorescence may distinguish monoclonal B-cell lymphomas from polyclonal hyperplastic lesions (68). In addition, the functional differentiation of neoplastic cells from cutaneous T-cell lymphomas into T-helper or T-suppressor populations can be accomplished in in vitro models of immunoglobulin synthesis (67). Recently, monoclonal antibodies to heavy $(\gamma,\mu,\alpha,\delta)$ and light chains (κ,λ) of human immunoglobulins, as well as to T lymphocytes and their functional helper-suppressor subsets, have extended the possibilities of typing lymphoid neoplasms by immunocytochemical methods (65). The use of surface markers in further defining groups of leukemia patients with differing prognoses is currently being assessed (69–71).

The Thomsen-Friedenreich (T) antigen (72) is related to normal blood group antigen MN and is found on normal cell membranes in a masked condition. However, the antigen may become unmasked in some cancers, eg, breast, lung, and pancreatic carcinomas, and elicit cellular and humoral immune responses in the host which can be assessed by delayed-type hypersensitivity or solid-phase immunofluorescent techniques, respectively (73). The unmasked antigen can be demonstrated on tumor cells in some cases of squamous cell carcinoma, adenocarcinoma, or small cell carcinoma of the lung, transitional cell carcinoma of the bladder, and melanoma (73). In combination with hyperdiploidy, expression of T antigen, detected by immunoperoxidase techniques, may have prognostic significance in patients with carcinoma of the urinary bladder through identification of patient subpopulations with high risk for deep muscle invasion (74).

Immune Parameters in the Cancer Patient

Assessment of immune competence in cancer patients may be directed either toward general immune functions or toward those immune functions that are related to tumor. Since general immune functions are nonspecific in regard to cancer, tumor-related parameters may more adequately assess the patient's clinical status. Although immune competence can be related to prognosis (75), the assays described below have, in general, not been adequately tested in large-scale clinical trials. Immunologic methods, however, have the potential to provide important information in a patient's clinical evaluation.

Nonspecific Parameters—In Vitro Assays

The humoral compartment of the immune system may be assessed by quantification of circulating immunoglobulins, complement proteins, and acute phase proteins, and by presence of suppressive factors in the serum (76). The complement proteins are discussed elsewhere in this volume (77). The immunoglobulins are readily quantitated by single radial immunodiffusion (78). The patient's serum is placed into a well cut in agar which contains antibodies to heavy chain (γ,α,μ,δ) of the immunoglobulin being assayed. Following incubation, a ring of antigen-antibody precipitate forms around the well as a result of diffusion. The diameter of the ring is related to Ig concentration and time of incubation. Quantitation of unknown is obtained by comparison with standards of known Ig content. IgE may be quantitated by solid-phase RIA (79). The large variation in Ig concentration in normal serum precludes the use of meaningful single point determinations, except in patients with monoclonal gammopathies. However, elevations in IgG and IgA have also been reported in several types of nonlymphoid cancers (80). Recently, Ig levels were used to develop an immunobiologic staging of patients with carcinoma of the head and neck (81). In this system elevated levels of IgA were correlated with poor prognosis; elevated levels of IgE and IgD indicated a more favorable prognosis. However, the immunobiologic approach to staging was effective only with patients who produced elevated levels of these immunoglobulins and was accurate only 60% of the time.

The acute phase proteins may also be quantitated by radial immunodiffusion. This group of proteins, which includes haptoglobin, fibrinogen, orosomucoid, α_1-acid glycoprotein, α-1 antitrypsin, transferrin, and C-reactive proteins, appears at high levels in serum from patients with extensive tissue damage or acute infections. At high concentrations, haptoglobin and fibrinogen inhibit phytohemagglutinin-induced mitogenesis in lymphocytes (82). In addition, these two proteins, as well as orosomucoid, inhibit the chemotaxis of monocytes (82). Reports of the immunomodulatory activity of C-reactive protein have not been confirmed (83). Assay of certain acute phase proteins may be useful as a prognostic indicator since levels can be related to extent of neoplastic disease (84–86). Plasmapheresis has been suggested as therapy to reverse immune depression in cancer patients with high levels of these humoral factors (87). Nevertheless, large-scale clinical studies are needed to determine the relationships between particular acute phase reactants and particular tumors and to evaluate their clinical utility in prognosis. Other humoral immunosuppressive factors have also been described (88), but their diagnostic (89) or prognostic (90) relevance has not been sufficiently studied.

The nonspecific cell-mediated immune compartment may be investigated in vitro by a number of techniques that assess either the numbers of immunologic cell types circulating in peripheral blood or the functional activity of these cells after separation from erythrocytes and plasma. The absolute number of circulating lymphocytes has been considered a general prognostic factor in Hodgkin's disease for many years, ie, lymphopenia is associated with poor prognosis (91). Similar observations have been reported for a number of solid tumors (81). In addition, elevated white blood cell counts, an indicator of infection, may reflect poor prognosis (92); however, in patients with nonsmall cell carcinoma of the lung, the Karnovsky score and levels of CEA have more clinical relevance than does the white blood cell count (93). Bruckner et al (94) recently reported that the absolute numbers of granulocytes, lymphocytes, and monocytes were three independent indicators of prognosis in metastatic gastric cancer. For patients with cancer of the head and neck, a prognostic index that combined total lymphocyte count with age and stage of disease accurately predicted results (follow-up of 3 years) 80% of the time (81).

Differentiation of lymphocyte populations on the basis of membrane receptors is routinely performed on peripheral blood mononuclear cells obtained by centrifugation on density gradients of Ficoll-sodium metrizoate (95). In a series of papers, Check et al (96–98) demonstrated that the percent of lymphocytes (% LG) in the mononuclear cell fraction obtained by centrifugation decreases with advancing stage of disease. The lower % LG resulted from decreases in total lymphocyte counts and the altered buoyant density of peripheral blood leukocytes in patients. The % LG correlated with survival and assessed prognosis more readily than other in vitro assays, ie, decreased % LG predicted for decreased survival.

T lymphocytes are thymus-dependent and responsible for delayed-type hypersensitivity reactions, homograft rejection, and regulation of immune responses via helper or suppressor functions. Enumeration of these cells and their helper-suppressor subsets may be accomplished by immunofluorescence with monoclonal anti-T-cell reagents (99). In addition, rosette formation with sheep erythrocytes has been used for many years to assess T-cell numbers. T lymphocytes bind sheep red blood cells forming spontaneous rosettes (E rosettes) of erythrocytes attached to a central mononuclear cell (100). Total T lymphocytes (determined by E rosette formation) and active T cells (determined by short-term incubation of mononuclear cells with sheep erythrocytes) (101) are decreased in number in several types of cancer (102–105). The depression in circulating rosette-forming lymphocytes may be related to the clinical state of the patient (101) and to the stage of disease (102,104,105). However, such observations are not consistent from one laboratory to another or within a particular type of tumor. High-affinity T-cell rosettes, an active subset of total T cells detected by incubation at 29 °C for 18 hours, have recently been suggested to differentiate between normal and cancer populations (106). On serial evaluation, a decline in this subset of T cells appeared to precede recurrence (106). The decline in rosetting cells may result either from an increase in low-affinity E rosettes (106) or from the presence of serum factors that block expression of high-affinity receptors (107). As more studies are performed with monoclonal antibodies to the T-cell subsets (99), the relevance, if any, of these T-lymphocyte subpopulations to prognosis or clinical management should become evident.

The assessment of other surface markers, eg, surface immunoglobulin and Fc or complement receptors, in mononuclear preparations from patients with solid tumors has not been particularly fruitful. However, surface receptors on lymphoma or leukemia cells are particularly important in differentiating these neoplastic diseases.

Lymphocyte proliferative (LP) assays are used to detect functional activity of lymphocyte populations that respond to incubation with nonspecific mitogens or specific antigens by undergoing a blastogenic transformation (95). Polyclonal mitogens, such as phytohemagglutinin or concanavalin A, and specific antigens, such as purified protein derivative or streptolysin-0, stimulate T lymphocytes and T lymphocytes from presensitized donors, respectively. Blastogenic responses of B lymphocytes may also be obtained following stimulation with the polyclonal activator, pokeweed mitogen. The use of irradiated or mitomycin C-treated allogeneic lymphocytes as stimulant in the mixed lymphocyte reaction is a sensitive indicator of T-cell blastogenesis, as well as the in vitro equivalent of a specific immune response. The degree of lymphoproliferation in these assays is usually determined by quantitating the amount of tritiated thymidine incorporated into cellular DNA during the last 4 to 18 hours of incubation.

Depressed LP responses have been demonstrated in mononuclear cell preparations from patients with lymphoid or nonlymphoid tumors (108). Although results of these assays may have a large variation, LP may be related to tumor burden (109), stage of disease, and period of survival (110,111). However, although the trend for decreased LP responses with advanced disease is apparent in several population studies, investigations on large numbers of patients with carcinoma of the lung or colorectum have shown that response to phytohemagglutinin is correlated with survival only in stage III disease (112).

The lack of general prognostic significance (111,113) in single-point determinations of LP reactivity in cancer patients may be related to the inherent variability of these assays or to the serum component in the incubation medium. To avoid the problems of day-to-day variation in LP tests, Dean et al introduced the relative proliferation index, comparing the result of the patient's test to that of three or more normal individuals tested simultaneously (114). This calculation more easily detected depressions in LP responses and permitted discrimination between cancer patients and normal individuals. An initial report using this index suggested that depressed LP response to allogeneic lymphocytes predicted poor prognosis in postoperative patients with stage I lung cancer more readily than did the tumor-node-metastases (TNM) staging system or histologic evaluation of the tumor (115). The incubation medium for LP assays includes serum, either fetal calf, autologous, or normal allogeneic AB+ human serum. Intrinsic cellular dysfunction can be detected in the presence of fetal calf serum or normal allogeneic human serum; however, incubation in autologous serum may detect humoral immunosuppressive factors. In assessing prognosis, the use of the patients' cells and serum in the assay may improve correlations with clinical outcome. For example, in a study of 501 patients with gastric carcinoma, Toge et al reported a highly significant relationship between LP responses to phytohemagglutinin in the presence of autologous serum and 5-year actuarial survival rates (116). Both of these technical factors should be considered in studies that attempt to correlate LP assays and clinical status of the patient.

Investigations of monocytes (117), natural killer cells (118,119), K cells that mediate antibody-dependent cellular cytotoxicity (120), and polymorphonuclear leukocytes (121) have demonstrated functional depression, especially in patients with advanced cancer. However, the clinical significance of these assays is unknown.

Nonspecific Parameters—In Vivo Assays

Although humoral antibody synthesis in cancer patients has been assessed in several studies (122), skin tests of delayed-type hypersensitivity have been more frequently used to evaluate the patient's ability to respond (a) to intradermal injections of microbial antigens that were previously encountered through natural exposure or immunization or (b) to *de novo* sensitization with a previously unencountered antigen, eg, dinitrochlorobenzene (DNCB) applied to the skin. Both assays reflect the functional capacity of the T-cell and inflammatory systems; however, *de novo* sensitization also assesses the patient's ability to recognize and react against a new foreign material, as well as to recall this ability on challenge.

Patients with lymphoid or nonlymphoid (solid) tumors have often shown a depression in skin test responses to recall antigens or to *de novo* sensitization with DNCB (122). Although early observations suggested that tests of delayed-type hypersensitivity might have prognostic value in surgical oncology (123,124), stratification of patients into more elaborate staging classifications, eg, the TNM system, may decrease the prognostic significance of skin test results (125). Indications that patients with anergy to recall antigens (123,124,126) or to DNCB (122,124,127,128) had a poorer prognosis suggested that skin tests might identify patients with greater risk of recurrence or decreased survival. However, more recent studies in patients with lung (93,112), breast (112,129), colorectal (112,129), or gastric (129) carcinomas did not produce a correlation with these clinical parameters, even in the presence of significant immune depression. Moertel et al (130) reported that general immune evaluation in patients with unresectable gastrointestinal carcinoma adds nothing to patient evaluation and that most general immune dysfunctions, including a correlation between response to recall antigens and survival, was related to performance status.

Tumor-Associated Parameters—In Vitro Assays

Although assays for tumor-associated immune reactivities have the greatest potential for diagnostic or prognostic value, development of clinically useful tests is proceeding slowly. Herberman (131) has cited the limitations of such techniques including (a) difficulties in discriminating between tumor-associated and normal-tissue antigens; (b) possible lack of a common tumor-associated antigen within tumors of one histologic type; and (c) the restraint to clinical usefulness if the specimens assayed must be autologous.

Relationships between levels of antibodies to tumor-associated antigens and the clinical status of patients have not been consistently well-correlated (131,132). However, in the case of the Epstein-Barr virus (EBV)-associated neoplasms, studies have begun to establish some useful relationships between serologic markers and clinical parameters. EBV, the causative agent of infectious mononucleosis, has been associated with, but not proven to be the etiologic agent of, African Burkitt's lymphoma and anaplastic nasopharyngeal carcinoma (133). Antibodies to viral capsid antigen (VCA), the virus-induced nonstructural early antigens (EA) found in infected cells, and membrane antigens (MA) found on the surface of productively infected cells are detected by direct or indirect immunofluorescent techniques (133). High levels of antibodies to VCA are present in sera from both types of tumors when compared with control populations (134), but these antibodies often do not discriminate sufficiently to serve as prognostic tools. In African Burkitt's lymphoma, high titers of antibodies to EA are related to poor prognosis (135), even in patients brought to remission (136); in nasopharyngeal carcinoma, levels of IgA antibodies to EA are related to tumor burden (137) and are considered prognostic in that the antibodies decline in successfully treated patients (138). Conversely, antibodies to MA may decline several months prior to recurrence in patients with African Burkitt's lymphoma (139). In population studies antibodies in patients' sera that reacted to high titer in antibody-dependent cell-mediated cytotoxicity (ADCC) reactions against EBV-infected Raji cells were associated with prolonged survival in cases of nasopharyngeal carcinoma (140) or were correlated with a significant response to therapy in cases of Burkitt's lymphoma (141). In this assay (142), antibodies, specific for EBV-related membrane antigen, coat the EBV-transformed target cells and impart specificity to the cytotoxic reaction effected by normal Fc receptor-bearing lymphocytes (K cells) contained in normal baboon mononuclear cell preparations. Although the ADCC reaction is prognostic in population studies, it is not useful in detecting changes in a patient's clinical condition. Recently, an IgA antibody that neutralized the LP effect of inactivated EBV on presensitized normal lymphocytes was detected in the sera of patients with nasopharyngeal carcinoma, but not in the sera of normal donors or patients with other head and neck tumors (143). The level of this antibody declined as patients entered remission and may, with further study, be found to have prognostic value.

In addition to humoral antibodies, sera from cancer patients have been tested for the presence of circulating immune (antigen-antibody) complexes. Several techniques have been used in these assays, including the Raji cell assay (144), Clq binding (145), and complement consumption (146). In each assay, complement (or a radiolabeled complement subunit, Clq) is added to human serum and is bound to immune complexes if they are present. The amount of complement (or subunit) bound is assessed by (a) adsorption of complement-antigen-antibody complexes to complement receptors on Raji cells, which may be detected by immunofluorescence or RIA using either fluorescein or radiolabeled antihuman IgG; (b) addition of polyethylene glycol to precipitate high molecular weight materials that have bound radiolabeled Clq; or (c) measuring residual functional activity of the added complement by quantitation of its hemolytic ability. A number of studies have demonstrated elevated levels of immune complexes in sera of cancer patients, and some studies demonstrated correlations between the levels of these complexes and clinical parameters (131). However, consistent results are not always obtained within (147) or between these assays (148). The use of three different methods to detect immune complexes in malignancies increased the rate of detection but did not enhance the ability to identify early cancer (148). Using complement consumption, Gupta et al reported that the degree of circulating immune complexes (as reflected by serum anticomplementary activity) is related to tumor burden, but not to clinical stage (146). In patients with untreated bronchogenic carcinoma, levels of immune complexes increased with stage of disease, but were not correlated with prognosis (149). In addition, the frequency and levels of immune complexes in patients with thoracic diseases other than cancer were similar to those found in patients with bronchogenic carcinoma (149). It is assumed that the presence of circulating immune complexes in the cancer patient results from the combination of antibody with tumor-associated antigen(s). However, these complexes can be found in a variety of autoimmune or infectious diseases and, therefore, their presence could be unrelated to the host response to neoplastic disease. Nevertheless, in a prospective study of patients with advanced malignant melanoma, the survival of patients with stage IV disease who produced immune complexes was decreased when compared with that of similar patients without circulating complexes (147).

Cell-mediated tumor-associated immune parameters have been assessed by (a) enumeration of tumor antigen-sensitive T lymphocytes, (b) functional assays such as response to autologous or allogeneic tumor cells in LP or cytotoxic assays, or (c) response to allogeneic tumor antigen(s) in the leukocyte migration inhibition or leukocyte adherence inhibition tests. Problems involved in these types of studies include the use of allogeneic tumor antigens, selection of appropriate normal tissue controls, the presence of cell-mediated reactivity in normal individuals, and, in the autologous situation, the logistical problems involved with obtaining materials from the patient to be tested.

Enumeration of tumor antigen-sensitive T lymphocytes has been attempted in small numbers of patients with breast (150) or lung (151) carcinoma. The assay assessed the percentage of active rosette-forming T cells following incubation in the presence of tumor antigen extracted by 3 molar potassium chloride (KCl). If antigen-sensitive T cells are present, the number of cells forming rosettes with sheep erythrocytes is increased. In patients with lung cancer the frequency of positive results decreased with clinical stage and, furthermore, suggested a correlation with survival (151). Further evaluation of the test on a large scale will determine its usefulness in prognosis.

LP responses to crude (152) and 3M KCl (153) extracts of tumor cells, as well as to irradiated (153) or mitomycin C-treated (154) tumor cells, have been reported. Use of allogeneic combinations of tumor cells in such studies may result in difficulties of interpretation because of histocompatibility differences between donors of the test mononuclear cell populations (whether normal or patient) and the donor of the tumor (and control) tissue sample. This problem is obviated when autologous tumor-lymphocyte combinations are tested. However, the tumor cell-directed specificity of the LP response is not clear. Early studies of autologous reactivities to tumor indicated a relationship between an LP response and good prognosis (155,156). In a more recent study of breast cancer patients following surgical resection (157), patients with LP responses to hypotonic membrane preparations of autologous tumor cells had significantly longer disease-free intervals than did patients with low responses. The LP response predicted clinical course more frequently than did histologic evidence of tumor in axillary lymph nodes. In retrospective studies of sarcoma (158) and lung carcinoma (159) patients, useful clinical information could be provided by autologous LP responses if the patient was free of metastasis at the time of surgery. A positive LP response was associated with a good prognosis (increased tumor-free periods and survival). Although a negative test indicated a bad prognosis, a positive test was a good prognostic sign which, however, lacked discriminatory ability. Thus, a positive LP response did not identify the 10% to 30% tumor-reactive patients with decreased tumor-free interval or decreased survival.

Cell-mediated cytotoxic reactions against tumor target cells (160) can be assayed in tests that measure (a) isotope release from radiolabeled target cells, (b) isotope incorporation into viable tumor cells following incubation with effector cells, or (c) the numbers of target cells visually destroyed by effector cells (161). Problems in the use of allogeneic effector-target combinations are similar to those discussed above; however, autologous effector-target combinations have also been investigated. Lymphocytes from patients who had metastatic disease in cases of breast (162) or lung (159) carcinoma or sarcoma (158) showed less frequent cytotoxic reactions to their autologous tumor. In contrast, patients with carcinoma of the colon had similar frequencies of cytotoxic activity in the presence or absence of metastasis (163). Autologous antitumor cytoxicity in patients with sarcomas (158) or lung (159) tumors was associated with prolonged disease-free intervals or prolonged survival and were better correlated with clinical state (absence of reaction in metastatic disease) than were LP assays (159).

Leukocyte migration inhibition (LMI) and leukocyte adherence inhibition (LAI) tests assess the presence of sensitized T lymphocytes in leukocyte preparations from cancer patients. In the presence of tumor antigen (usually organ-specific), sensitized T cells release lymphokines that either inhibit the migration of leukocytes from a capillary tube (164) or agarose droplet (165) or inhibit the adherence of leukocytes to hemocytometer coverslips (166). The LAI may be related to the LMI, but is more rapid. Both tests have been used extensively in tumor immunology (167). Addition of patient's serum to either test can be used to detect presence of blocking factors. Correlations between LMI assays and the clinical condition of the patient have produced discordant results (131,168), and the value of LMI in diagnosis and prognosis is currently being evaluated. The LAI may have diagnostic value for tumors such as colorectal carcinoma (169) or melanoma (170). However, since the reactivity is unrelated to stage of disease, it has no prognostic value.

The tube LAI is mediated by cytophilic IgG antitumor antibodies bound to the Fc receptors of monocytes (171,172). On exposure to antigen (organ-specific tumor extracts), the adherence of monocytes to the tube is decreased (173). The assay may prove to be useful in immunodiagnosis of tumors (174), and in colorectal cancer the detection of tumor by tube LAI was not statistically different from detection by barium enema (175). The test becomes negative in advanced disease, possibly as a result of excess circulating tumor antigen (172). Reincubation of the primary tube in a second test (172) or treatment of leukocytes with prostaglandin E_2 (176) may increase the sensitivity of tumor detection in more advanced disease. As in any assay of immune reactivity against tumor-associated antigens, problems with extraction and standardization of antigens have not been completely overcome (177,178).

Tumor-Associated Parameters—In Vivo Assays

Delayed-type hypersensitivity reactions to tumor-associated antigens have been assessed by intradermal injection of tumor extracts (179) or by application of cryostat-sectioned autologous tumor to abraded skin (180). The varying antigenicity and specificity of different tumor extracts are a problem in these studies (181). Intradermal injection of crude tumor extracts into control populations, both normal individuals and patients without malignancy, encounter ethical problems. In addition, injection of normal tissue extracts as a control challenge may result in positive responses in patients (181). The investigation of purified tumor-associated antigen(s) in studies of delayed hypersensitivity may reduce some of these difficulties (182).

Serial Testing of Immune Parameters

Although most, but not all, of the investigations cited were population studies using single-point determinations of immune parameters, Braun and Harris (183) have recently reviewed the problems in, and emphasized the importance of, serially testing immune function in cancer patients. Such serial evaluation in individual patients provides possible identification of immunologic markers for recurrent disease and for evaluation of changes in immune function during immunotherapy. For example, the presence of indomethacin-sensitive suppressor activity (184,185) was found to develop prior to recurrence in surgically resected lung cancer patients on serial testing of LP responses to phytohemagglutinin (186). The differentiation of the most important immune markers and the development of suitably standardized laboratory procedures should enhance the value of such studies.

Comment

This methodologic overview has demonstrated the importance of sensitive and specific immunologic techniques in histopathologic diagnosis and assessment of tumor burden. Future studies should, in addition, bring important contributions to radioimmunoimaging procedures. In these areas, immunology has provided the tools for progress. The complexities of host-tumor interactions have prevented the ready identification of markers of human immune functions that are consistently of value in diagnosis and prognosis. However, the basic techniques in evaluation of general or tumor-associated immune functions have been developed. The necessity of and the difficulties in applying these assays in large-scale prospective clinical trials are obvious. Nevertheless, the relationship of certain of the assays to clinical status or course and to diagnosis suggest that they may become important clinical tools. Combinations of immune and other clinical parameters (81,187) might provide prognostic differentiation of patients. Whether the immune dysfunction is primary or covariable with neoplastic disease, immune evaluations may, in the future, aid in individualizing therapy for the cancer patient.

References

1. Herberman RB, Thurman GB: Approaches to the immunological monitoring of cancer patients treated with natural or recombinant interferons. *J Biol Response Mod* 2:548–562, 1983.
2. Currie GA: Immunological aspects of human cancer, in Lachmann PJ, Peters DK (eds): *Clinical aspects of immunology,* ed 4. Oxford, Blackwell Scientific Publ, 1982, pp 1279–1298.
3. Field EJ, Caspary EA: Lymphocyte sensitization: an *in vitro* test for cancer? *Lancet* ii:1337–1341, 1970.
4. Ax W: Tumor diagnosis using electrophoretic mobility test (EMT). Review on state of the art with references to the use of stabilized erythrocytes as indicator particles, in Flad HD, Herfath C, Betzler M (eds): *Immunodiagnosis and immunotherapy of malignant tumors. Relevance to surgery.* Berlin, Springer-Verlag, 1979, pp 169–183.
5. Pritchard JAV, Moore JL, Sutherland WH, Joslin CAF: Evaluation and development of the macrophage electrophoretic mobility (MEM) test for malignant disease. *Br J Cancer* 27:1–9, 1973.
6. Dyson JED, Watkinson AP, Jones WG, Corbett PJ, Joslin CAF: Lymphocyte supernatants and the electrophoretic mobility of erythrocytes: further experience of cancer diagnosis. *Br J Cancer* 42:448–454, 1980.
7. Kast RE: Cancer diagnostic test of Field and Caspary: Part II. A review and interpretation of the collected data. *Med Hypoth* 6:63–72, 1980.
8. Pritchard JAV, Moore JL, Sutherland WH, Joslin CAF: Technical aspects of the macrophage electrophoretic mobility (MEM) test for malignant disease. *Br J Cancer* 28 Suppl 1:229–236, 1973.
9. Whitehead RH: Discussion, in Flad H-D, Herfath C, Betzler M (eds): *Immunodiagnosis and immunotherapy of malignant tumors. Relevance to surgery.* Berlin, Springer-Verlag, 1979, pp 184–185.
10. Cercek L, Cercek B, Franklin CIV: Biophysical differentiation between lymphocytes from healthy donors, patients with malignant diseases and other disorders. *Br J Cancer* 29:345–352, 1974.
11. Mitchell II, Wood P, Pentycross CR, Abel E, Bagshawe KD: The SCM test for cancer. An evaluation in terms of lymphocytes from healthy donors and cancer patients. *Br J Cancer* 41:772–777, 1980.
12. Bagshawe KD: Workshop on macrophage electrophoretic mobility (MEM) and structuredness of cytoplasmic matrix (SCM) tests. *Br J Cancer* 35:701–704, 1977.
13. Schnuda ND: Evaluation of fluorescence polarization of human blood lymphocytes (SCM test) in the diagnosis of cancer. *Cancer* 46:1164–1173, 1980.
14. Atkinson RJ, Lowry WS, Strain P: An analysis of the SCM test in cancer diagnosis. *Cancer* 52:91–100, 1983.
15. Cercek L, Cercek B: Comments on "the SCM test for cancer. An evaluation in terms of lymphocytes from healthy donors and cancer patients". *Br J Cancer* 42:947–948, 1980.
16. Pritchard JAV, Sutherland, WH, Siddal JE, Bater AJ, Kerby IJ, Deeley TJ, Griffith G, Sinclair R, Davies BH, Rimmer A, Webster DJT: A clinical assessment of fluorescence polarization changes in lymphocytes stimulated

by phytohaemagglutinin (PHA) in malignant and benign diseases. *Eur J Cancer Clin Oncol* 18:651–659, 1982.

17. Hocking GR, Rolland JM, Nairn RC, Pihl E, Cuthbertson AM, Hughes ESR, Johnson WR: Lymphocyte fluorescence polarization changes after phytohemagglutinin stimulation in the diagnosis of colorectal carcinoma. *J Natl Cancer Inst* 68:579–583, 1982.

18. Vecchio TJ: Predictive value of a single diagnostic test in unselected populations. *N Engl J Med* 274:1171–1173, 1966.

19. Casscells W, Schoenberger A, Graboys TB: Interpretations by physicians of clinical laboratory results. *N Engl J Med* 299:999–1001, 1978.

20. Bagshawe KD: Tumour markers—where do we go from here? *Br J Cancer* 48:167–175, 1983.

21. Hewitt HB: Animal tumor models and their relevance to human tumor immunology. *J Biol Response Mod* 1:107–119, 1982.

22. Gold P, Shuster J: Historical development and potential uses of tumor antigens as markers of human cancer growth. *Cancer Res* 40:2973–2976, 1980.

23. Kyle RA: Classification and diagnosis of monoclonal gammopathies, in Rose NR, Friedman H (eds): *Manual of clinical immunology*, ed 2. Washington, Am Soc Microbiol, 1980, pp 135–150.

24. Durie BG, Salmon SE: A clinical staging system for multiple myeloma: Correlation of measured myeloma cell mass with presenting clinical features, response to treatment, and survival. *Cancer* 36:842–854, 1975.

25. Merlini G, Waldenström JG, Jayakar SD: A new improved clinical staging system for multiple myeloma based on analysis of 123 treated patients. *Blood* 55:1011–1019, 1980.

26. Bettini R, Steidl L, Rapazzini P, Giardina G: Prognostic value of the staging system proposed by Merlini, Waldenström and Jayakar for multiple myeloma. *Acta Haemat* 70:379–385, 1983.

27. Berson SA, Yalow R: Radioimmunoassay, in Berson SA, Yalow R (eds): *Methods in investigative and diagnostic endocrinology*. Amsterdam, North Holland, 1973, pp 84–119.

28. Zamcheck N, Kupchik HZ: Summary of clinical use and limitations of the carcinoembryonic antigen assay and some methodological considerations, in Rose NR, Friedman H (eds): *Manual of clinical immunology*, ed 2. Washington, Am Soc Microbiol, 1980, pp 919–935.

29. McIntire KR, Waldmann TA: Measurement of alpha-fetoprotein, in Rose NR, Friedman H (eds): *Manual of clinical immunology*, ed 2. Washington, Am Soc Microbiol, 1980, pp 936–943.

30. Choe BK, Pontes EJ, Rose NR: Methods for the detection of human prostatic acid phosphatase, in Rose NR, Friedman H (eds): *Manual of clinical immunology*, ed 2. Washington, Am Soc Microbiol, 1980, pp 951–962.

31. Hirsch PF, Gauthier GF, Munson PL: Thyroid hypocalcemic principle and recurrent laryngeal nerve injury as factors affecting the response to parathyroidectomy in rats. *Endocrinol* 73:244–252, 1963.

32. Vaitukaitis JL: Human chorionic gonadotropin as a tumor marker. *Ann Clin Lab Sci* 4:276–280, 1974.

33. Lange PH, McIntire KR, Waldman TA, Hokala TR, Fraley EE: Serum alpha fetoprotein and human chorionic gonadotropin in the diagnosis and management of nonseminomatous germ cell testicular cancer. *N Engl J Med* 295:1237–1240, 1976.

34. Voller A, Bidwell D, Bartlett A: Enzyme-linked immunosorbent assay, in Rose NR, Friedman H (eds): *Manual of clinical immunology,* ed 2. Washington, Am Soc Microbiol, 1980; pp 359–371.

35. Dilley WG, Wells SA Jr, Cooper CW: Calcitonin radioimmunoassay, in Rose NR, Friedman H (eds): *Manual of clinical immunology,* ed 2. Washington, Am Soc Microbiol, 1980; pp 944–950.

36. Fleischmann J, Catalona WJ, Fair WR, Heston WDW, Menon M: Lack of value of radioimmunoassay for prostatic acid phosphatase as a screening test for prostatic cancer in patients with obstructive prostatic hyperplasia. *J Urol* 129:312–314, 1983.

37. McIntire KR: Tumor markers for radioimmunodetection of cancer. *Cancer Res* 40:3083–3085, 1980.

38. Sugarbaker PH: Clinical use of carcinoembryonic antigen in the management of patients with cancer, in Prasad N (ed): *Radiotherapy and cancer immunology,* Vol 1. Boca Raton, CRC Press, 1981, pp 155–173.

39. Teichmann RK, Spelsberg F, Heberer G: Intraoperative biochemical localization of insulinomas by quick radioimmunoassay. *Am J Surg* 143:113–115, 1982.

40. Herberman RB (ed): *Compendium of assays for immunodiagnosis of human cancer.* New York, Elsevier/North Holland, 1979.

41. Sell S, Wahren B (eds): *Human cancer markers.* Clifton NJ, Humana Press, 1982.

42. Pohl AL, Graninger W, Francesconi M, Lenzhofer RS, Ganzinger UC, Moser KV: Present value of tumor markers in the clinic. *Cancer Detect Prevent* 6:7–20, 1983.

43. Pressman D: The development and use of radiolabeled antitumor antibodies. *Cancer Res* 40:2960–2964, 1980.

44. Mach J-P, Carrel S, Merenda C, Sordat B, Cerottini J-C: *In vivo* localization of radiolabelled antibodies to carcinoembryonic antigen in human colon carcinoma grafted into nude mice. *Nature* 248:704–706, 1974.

45. Primus FJ, Bennett SJ, Kim EE, DeLand FH, Zahn MC, Goldenberg DM: Circulating immune complexes in cancer patients receiving goat radiolocalizing antibodies to carcinoembryonic antigen. *Cancer Res* 40:497–501, 1980.

46. Goldenberg DM, DeLand F, Kim E, Bennett S, Primus FJ, VanNagell JR Jr, Estes N, DeSimone P, Rayburn P: Use of radiolabeled antibodies to carcinoembryonic antigen for the detection and localization of diverse cancers by external photoscanning. *N Engl J Med* 298:1384–1388, 1978.

47. Goldenberg DM, Kim EE, DeLand F, Spremulli E, Nelson MO, Gockerman JP, Primus FJ, Corgan RL, Alpert E: Clinical studies on the radioimmunodetection of tumors containing alpha-fetoprotein. *Cancer* 45:2500–2505, 1980.

48. Goldenberg DM, DeLand FH: History and status of tumor imaging with radiolabeled antibodies. *J Biol Response Mod* 1:121–136, 1982.

49. Burchiel SW, Rhodes BA (eds): *Radioimmunoimaging and radioimmunotherapy.* New York, Elsevier, 1983.

50. Lyerla HC, Forrester FT: *Immunofluorescence methods in virology.* Atlanta, US Dept Health, Education, and Welfare, 1979.

51. Kurman RJ, Casey C: Immunoperoxidase techniques in surgical pathology: principles and practice, in Rose NR, Friedman H (eds): *Manual of clinical immunology,* ed 2. Washington, Am Soc Microbiol, 1980, pp 60–69.

52. Taylor CR: Immunoperoxidase techniques: practical and theoretical aspects. *Arch Pathol Lab Med* 102:113–121, 1978.
53. Gregoire KE, Goldschneider I, Barton RW, Bollum FJ: Intracellular distribution of terminal deoxynucleotidyl transferase in rat bone marrow and thymus. *Proc Natl Acad Sci USA* 74:3993–3996, 1977.
54. Stass SA, Peiper SC, Bollum FJ: Immunoassay of circulating terminal transferase in patients with acute lymphoblastic leukemia: a new technique for diagnosis. *Am J Hematol* 9:429–433, 1980.
55. Sienski W, Dorsett B, Ioachim HL: Identification of prekeratin by immunofluorescence staining in the differential diagnosis of tumors. *Human Pathol* 12:452–457, 1981.
56. Kallioinen M, Dammert K: β-2-microglobulin in primordial and differentiated basocellular carcinomas and basosquamous carcinomas. *Acta path microbiol immunol Scand Sect A* 91:217–222, 1983.
57. Jobsis AC, DeVries GP, Anholt RRH, Sanders GTB: Demonstration of the prostatic origin of metastases. *Cancer* 41:1788–1793, 1978.
58. Javadpour N: Immunocytochemical localization of various markers in cancer cells and tumors. Diagnostic and therapeutic strategy in urologic cancers. *Urology* 21:1–7, 1983.
59. Pinkus GS, Said JW: Profile of intracytoplasmic lysozyme in normal tissues, myeloproliferative disorders, hairy cell leukemia, and other pathologic processes: an immunoperoxidase study of paraffin sections and smears. *Am J Pathol* 89:351–366, 1977.
60. Pinkus GS, Said JW: Intracellular hemoglobin—a specific marker for erythroid cells in paraffin sections: an immunoperoxidase study of normal, megaloblastic, and dysplastic erythropoiesis, including erythroleukemia and other myeloproliferative disorders. *Am J Pathol* 102:308–313, 1981.
61. Espinoza CG, Pillarisetti SG, Azar HA: Selected applications of immunoperoxidase techniques in surgical pathology. *Ann Clin Lab Sci* 13:240–248, 1983.
62. Nadji M, Morales AR: Immunoperoxidase: Part II. Practical applications. *Lab Med* 15:33–37, 1984.
63. Köhler G, Milstein C: Continuous cultures of fused cells secreting antibody of predefined specificity. *Nature* 256:495–497, 1975.
64. Ghosh AK, Mason DY, Spriggs AI: Immunocytochemical staining with monoclonal antibodies in cytologically "negative" serous effusions from patients with malignant disease. *J Clin Pathol* 36:1150–1153, 1983.
65. Gatter KC, Cordell JL, Falini B, Ghosh AK, Heryet A, Nash JRG, Pulford KA, Moir DJ, Erber WN, Stein H, Mason DY: Monoclonal antibodies in diagnostic pathology: techniques and applications. *J Biol Response Mod* 2:369–395, 1983.
66. Thierfelder S, Rodt H, Thiel E (eds): *Immunological diagnosis of leukemias and lymphomas*. New York, Springer-Verlag, 1977.
67. Ford RJ, Maizel AL: Immunobiology of lymphoreticular neoplasms, in Twomey JJ (ed): *The pathophysiology of human immunologic disorders*. Baltimore, Urban and Schwarzenberg, 1982, pp 199–217.
68. Levy R, Warnke R, Dorfman RF, Haimovich J: The monoclonality of human B-cell lymphomas. *J Exp Med* 145:1014–1028, 1977.
69. Mellstedt H, Pettersson D, Holm G: Lymphocyte subpopulations in chronic lymphatic leukemia (CLL). *Acta Med Scand* 204:485–489, 1978.

70. Sallan SE, Ritz J, Pesandro J, Gelber R, O'Brien C, Hitchcock S, Coral F, Schlossman SF: Cell surface antigens: prognostic implications in childhood acute lymphoblastic leukemia. *Blood* 55:395–402, 1980.
71. Miale TD, Stenke LAL, Lindblom JB, Sjögren A-M, Reizenstein PG, Udén A-M, Lawson DL: Surface Ia-like expression and MLR-stimulating capacity of human leukemic myeloblasts: implications for immunotherapy and prognosis. *Acta Haemat* 68:3–13, 1982.
72. Springer GF, Desai PR, Yang HJ, Murthy MS: Carcinoma-associated blood group MN precursor antigens against which all humans possess antibodies. *Clin Immunol Immunopathol* 7:426–441, 1977.
73. Springer GF, Desai PR, Fry WA, Goodale RL, Shearen JG, Scanlon EF: T antigen, a tumor marker against which breast, lung and pancreas carcinoma patients mount immune responses. *Cancer Detect Prevent* 6:111–118, 1983.
74. Summers JL, Coon JS, Ward RM, Falor WH, Miller AW III, Weinstein RS: Prognosis in carcinoma of the urinary bladder based upon tissue blood groups ABH and Thomsen-Friedenreich antigen status and karyotype of the initial tumor. *Cancer Res* 43:934–939, 1983.
75. Hersh EM, Gutterman JU, Mavligit GM, Mountain CW, McBride CM, Burgess MA, Lurie PM, Zelen M, Takita H, Vincent RG: Immunocompetence, immunodeficiency and prognosis in cancer. *Ann NY Acad Sci* 276:386–406, 1976.
76. McCormick KJ: Host-tumor interactions and methods of evaluating immunocompetence in humans, in Prasad N (ed): *Radiotherapy and cancer immunology*, Vol I. Boca Raton, CRC Press, 1981, pp 21–49.
77. Cooper PD: in Ray PK (ed): *Advances in immunity and cancer therapy*, Vol I. New York, Springer-Verlag, 1985, pp 125–166.
78. Jackson AL, Davis NC: Quantitation of immunoglobulins, in Rose NR, Friedman H (eds): *Manual of clinical immunology*, ed 2. Washington, Am Soc Microbiol, 1980, pp 109–120.
79. Stevens RH: Quantitative radioimmunoassays for antibodies and immunoglobulin produced *in vitro*, in Rose NR, Friedman H (eds): *Manual of clinical immunology*, ed 2. Washington, Am Soc Microbiol, 1980, pp 157–162.
80. Cochran AJ, Mackie RM, Grant RM, Ross CE, Connell MD, Sandilands G, Whaley K, Hoyle DE, Jackson AM: An examination of the immunology of cancer patients. *Int J Cancer* 18:298–309, 1976.
81. Katz AE: Immunobiologic staging of patients with carcinoma of the head and neck. *Laryngoscope* 93:445–463, 1983.
82. Samak R, Edelstein R, Israël L: Immunosuppressive effect of acute-phase reactant proteins in vitro and its relevance to cancer. *Cancer Immunol Immunother* 13:38–43, 1982.
83. Pepys MB, Baltz ML: Acute phase proteins with special reference to C-reactive protein and related proteins (pentaxins) and serum amyloid A protein. *Adv Immunol* 34:141–212, 1983.
84. Latner AL, Turner GA, Lamin MM: Plasma alpha-l-antitrypsin levels in early and late carcinoma of the cervix. *Oncology* 33:12–14, 1976.
85. Ward AM, Cooper EH, Turner R, Anderson JA, Neville AM: Acute-phase reactant protein profile: an aid to monitoring large bowel cancer by CEA and serum enzymes. *Br J Cancer* 35:170–178, 1977.
86. te Velde ER, Berrens L, Zegers BJM, Ballieux RE: Acute phase reactants

and complement components as indicators of recurrence in human cervical cancer. *Eur J Cancer* 15:893–899, 1979.

87. Israël L, Edelstein R, Samak R: Some new approaches to cancer immunotherapy in man, in *Immunotherapy of human cancer*. New York, Raven Press, 1978, pp 363–374.

88. Kamo I, Friedman H: Immunosuppression and the role of suppressive factors in cancer. *Adv Cancer Res* 25:271–321, 1977.

89. Izumi T, Nagai S, Suginoshita T: Serum immunosuppression test as a new tool for immunodiagnosis of lung cancer. *Cancer Res* 40:444–447, 1980.

90. Sugden PJ, Lilleyman JS: Prognosis in lymphoblastic leukaemia related to plasma mediated inhibition of incorporation of tritiated thymidine by transformed lymphocytes. *Leuk Res* 4:333–336, 1980.

91. Rafla S, Yang S-J: Radiotherapy and immune response in malignant lymphomas, in Prasad N (ed): *Radiotherapy and cancer immunology*, Vol I. Boca Raton, CRC Press, 1981, pp 73–91.

92. Check IJ, DeMeester T, Vardiman J, Hunter RL: Differential counts and survival in lung cancer. *Lancet* ii:1317–1318, 1978.

93. Oldham RK, Gail MH, Baker MA, Forbes JT, Heineman W, Hersh E, Holmes EC, Ritts RE, Wright PW and the Lung Cancer Study Group: Immunological studies in a double blind randomized trial comparing BCG against placebo in patients with resected Stage I non-small cell lung cancer. *Cancer Immunol Immunother* 13:164–173, 1982.

94. Bruckner HW, Lavin PT, Plaxe SC, Storch JA, Livstone EM for the Gastrointestinal Tumor Study Group: Absolute granulocyte, lymphocyte, and monocyte counts. Useful determinants of prognosis for patients with metastatic cancer of the stomach. *J Am Med Assoc* 247:1004–1006, 1982.

95. Oppenheim JJ, Schecter B: Lymphocyte transformation, in Rose NR, Friedman H (eds): *Manual of clinical immunology*, ed 2. Washington, Am Soc Microbiol, 1980, pp 233–245.

96. Check IJ, Hunter RL, Rosenberg KD, Herbst AL: Prediction of survival in gynecological cancer based on immunological tests. *Cancer Res* 40:4612–4616, 1980.

97. Check IJ, Hunter RL, Lounsbury B, Rosenberg K, Matz G: Prediction of survival in head and neck cancer based on leukocyte sedimentation in Ficoll-Hypaque gradients. *Laryngoscope* XC: 1281–1290, 1980.

98. Check IJ, Hunter RL, Karrison T, DeMeester TR, Golomb HM, Vardiman J: Prognostic significance of immunological tests in lung cancer. *Clin Exp Immunol* 43:362–369, 1981.

99. Haynes BF: Human T lymphocyte antigens as defined by monoclonal antibodies. *Immunological Rev* 57:127–161, 1981.

100. Ross GD, Winchester RJ: Methods for enumerating lymphocyte populations, in Rose NR, Friedman H (eds): *Manual of clinical immunology*, ed 2. Washington, Am Soc Microbiol, 1980, pp 213–228.

101. Wybran J, Fudenberg HH: Thymus-derived rosette-forming cells in various human disease states: cancer, lymphoma, bacterial and viral infections, and other diseases. *J Clin Invest* 52:1026–1032, 1973.

102. Catalona WJ, Potvin C, Chretien PB: T-lymphocytes in bladder and prostatic cancer patients. *J Urol* 112:378–382, 1974.

103. Wybran J, Fudenberg HH: T-cell rosettes in human cancer, in Wybran J,

Staquet MJ (eds): *Clinical tumor immunology*. New York, Pergamon Press, 1976, pp 31–40.

104. Woodruff MFA: *The interaction of cancer and host. Its therapeutic significance*. New York, Grune and Stratton, 1980, pp 81–82.

105. Wig U, Saini AS, Gupta VK: E-rosette forming cells (E-RFC) in squamous cell carcinoma of the larynx and laryngopharynx. *J Laryngol Otol* 97:527–530, 1983.

106. Weese JL, West WH, Herberman RB, Payne SM, Siwarski JW, Turcotte JG: "High-affinity" T-cell rosettes: the effects of clinical manipulations and potential prognostic significance. *J Surg Oncol* 13:145–153, 1980.

107. Bashford J, Gough IR: Depression of high-affinity rosette formation in dysplasia and carcinoma *in situ* of the uterine cervix: mediation by serum factors. *Cancer Res* 43:3959–3962, 1983.

108. Woodruff MFA: *The interaction of cancer and host. Its therapeutic significance*. New York, Grune and Stratton, 1980, pp 82–83.

109. Catalona WJ, Tarpley JL, Chretien PB, Castle JR: Lymphocyte stimulation in urologic cancer patients. *J Urol* 112:373–377, 1974.

110. Jenkins VK, Griffiths CM, Ray P, Perry RR, Olson MH: Radiotherapy and head and neck cancer. Role of lymphocyte response and clinical stage. *Arch Otolaryngol* 106:414–418, 1980

111. Dalbow MH, Concannon JP, Eng CP, Weil CS, Conway J, Nambisan PTN: Lymphocyte mitogen stimulation studies for patients with lung cancer: evaluation of prognostic significance of preirradiation therapy studies. *J Lab Clin Med* 90:295–302, 1977.

112. Wanebo HJ, Pinsky CM, Beattie EJ, Oettgen HF: Immunocompetence testing in patients with one of the common operable cancers—a review, in Flad H-D, Herfath C, Betzler M (eds): *Immunodiagnosis and immunotherapy of malignant tumors. Relevance to surgery*. Berlin, Springer-Verlag, 1979, pp 103–114.

113. Kovarik J, Ninger E, Zemanova D, Lauerova L: A prospective study of lymphocyte responses to phytohemagglutinin in melanoma patients. (Lack of prognostic value of correlation with minimal tumor burden.) *Neoplasma* 27:575–582, 1980.

114. Dean JH, Connor R, Herberman RB, Silva J, McCoy JL, Oldham RK: The relative proliferative index as a more sensitive parameter for evaluating lymphoproliferative responses of cancer patients to mitogens and alloantigens. *Int J Cancer* 20:359–370, 1977.

115. Cannon GB, Dean JH, Herberman RB, Perlin E, Reid J, Miller C, Lang NP: Association of depressed postoperative lymphoproliferative responses to alloantigens with poor prognosis in patients with stage I lung cancer. *Int J Cancer* 25:9–17, 1980.

116. Toge T, Oride M, Yanagawa E, Hamamoto S, Kohno H, Nakanishi K, Hattori T: Prognostic significance of lymphocyte proliferative responses to mitogen in gastric cancer patients. *Jap J Surg* 12:424–428, 1982.

117. Jerrells TR, Dean JH, Richardson G, Cannon GB, Herberman RB: Increased monocyte-mediated cytostasis of lymphoid cell lines in breast and lung cancer patients. *Int J Cancer* 23:768–776, 1979.

118. Pross HF, Baines MG: Natural killer cells in tumor-bearing patients, in Herberman RB (ed): *Natural cell-mediated immunity against tumors*. New York, Academic Press, 1980, pp 1063–1072.

119. Hajto T, Lanzrein C: Frequency of large granular lymphocytes in peripheral blood of healthy persons and breast cancer patients. *Cancer Immunol Immunother* 16:65–66, 1983.

120. McCredie JA, MacDonald HR: Antibody-dependent cellular cytotoxicity in cancer patients: lack of prognostic value. *Br J Cancer* 41:880–885, 1980.

121. Korec S: The role of granulocytes in host defense against tumors, in Herberman RB (ed): *Natural cell-mediated immunity against tumors.* New York, Academic Press, 1980, pp 1301–1307.

122. Woodruff MFA: *The interaction of cancer and host. Its therapeutic significance.* New York, Grune and Stratton, 1980, pp 80–81.

123. Eilber FR, Morton DL: Impaired immunologic reactivity and recurrence following cancer surgery. *Cancer* 25:362–367, 1970.

124. Eilber FR, Morton DL, Ketcham AS: Immunologic abnormalities in head and neck cancer. *Am J Surg* 128:534–538, 1974.

125. Johns ME: Immunological considerations in head and neck cancer, in Batsakis JG: *Tumors of the head and neck. Clinical and pathological considerations,* ed 2. Baltimore, Williams and Wilkins, 1979, pp 501–513.

126. Wells SA Jr, Burdick JF, Joseph WL, Christiansen CL, Wolfe WG, Adkins PC: Delayed cutaneous hypersensitivity reactions to tumor cell antigens and to nonspecific antigens: prognostic significance in patients with lung cancer. *J Thorac Cardiovasc Surg* 66:557–562, 1973.

127. Liebler GA, Concannon JP, Magovern GJ, Dalbow MH, Hodgson SE: Immunoprofile studies for patients with bronchogenic carcinoma. I. Correlation of pretherapy studies with survival. *J Thorac Cardiovasc Surg* 74:506–518, 1977.

128. Oldham RK, Weese JL, Herberman RB, Perlin E, Mills M, Heim W, Blom J, Green D, Reid J, Bellinger, S, Law, I, McCoy JL, Dean JH, Cannon GB, Djeu J: Immunological monitoring and immunotherapy in carcinoma of the lung. *Int J Cancer* 18:739–749, 1976.

129. Hughes LE, Teasdale C, Forbes JF, Hillyard JW, Whitehead RH: Correlation between nonspecific immune competence and clinical outcome of breast, colon, and stomach cancer, in Flad H-D, Herfath C, Betzler M (eds): *Immunodiagnosis and immunotherapy of malignant tumors. Relevance to surgery.* Berlin, Springer-Verlag, 1979, pp 95–102.

130. Moertel CG, Ritts RE Jr, O'Connell MJ, Silvers A: Nonspecific immune determinants in the patient with unresectable gastrointestinal carcinoma. *Cancer* 43:1483–1492, 1979.

131. Herberman RB: Immunologic defenses against cancer, in Twomey JJ (ed): *The pathophysiology of human immunologic disorders.* Baltimore, Urban and Schwarzenberg, 1982, pp 219–257.

132. Woodruff MFA: *The interaction of cancer and host. Its therapeutic significance.* New York, Grune and Stratton, 1980, pp 98–99.

133. zur Hausen H: Oncogenic herpesviruses, in Tooze J (ed): *DNA tumor viruses: Molecular biology of tumor viruses,* ed 2 (part 2/revised). Cold Spring Harbor, Cold Spring Harbor Laboratory, 1980, pp 747–795.

134. Ablashi DV, Easton JM, Guegan JH: Herpesviruses and cancer in man and subhuman primates. *Biomedicine* 24:286–305, 1976.

135. Henle G, Henle W, Klein G, Gunvén P, Clifford P, Morrow RH, Ziegler JL: Antibodies to early Epstein-Barr virus-induced antigens in Burkitt's lymphoma. *J Natl Cancer Inst* 46:861–871, 1971.

136. Henle W, Henle G, Gunvén P, Klein G, Clifford P, Singh S: Patterns of antibodies to Epstein-Barr virus-induced early antigens in Burkitt's lymphoma. Comparison of dying patients with long-term survivors. *J Natl Cancer Inst* 50:1163–1173, 1973.

137. Callaghan DJ, Conner BR, Strauss M: Epstein-Barr virus antibody titers in cancer of the head and neck. *Arch Otolaryngol* 109:781–784, 1983.

138. Henle W, Ho JHC, Henle G, Chau JCW, Kwan HC: Nasopharyngeal carcinoma: significance of changes in Epstein-Barr virus-related antibody patterns following therapy. *Int J Cancer* 20:663–672, 1977.

139. Gunvén P, Klein G, Clifford P, Singh S: Epstein-Barr virus-associated membrane-reactive antibodies during long-term survival after Burkitt's lymphoma. *Proc Natl Acad Sci USA* 71:1422–1426, 1974.

140. Pearson GR, Johansson B, Klein G: Antibody-dependent cellular cytotoxicity against Epstein-Barr virus-associated antigens in African patients with nasopharyngeal carcinoma. *Int J Cancer* 22:120–125, 1978.

141. Pearson GR, Qualtiere LF, Klein G, Norin T, Bal IS: Epstein-Barr virus-specific antibody-dependent cellular cytotoxicity in patients with Burkitt's lymphoma. *Int J Cancer* 24:402–406, 1979.

142. Pearson GR: *In vitro* and *in vivo* investigations on antibody-dependent cellular cytotoxicity. *Curr Topics Microbiol Immunol* 80:65–96, 1978.

143. Kamaraju CS, Levine PH, Sundar SK, Ablashi DV, Faggioni A, Armstrong GR, Bertram G, Krueger GRF: Epstein-Barr virus-related lymphocyte stimulation inhibitor: a possible prognostic tool for undifferentiated nasopharyngeal carcinoma. *J Natl Cancer Inst* 70:643–647, 1983.

144. Theofilopoulos AN, Dixon FJ: Immune complexes in human sera detected by the Raji cell radioimmune assay, in Bloom BR, David JR (eds): *In vitro methods in cell-mediated and tumor immunity*. New York, Academic Press, 1976, pp 555–563.

145. Zubler RH, Lambert P-H: The ^{125}I-C1q binding test for the detection of soluble immune complexes, in Bloom BR, David JR (eds): *In vitro methods in cell-mediated and tumor immunity*. New York, Academic Press, 1976, pp 565–572.

146. Gupta RK, Golub SH, Morton DL: Correlation between tumor burden and anticomplementary activity in sera from cancer patients. *Cancer Immunol Immunother* 6:63–71, 1979.

147. Rossen RD, Crane MM, Morgan AC, Giannini EH, Giovanella BC, Stehlin JS, Twomey JJ, Hersh EM: Circulating immune complexes and tumor cell cytotoxins as prognostic indicators in malignant melanoma: a prospective study of 53 patients. *Cancer Res* 43:422–429, 1983.

148. Krapf F, Renger D, Schedel I, Fricke M, Kemper A, Deicker H: Circulating immune complexes in malignant diseases. Increased detection rate by simultaneous use of three assay methods. *Cancer Immunol Immunother* 15:138–143, 1983.

149. Ruiz-Arguelles A, Jett JR, Ritts RE Jr: Stage-associated incidence of serum circulating immune complexes in patients with untreated bronchogenic carcinoma. *Cancer Immunol Immunother* 12:197–201, 1982.

150. Ramey WG, Hashim GA, Burrows WB, Swistel AJ, Munther A, Fitzpatrick H: Detection of breast tumor antigen-sensitive circulating T-lymphocytes by antigen-stimulated active rosette formation. *Cancer Res* 39:4796–4801, 1979.

151. Ramey WG, Fitzpatrick HF, Hashim GA, Munther AS, Swistel AJ, Burrows WB: Diagnosis, stage, and prognosis of lung carcinoma by preoperative assay of lung tumor antigen-sensitive T lymphocytes. *J Thorac Cardiovasc Surg* 80:656–660, 1980.
152. Savel H: Effect of autologous tumor extracts on cultured human peripheral blood lymphocytes. *Cancer* 24:56–63, 1969.
153. Gutterman JU, Mavligit GM, Hunter CY, Hersh EM: Lymphocyte transformation against human tumor antigens, in Bloom BR, David JR (eds): *In vitro methods in cell-mediated and tumor immunity.* New York, Academic Press, 1976, pp 587–596.
154. Vanky F, Stjernswärd J: Lymphocyte stimulation test for detection of tumor-specific reactivity in humans, in Bloom BR, David JR (eds): *In vitro methods in cell-mediated and tumor immunity.* New York, Academic Press, 1976, pp 597–606.
155. Gutterman JU, Hersh EM, Mavligit GM, Freireich EJ, Rossen RD, Butler WT, McCredie KB, Bodey GP Sr, Rodriguez V: Cell-mediated and humoral immune response to acute leukemia cells and soluble leukemia antigen-relationship to immunocompetence and prognosis. *Natl Cancer Inst Monogr* 37:153–165, 1973.
156. Mavligit GM, Gutterman JU, McBride CM, Hersh EM: Cell-mediated immunity to human solid tumors: *in vitro* detection by lymphocyte blastogenic responses to cell-associated and solubilized tumor antigens. *Natl Cancer Inst Monogr* 37:167–176, 1973.,
157. Cannon GB, Dean JH, Herberman RB, Keels M, Alford C: Lymphoproliferative responses to autologous tumor extracts as prognostic indicators in patients with resected breast cancer. *Int J Cancer* 27:131–138, 1981.
158. Vanky F, Willems J, Kreicbergs A, Aparisi T, Andréen M, Broström L-A, Nilsonne U, Klein E, Klein G: Correlation between lymphocyte-mediated auto-tumor reactivities and clinical course. I. Evaluation of 46 patients with sarcoma. *Cancer Immunol Immunother* 16:11–16, 1983.
159. Vanky F, Péterffy A, Böök K, Willems J, Klein E, Klein G: Correlation between lymphocyte-mediated auto-tumor reactivities and the clinical course. II. Evaluation of 69 patients with lung carcinoma. *Cancer Immunol Immunother* 16:17–22, 1983.
160. Woodruff MFA: *The interaction of cancer and host. Its therapeutic significance.* New York, Grune and Stratton, 1980, pp 100–102.
161. Bean MA, Bloom BR, Cerottini J-C, David JR, Herberman RB, Lawrence HS, MacLennen ICM, Perlmann P, Stutman O: Evaluation of *in vitro* methods for assaying tumor immunity, in Bloom BR, David JR (eds): *In vitro methods in cell-mediated and tumor immunity.* New York, Academic Press, 1976, pp 27–65.
162. Deodhar SD, Crile G Jr, Esselstyn CB Jr: Study of the tumor cell-lymphocyte interaction in patients with breast cancer. *Cancer* 29:1321–1325, 1972.
163. Vose BM, Gallagher P, Moore M, Schofield PF: Specific and non-specific lymphocyte cytotoxicity in colon carcinoma. *Br J Cancer* 44:846–855, 1981.
164. McCoy JL, Jerome LF, Dean JH, Cannon GB, Connor RJ, Herberman RB: Direct capillary tube leukocyte migration inhibition assay for detection of cell-mediated immunity to human tumor-associated antigens, in Bloom BR, David JR (eds): *In vitro methods in cell-mediated and tumor immunity.* New York, Academic Press, 1976, 607–612.

165. McCoy JL, Dean JH, Herberman R: Human cell-mediated immunity to tuberculin as assayed by the agarose micro-droplet leukocyte migration inhibition technique: comparison with the capillary tube assay. *J Immunol Meth* 15:355–371, 1977.

166. Halliday WJ: Leukocyte-adherence inhibition test and blocking factors in cancer, in Bloom BR, David JR (eds): *In vitro methods in cell-mediated and tumor immunity*. New York, Academic Press, 1976, pp 547–554.

167. Woodruff MFA: *The interaction of cancer and host. Its therapeutic significance*. New York, Grune and Stratton, 1980, pp 102–103.

168. McCoy JL: Clinical applications of assay of leukocyte migration inhibition, in Herberman RB, McIntire KR (eds): *Immunodiagnosis of cancer, Part 2*. New York, Marcel Dekker, 1979, pp 979–998.

169. Maluish AE, Halliday WJ: in Herberman RB (ed): *Compendium of assays for immunodiagnosis of human cancer*. New York, Elsevier-North Holland, 1979, pp 251–255.

170. Halliday WJ, Maluish AE: in Herberman RB (ed): *Compendium of assays for immunodiagnosis of human cancer*. New York, Elsevier-North Holland, 1979, pp 619–623.

171. Shuster J, Thomson DMP, Fuks A, Gold P: Diagnostic immunologique des neoplasies malignes. *L'Union Med Can* 109:902–909, 1980.

172. Morizane T, Kumagai N, Tsuchimoto K, Watanabe T, Tsuchiya M: Specific immunodiagnosis of hepatoma by tube leukocyte adherence inhibition assay and a modified method of repeated tube leukocyte adherence inhibition assay. *Cancer Res* 40:2928–2934, 1980.

173. Grosser N, Marti JH, Proctor JW, Thomson CMP: Tube leukocyte adherence inhibition assay for the detection of anti-tumor immunity. I. Monocyte is the reactive cell. *Int J Cancer* 18:39–47, 1976.

174. Hašek M, Holáň V, Kousalova M: Tube LAI assay in diagnosis and monitoring of a cancer disease. *Biomedicine* 35:207–208, 1981.

175. Ayeni AO, Thomson DMP, MacFarlane JK, Daley D: A comparison of tube leukocyte adherence inhibition assay and standard physical methods for diagnosing colorectal cancer. *Cancer* 48:1855–1862, 1981.

176. MacFarlane JK, Thomson DMP, Phelan K, Shenouda G, Scanzano R: Predictive value of tube leukocyte adherence inhibition (LAI) assay for breast, colorectal, stomach and pancreatic cancer. *Cancer* 49:1185–1193, 1982.

177. Fritze D, Fedra G, Kaufmann M: Prospective evaluation of the leukocyte adherence inhibition (LAI) test in breast cancer using a panel of extracts from known and unknown primary tumors. *Int J Cancer* 29:261–264, 1982.

178. Kovarik J, Lauerová L, Feit J, Ninger E, Munzarová M, Zemanová D, Hlávková J: Leukocyte adherence inhibition responses obtained with various tumor extracts in breast cancer patients. *Cancer Detect Prevent* 6:215–219, 1983.

179. Woodruff MFA: *The interaction of cancer and host. Its therapeutic significance*. New York, Grune and Stratton, 1980, pp 104–105.

180. Black MM, Leis HP Jr: Cellular responses to autologous breast cancer tissue: sequential observations. *Cancer* 32:384–389, 1973.

181. Weese JL, Herberman RB, Hollinshead AC, Cannon GB, Keels M, Kibrite A, Morales A, Char DH, Oldham RK: Specificity of delayed cutaneous hypersensitivity reactions to extracts of human tumor cells. *J Natl Cancer Inst* 60:255–263, 1978.

182. Hollinshead A: in Herberman RB (ed): *Compendium of assays for immuno-diagnosis of human cancer*. New York, Elsevier-North Holland, 1979, pp 335–343; 461–466.
183. Braun DP, Harris JE: Serial immune function testing to predict clinical disease relapse in patients with solid tumors. *Cancer Immunol Immunother* 15:165–171, 1983.
184. Maca RD, Panje WR: Indomethacin sensitive suppressor cell activity in head and neck cancer patients pre- and postirradiation therapy. *Cancer* 50:483–489, 1982.
185. Murray JL, Springle C, Ishmael DR, Lee ET, Longley R, Kollmorgen GM, Nordquist RL: Adherent indomethacin-sensitive suppressor cells in malignant melanoma. Correlation with clinical status. *Cancer Immunol Immunother* 11:165–172, 1981.
186. Braun DP, Nisius S, Hollinshead A, Harris JE: Serial immune testing in surgically resected lung cancer patients. *Cancer Immunol Immunother* 15:114–120, 1983.
187. Payne JE, Meyer JH, Macpherson JG, Nelson DS, Walls RS, Pheils MT: The value of lymphocyte transformation in carcinoma of the colon and rectum. *Surg Gyn Obst* 150:687–693, 1980.

Chapter 4

Complement and Cancer: Activation of the Alternative Pathway as a Theoretical Base for Immunotherapy

PETER D. COOPER

Contents

(*continued*)

Active immunotherapy or immunopotentiation against human cancer is an attractive possibility because it suggests a natural treatment in which the body's own defenses can be mobilized. A treatment modality that could be less mutilating for the patient than many currently employed is offered. If regularly used as an adjunct to these existing treatments, there is, with minimal extra morbidity, the chance of reducing the tumor burden to levels so low that a cure routinely becomes a practical possibility. In fact, although it may only be able to cope with a relatively small number of tumor cells, active immunotherapy has the potential of identifying and killing the "last remaining (foreign) cell" (1), which surgery, chemotherapy, and radiotherapy together generally do not.

This approach was started at the turn of the century, and since 1960 many laboratory and clinical studies have been concerned with it, particularly its nonspecific form. Both laboratory and clinical applications (1–5) have been sufficiently effective on many occasions to make it fairly certain that some fundamental immune system or principle exists that might be consistently exploited with benefit to cancer patients. Unfortunately, such a principle has not yet clearly emerged, despite the time interval. Perhaps because of this, the plethora of preparations used and their usually complex and poorly defined nature have led to difficulties of reproducibility and of optimizing the response, so that effort has been diluted and this treatment modality constrained in a prolonged experimental stage. Such treatment is still not available on a regular basis for cancer patients.

This article points out that there is, in fact, a strongly supported common factor in the many varieties of nonspecific active immunotherapy that have given some clinical response. This common factor is the predicted activation of the alternative pathway of complement (APC), either free in plasma or as a component of leukocytes, that occurs at the beginning of or very early in a chain of events resulting from administration of all sufficiently studied immunopotentiating regimes. APC activation could provide the fundamental principle or theoretical base that is so far lacking for this treatment modality and that one could then exploit for a rational clinical treatment that is relatively easy and safe to apply and accurate to monitor.

Outline of the Pathways of Complement Activation

The immune principle known as "complement" is a complex system of 14 proteins highly interlinked in precursor-activated product, enzyme-cofactor or enzyme-substrate relationships, with an additional number of specific regulator proteins. Current information has been authoritatively summarized in several comprehensive reviews (6–11).

This system really operates through three connected pathways (Fig. 4-1), of which two (the "classical" and the "alternative") are recognition, activation and amplification pathways converging on two different complexes with an identical enzymic activity: the ability to cleave C5 specifically to C5a and C5b (C5 convertases). Both pathways amplify by cascade reactions, the classical being linear and the alternative cyclic (see below). Their working principle is the same, namely that a very small "trigger," perhaps a single initiating molecule, can activate the first component of one or the other cascade (C1q or C3, respectively) to create a highly specific protease whose substrate is the next member of the chain, the cleavage of which creates a second specific protease, and so on. Specific cofactor proteins, often also activated by cleavage, are usually required. As each product is an enzyme that can cleave many substrate molecules, the number of molecules involved increases explosively at each step, with

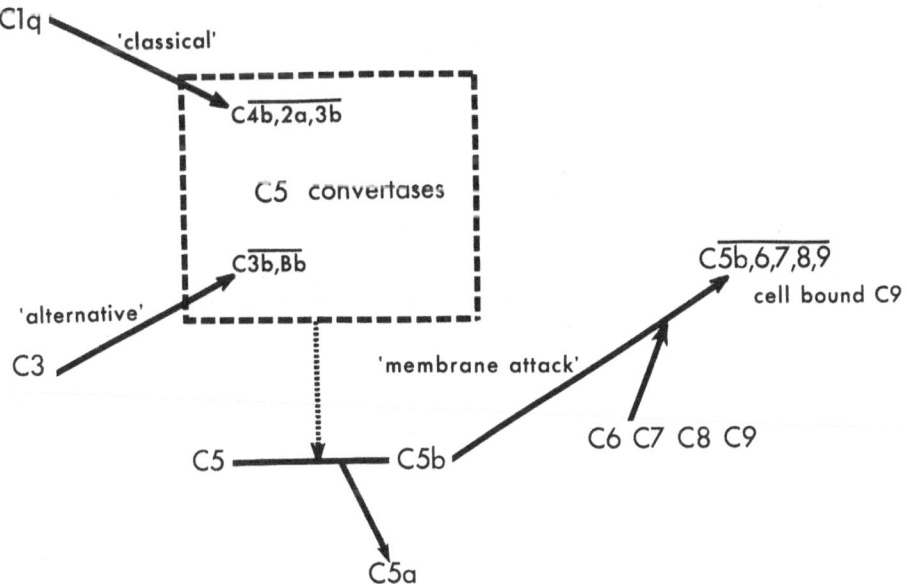

Figure 4-1. Relations between the "classical," "alternative," and "membrane attack" pathways of complement. *Broken-line arrow* denotes action on a step by proteolytic cleavage.

ultimately a very large number of the end products of the cascades, the C5 convertases, being produced rapidly in high local concentration. A crucial step is the transfer of the C5 convertase from solution to an organic surface, where it is anchored by a covalent bond to become an insoluble enzyme complex.

The third or terminal pathway, also called the membrane attack pathway, creates an activated complex of the molecules C5b, C6, C7, C8, noncovalently bound to the surface due for attack, in association with a number of C9 molecules. This complex is formed by a self-assembly process and becomes inserted into the membrane and then kills, say, an invading bacterium or a tumor cell recognized as "foreign" by the initiating step of the amplifying pathway.

These pathways are now understood in very substantial detail, with the possible exception of the last step (the function of C9). All components of complement have been isolated and characterized and the complement pathways completely reassembled from these isolated components. Interestingly, the "classical" pathway, so-called because it was discovered first, probably arose phylogenetically (and is recapitulated ontogenetically) later than the "alternative" pathway (12a,12b), and it might, indeed, have been more apt if the accident of history had allowed their names to be reversed. The significance of their evolution is that the specifically initiated classical pathway and specific IgG responses are likely to have evolved together, whereas the more primitive alternative pathway has retained a role that is relatively nonspecialized and accordingly might be expected to be more relevant to a nonspecific immunotherapy.

The Alternative Pathway of Complement

This chapter is primarily concerned with the alternative pathway, sometimes still called the "properdin" pathway, as it was the discovery of this component that gave the first indication that an alternative pathway existed. However, properdin itself is now known to play only a minor role.

Figure 4-2 illustrates the cyclic amplification cascade of the alternative pathway. The central role is played by the complex C3b,Bb, the C3 convertase that is also a C5 convertase. This enzyme is able to cleave fresh C3—which, as the most numerous complement molecule in serum (approximately 1 g/L), comprises a very large reservoir—to make C3b with liberation of the anaphylatoxin C3a. C3b then combines with factor B to make the complex C3b,B, which is enzymatically almost inactive but which is cleaved by factor $\bar{D}$ (itself activated by enzymic cleavage of factor D) to make more of the active convertase C3b,Bb (with liberation of Ba), which again interacts with fresh C3. Properdin (now known as factor P) stabilizes the complex C3b,B,$\bar{D}$. Unless it is stopped by regulation (see below), this cyclic amplification very rapidly cleaves C3 and

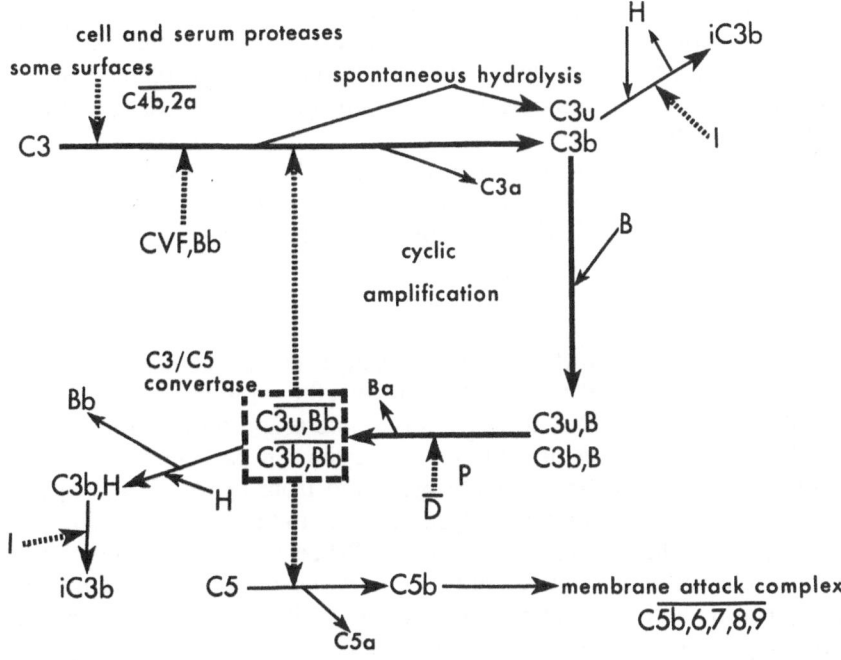

Figure 4-2. The alternative pathway of complement. *Broken-line arrows* denote action on a step by proteolytic cleavage.

factor B to exhaustion, when the activated enzyme decays in due course mainly by loss or inactivation of the heat-labile Bb.

When C3b is produced by cleavage of C3, an internal thioester bond is exposed which, through conformational changes in the bulk of the molecule, becomes stressed or "metastable," ie, highly reactive. It is rapidly hydrolyzed, reacting within microseconds mainly with water but occasionally with other nearby nucleophilic groups ($-OH$ and $-NH_2$) on organic molecules. When these occur on an insoluble surface, eg, of a tumor cell, the C3b becomes covalently bonded to, and forms an insoluble C3/C5 convertase on, that surface. Thus is provided an irreversibly attached surface marker that either opsonizes that surface for phagocytosis (discussed later in this chapter) or provides a nucleus for more enzyme activity. Such an active nucleus rapidly increases the number of C3/C5 convertase molecules attached locally to that surface.

As shown in Fig. 4-2, a number of proteases can cleave C3 in vivo. However, the cycle is thought to be initiated by a very slow spontaneous hydrolysis of the internal thioester bond of C3 to make a constant small number of molecules of C3u, otherwise known as $C3(H_2O)$. Although it differs from C3b in that it remains uncleaved, C3u is like C3b in that it can combine with factor B to make an active C3/C5 convertase, $\overline{C3u,Bb}$; however, as it lacks the thioester bond, it must remain soluble and cannot lyse a sheep erythrocyte in a standard complement test, so that it is hemolytically inactive.

Continual generation of C3u is enough to keep the cycle constantly primed in what has been termed the "tick-over" model (8). Small amounts of C3b and $\overline{C3b,Bb}$ are continually produced, presumably balanced by regular synthesis of C3 and factor B in liver and by leukocytes. The cycle is kept under control by combination of C3b or C3u with factor H in plasma, which is able if necessary to displace factor Bb. Factor I is then able to combine with the C3b,H or C3u,H complex and acts to cleave the C3b moiety to the inactive iC3b by specific proteolysis.

However, if the surface to which it is bound is appropriate, for example the beta-1,3 glucan on the surface of a zymosan particle, the complex $\overline{C3,Bb}$ is thought to be relatively protected from factor H, perhaps by steric factors provided by the polysaccharide. In this situation it can react with more C3 faster than with factor I. When this occurs, the cascade begins to cycle and thus to amplify on the zymosan surface, and the APC is said to be activated. During activation highly reactive C3b is created and may interact with other surfaces or cells, but if activation goes to completion, all available C3 and factor B have been depleted and $\overline{C3b,Bb}$ decays or is inactivated by factors H and I.

Needless to say, this local protection of $\overline{C3b,Bb}$ cannot, in general, occur on the surface of normal cells, and the body appears to have engineered the structure of its polysaccharides, etc, accordingly. Such protection therefore affords a form of nonspecific recognition of "nonself" in the presence of "self" that seems in practice to be highly effective. It is interesting that this constraint on normal cell surface components need not apply to antigens expressed in the embryo before the alternative pathway has developed, nor to antigens not normally present on surfaces. It is perhaps such antigens expressed on the surface of cancer cells that enable them to be recognized as "nonself" by the APC. "Successful" tumors are by definition not attacked by the APC in its normal low state of activation. In this case it may be that the surface protection of $\overline{C3b,Bb}$ from factor H is only partial, and when the local concentration of C3b is raised sufficiently, the balance between amplification and inactivation is tipped in favor of the former, rendering the tumor sensitive to APC attack (see below).

Cobra venom factor (CVF) is able to activate the APC because it appears to be the cobra analog of C3b (cobra C3a is the venom neurotoxin), which, in combination with mammalian Bb, happens to be enzymatically active but highly resistant to inactivation by factors H and I. CVF activation of the APC is potent and highly specific.

The Classical Pathway of Complement

The recognition component of the classical pathway is the molecule C1q (Fig. 4-3), a unique hexamer of subunits having a globular head with moderate affinity for the Fa region of IgG and a collagen-like tail. The subunits are held together by the interaction of the tail-fibers, and the heads interact with aggregates of IgG. C1q is thus able to recognize and bind to IgG clustered on, say, a bacterial cell surface. C1q normally forms in plasma a reversible complex, "C1" (mediated by Ca^{2+} ions) with a subunit comprising one each of the molecules C1r and C1s. Binding of C1q to IgG aggregates is considered to induce a conformational change in C1q that induces a corresponding change in the associated C1r, which allows an autocatalytic cleavage of C1r to $\overline{C1r}$ with liberation of a small peptide. Activated $\overline{C1r}$ now specifically cleaves the associated C1s to the activated form $\overline{C1s}$, another specific protease whose substrate is C4. C4 (and C5) has structural homologies with C3 and may have evolved by duplication of the C3 gene; they both contain an internal thioester bond that is activated by specific cleavage to C4b or C3b, with liberation of the anaphylatoxins C4a and C3a. Activation of C4 to C4b by cleavage with C1s allows the $\overline{C4b,C1s}$ complex to bind C2, when the $\overline{C1s}$ cleaves C2 to C2a, with liberation of C2b and $\overline{C1s}$. The activated complex $\overline{C4b,2a}$ is a

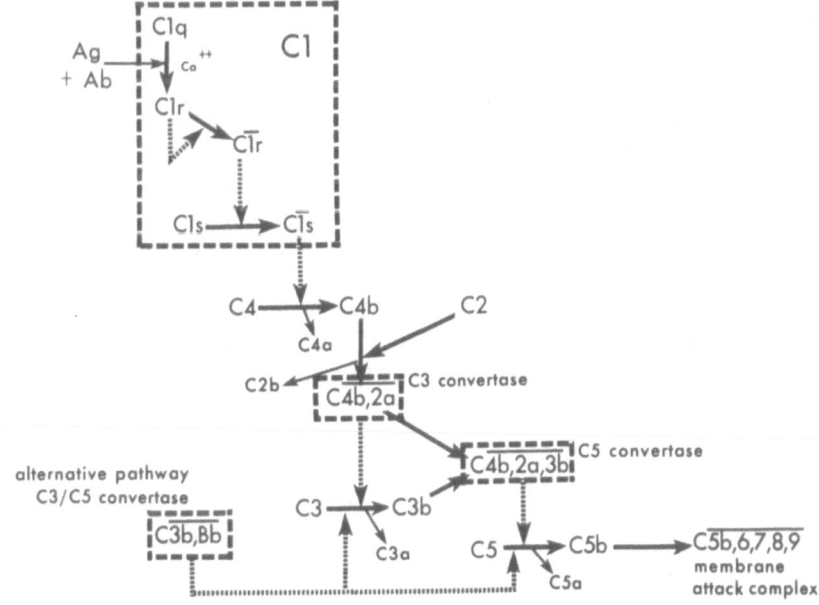

Figure 4-3. The classical pathway of complement. *Broken-line arrows* denote action on a step by proteolytic cleavage.

specific C3 convertase, binding C3 and creating (with liberation of the anaphylatoxin C3a) the complex $\overline{C4b,2a,3b}$ that now has the desired C5 convertase specificity. Both C4b and C3b of these various complexes can irreversibly attach to surfaces via their internal thioester bond, thus opsonizing them for phagocytosis and creating insoluble enzyme complexes, usually very close to their points of initiation. The C3 convertase $\overline{C4b,2a}$ also can activate the APC (Fig. 4-2). Like the APC, activation of the classical pathway is controlled by regulator proteins, notably $\overline{C1}$ inhibitor, C4-binding protein, and others.

Biologic Involvement of the Alternative Pathway of Complement

Complement, through either the classical or the alternative pathway, is involved in a large variety of disease states and generates a substantial variety of biologic activities (13,14). Central to all these is the molecule C3. The APC also interacts with a large proportion of the components of the immune response, and some biologic activities of the APC pertinent to cancer-related immune reactions are summarized below.

Macrophage Activation

For our purposes the most significant role of the APC may be that elucidated mainly by Schorlemmer and colleagues (23–29) for the activation of macrophages. Such activation, defined as acquisition of marked metabolic changes (15) including ability to kill neoplastic cells or microbes (16), release of lysosomal enzymes, and a variety of physiologic activities (17–19), comprises at least two steps. After a stage of precursor-cell differentiation into a responsive state, the still immature monocytes are sensitive to priming by lymphokines induced by antigen or mitogen from T or occasionally B lymphocytes accumulated at inflammatory sites (20,21). The primed cells are then, for a time, sensitive to triggering by various stimuli, including immune complexes, $F(ab')_2$ and several lymphokines (22), but most significantly by any of a wide variety of substances (23–25) that confer nonspecific immunity to the host (15), most or all of which are able to activate the APC (26). Examples are endotoxin, zymosan, collagen type II, and dextran sulfate. An important instance is the activation of macrophages by exogenous C3b (27,28), which is specific for the APC. Exogenous C3b in a serum-free medium elicited a dose-dependent release of several hydrolases (29), but not lactate dehydrogenase, which is a measure of cell death. Such activated macrophages concurrently acquired the ability to lyse added tumor cells.

Many of the components of the APC (especially C3 and factors B, D, and P) are synthesized by normal macrophages (30), and macrophages have C3b receptors on their surface (31,32). Macrophages contain proteases in their lysosomes that are secreted on activation (33), and it is therefore feasible for macrophages to cleave their own C3 and present their own C3b on their surface via these receptors. Their own factors B, D, and P allow them to form their own C3/C5 convertase, and Schorlemmer and Allison (27) have shown that supernatants of activated but not nonactivated macrophages were indeed able to cleave added C3. Macrophages stimulated by various agents secrete a factor that is pharmacologically and immunologically indistinguishable from C3a (29), as is required of a functioning C3 convertase. There is, indeed, evidence that macrophages do cleave their own C3, and via their surface C3b receptors present this to the external environment in the presence of Mg^{2+} in the form of an active C3/C5 convertase $\overline{C3b,Bb}$ (29). They also secrete a factor, indistinguishable from C3b, that can activate other macrophages. These activities occur in the absence of serum. Clearly, macrophages express all the activities necessary for cell-mediated amplification of the APC cyclic cascade and do function as important, self-mobile, and self-sufficient amplifiers of this pathway (15).

There thus appears to have accumulated persuasive evidence that macrophage activation in vitro can actually occur via activation of its endogenous APC. At all events, the two processes appear to be very closely linked biochemically, so that activation of one in vivo is unlikely to occur without some activation of the other. This is important in view of the known ability of activated macrophages to kill tumor cells.

Interaction with Lymphocytes

Normal B lymphocytes and a small proportion of T cells also carry surface receptors for complement components, notably C1q and C3 (34), and can be shown to carry C3b on their surface (35). Lymphocytes actually have two species of C3b receptors (36), one of which resembles the primate erythrocyte immune adherence receptor (37), and the other appears to be related to the in vitro response to antigen (38). These are carried by B cells (39). Fixed C3 interacts between macrophages and B cell C3 receptors to mediate T-dependent presentation of antigen to B cells (40,41).

B cells are themselves able to activate the APC (42,43), with deposition of C3b on their surface. Cell-free C3b is able to stimulate B cells but not T cells to produce a chemotactic lymphokine (44). C3 may be involved in B-cell triggering (45). A variety of other roles for complement in the functions of lymphocytes have been documented (34).

Like the macrophage, current information suggests that activation on the lymphocyte surface of complement, particularly of the APC, can lead to cellular activation. It appears feasible that nonspecific stimulation of the lymphocyte in this way is important for the development of lymphocyte antitumor immune responses.

Production of Anaphylatoxins C3a, C4a, and C5a

Activation of the APC, as well as of the classical pathway, leads crucially to enzymic cleavage of C3 with production of C3a (9,000 molecular weight) and C3b and then to cleavage of C5 with production of C5a (15,000 molecular weight) and C5b. As summarized earlier, C3b and C5b play direct roles in the complement pathway, but the apparent by-products C3a and C5a also have multiple biologic activities of their own (reviewed in ref. 46). They, along with C4a produced via the classical pathway, are spasmogens having effects on blood vessels and smooth muscle and stimulating production and release of leukotrienes in tissue (47). They interact with mast cells and basophils to liberate vasoactive amines and activate neutrophils to secrete lysosomal enzymes. Human leukocytes generate the cytotoxic superoxide (O_2^-) after contact with human C5a (48). C5a chemotactically attracts basophils (49), neutrophils (50), and mononuclear phagocytes (51), but C3a does not attract neutrophils (50). The body regulates the concentration of these very active substances by specific proteinase inactivators, so that they are normally short-lived and in low concentration in plasma, but not in their local region of production.

It can be seen that anaphylatoxins act as cell-modifying amplifiers of the complement pathways by recruiting to the regions of "foreign" invasion (and then activating) more leukocytes that are able to increase the local pool of complement resource. They thus play an important role in inflammation and are likely to be equally significant in any antitumor response in which complement is active.

In addition, C3a and other C3 fragments have major suppressor effects on components of the humoral and cellular responses, while C5a enhances others (52,53). It appears that the anaphylatoxins when present in high local concentrations have important functions in regional regulation of the immune response.

However, anaphylatoxins have also been implicated in acute hypotensive shock, although the role of complement was not clear at the time of the review of Hugli and Müller-Eberhard (46). Acute respiratory distress may result from granulocyte accumulation in the lungs as a response to C5a production, and the impact of the anaphylatoxins may possibly be the major clinical concern in deliberate complement manipulation (see below).

Opsonization

When C3 is cleaved to produce C3a and C3b, the internal thioester bond (in the C3b moiety) is exposed and at the same time stressed by conformational change in the peptide backbone. This highly reactive bond then reacts with the nearest nucleophilic groups, a small proportion of which are —OH or —NH$_2$ residues on organic molecules, perhaps on the surface of a foreign particle. If this surface is appropriate ("nonself" and often exogenous polysaccharide in nature), the C3b now covalently bound to the particle will be relatively protected from binding to factor H (which would prime it for proteolytic cleavage by factor I to iC3b). It is then capable of binding to the C3b receptors found on the surface of all mononuclear and polymorphonuclear phagocytes (54,55), as well as on some lymphocytes and other cells, and is opsonized (56), ie, sensitized for phagocytosis. C3b and IgG are the only significant opsonins (54). If the phagocytes are activated, these bound opsonized particles are then ingested, in which process C3b may also play a role (57,58). In the opsonized state the surface C3b can also form the C3/C5 convertase, $\overline{C3b,Bb}$, and activate the APC. If the C3b is degraded to iC3b or other fragments, the phagocytes or other leukocytes have specific surface receptors for many of these also (55).

Role of Complement in Host Defenses Against Cancer

Complement, as an integral part of the body's defense mechanism, has so many diverse activities that it is not surprising to find it involved in defense against tumors. An example that it can be a limiting factor in host defense is the observation that normal serum from a variety of species, including mouse, can temporarily reverse the spontaneous leukemia of AKR mice (59), which are C5-deficient. Serum from AKR mice usually cannot. Heating (56 °C for 30 min) or treatment with cobra venom factor [which depletes C3-C9 (60)] abolished the activity; nine complement components tested separately showed that only C5 (highly purified) was effective in replacing it. It is likely that cytotoxic antibody was involved in this regression, as in many other studies (some reviewed in ref. 61), and consequently may be mediated via either the APC or the classical pathway of complement, or conceivably both.

Changes in Complement Levels in Sera of Tumor-Bearing Animals and Humans

If complement were consistently involved in defense against tumors, one might expect to see consistent variations in serum complement levels during growth of malignancies. Many such changes have indeed been found (61), but as these reviewers point out, they are conflicting and difficult to evaluate. A frequent finding is of higher levels than normal in the active phase of malignant disease (62) and a lower level than normal with growing tumor burden (63). The latter may result from, eg, C1q binding by immune complexes (64) or C3b fixation of their Fd regions (65), as well as consumption by APC (66) and other defense mechanisms. There may be inhibitors of C3 or C3b in sera of cancer patients (67,68).

There was a link between the gene for factor B and acute lymphocytic leukemia (69) and melanoma (70).

One important lesson from all these findings may be that any attempt at deliberate complement activation therapy should include an assessment of the patient's complement status, eg, as to whether there is, in fact, enough endogenous complement to activate.

Direct Cytotoxicity of the APC for Neoplastic Cells

If the neoplastic cells do carry surface antigens that differ from normal cells, then (like bacteria and other "nonself" parasites) these antigens may be able to protect bound C3b from the plasma inactivators H and I enough to allow local amplification of the APC, leading to C5b fixation and attack by the membrane attack complex. Such attack has indeed been found with purified APC components (71). These can directly lyse Raji cells, which are a continuous human lymphoblastoid cell line derived from a patient with Burkitt's lymphoma. Other findings with serum are similar (72–74), but the effect appears to be limited to Burkitt-related cells, perhaps because they carry surface Epstein-Barr virus (EBV) antigens (75). The APC activation by leukemic cells from the carrier AKR line (76) may also be due to surface viral antigens. Among human leukemia cells, only Schilling-type acute monocytic leukemias and cells from a generalized reticulohistiocytosis were able to activate the APC via surface components (77).

A variety of foreign cells (normal and malignant murine cells) are lysed by cell-free human serum via the APC, independently of natural or induced antibodies (78). C3a is directly cytolytic, tumor cells being more sensitive than normal cells (79).

Cytotoxicity Mediated by Macrophages

There is a wealth of evidence to implicate the macrophage as important or even crucial, in collaboration with B and T cells, in the rejection of malignant disease (80–82). In brief, (a) macrophages comprise a significant proportion of the cells of tumors undergoing rejection, and cytolytically activated macrophages can be isolated from them. Normal cells are much less sensitive to activated macrophages than tumor cells. (b) Agents that inhibit or remove macrophages enhance tumor survival, and agents that promote macrophages enhance tumor destruction. (c) Macrophages are obligate in the destruction of some tumors, where they seem to act as effectors after they have been attracted there and activated. Indeed, macrophages are equipped with an armory very suitable for dealing with tumor rejection. It has been postulated that they may be the effector cells involved in immune surveillance against tumors, since it now seems unlikely that lymphocytes can play this role (83).

As mentioned earlier, the APC appears to play a crucial role in the activation of macrophages in vitro, and it appears likely that the mechanism of activation in vivo is essentially the same (15).

Once activated, the macrophage then has the interestingly selective ability to kill tumor cells, as well as, eg, bacteria. It is likely that the surface of tumor cells themselves are able to trigger the activation (20,84) once the macrophage is primed by lymphokine. The killing occurs both specifically and nonspecifically. "Specific" in this sense means that it is specific antibody-dependent, but this action is nonselective in the sense that it can occur with normal as well as neoplastic cells. Specific killing of tumor cells may be important in vivo because antitumor antibodies have often been found in spontaneous neoplasms (85) and may well involve the APC, but it will not be considered here. In addition, a third natural-killer-like activity has been proposed (20).

Nonspecific cytotoxicity of activated macrophages for neoplastic cells (86) is selective for such cells and is slow, contact-dependent, and antibody-independent. There is an initial, rapid contact and binding step, which at 37° becomes extremely firm and requires metabolic activity and which does not occur with nonneoplastic cells. This is followed by a secondary release of lytic substances (87), including reactive oxygen intermediates (88). Target cell death may occur by induction of cell division with restricted DNA replication so that progeny cells have insufficient DNA for viability (89), or through mitochondrial injury (90).

Exogenous C3b in a serum-free medium produced in macrophages a dose-dependent acquisition of the ability to lyse added tumor cells (25,29), possibly by production of C3a (91). In vivo procedures that can be shown to activate macrophages, eg, chronic infection with BCG vaccine (92) or with *Toxoplasma* (93), gave rise to macrophage populations that for months retained their in vitro cytotoxicity for tumor cells. Specific macrophage activation has been attempted in vivo using muramyl dipeptide [the minimal unit of adjuvant activity that can replace mycobacteria in Freund's adjuvant (94)]. Free muramyl dipeptide was ineffective, but when encapsulated in liposomes (95) it was able to elicit cytotoxicity in alveolar macrophages for several tumor cell lines in vitro. Lymph node and pulmonary metastases from a melanoma in C57BL mice were eradicated.

Tumor Cell Chemotaxis

C5a generated in vitro or in vivo is able to chemotactically attract certain tumor cells (96–98), and it was argued that chemotactic mechanisms might contribute to formation of metastases. This might be a concern for complement activation therapy. However, where metastases already exist, it may also have the beneficial effect of opening up tumor nodules to attack by other treatment modalities and may be related to such an effect from delayed-type hypersensitivity (DTH) reactions induced in such nodules by vaccination (99).

Agents Active in Nonspecific Immunotherapy Against Cancer

Treatment of cancer patients with microbial vaccines dates back to the last century when Coley (100) treated with considerable success (2,3) a large number of inoperable cancer patients with a mixture of killed *Streptococcus* and *Bacillus prodigiosus* (*Serratia marcescens*). Many different types of preparation have been used since (1,4) in human and animal studies to attempt a nonspecific immunopotentiation or stimulation of the immune system in the hope of reversing the malignant process. "Nonspecific" in this sense means not deliberately administering a tumor antigen, although because these preparations all have adjuvant activity, one effect may be to increase the antigenicity of a weak tumor antigen already present. In addition, nonspecific immunopotentiation has been used in conjunction with tumor products in a classical immune adjuvant situation. Interest in this approach has been increasing since the 1960s and has now resulted in a very large literature.

In this section two agents (*Corynebacterium parvum* and *Staphylococcus aureus* protein A) are considered in some detail, and a number of other agents summarized (Table 4-1).

C parvum (Propionibacterium acnes) and *C granulosum*

The material administered is a killed whole bacterial vaccine consisting of gram-positive rods treated with heat and formalin. It is a typical adjuvant for the humoral response and a stimulator of cell-mediated immunity (165); toxic reactions are, in general, minimal.

In our hands, references to *C parvum* comprised the majority of recoveries from a computer search for articles on immune potentiation over the last ten years. Many studies have shown pronounced antitumor effects in experimental animals (although the results were not consistently favorable). *C parvum* could be active systemically against various murine tumors—eg, vaccine given intravenously (IV) or intraperitoneally (IP) inhibited the growth of tumor cells given subcutaneously (SC) (166)—and could reduce metastases (167). Multiple intralesional injections of *C parvum* and other bacterial vaccines caused complete regression of hepatomas in the majority of guinea pigs (109). Treatment of animals with *C parvum* can advantageously be combined with chemotherapy (168), but certain rules emerged (4). The relative timing of vaccine and drug is critical, perhaps because many of the drugs used are immunosuppressants. The dose of vaccine is also critical, very low and very high doses being less effective. Route of administration is important, the SC route giving the poorest response and the IV route (with proper dose and timing) markedly augmenting the response. Intratumor or regional application was also favorable, but the oral route was ineffective (169).

In vitro *C parvum* has a macrophage-chemotactic and a macrophage-activating effect (170), even in the absence of serum (26), and macrophages from *C parvum*-treated animals have enhanced thymus-independent cytotoxicity for tumor cells (171,172). In vivo, the effect is independent of T or B cells and hence may depend only on macrophages (4), although some *C parvum*-elicited cells cytolytic for tumor cells were not phagocytic but had the character of natural killer cells (173). In a study of chronic lymphocytic leukemia patients (174), killer cell activity was found to be associated with a cell population carrying receptors for C3b.

A malignancy lacking tumor-specific transplantation antigens was inhibited by IV injections of *C parvum,* again suggesting macrophage activation (175). The tumor-infiltrating macrophages after *C parvum* treatment of a murine fibrosarcoma were consistently in the activated state (176), as were peritoneal macrophages from a *C parvum*-treated leukemia cell tumor (P388) inoculated intraperitoneally, provided that the tumor cell yield was decreased (108,177). The antitumor effect might generalize against existing or soon-arising spontaneous microfoci, as later spontaneous tumors were also reduced by *C parvum* treatment (178).

A very significant correlation may be that given by Sadler et al (103), who showed that one strain of *C parvum* that had antitumor activity in the mouse was able to bind to macrophages in vitro and activated the APC of guinea pig serum, whereas another strain that failed to show antitumor activity did not bind to macrophages and did not activate the APC. Similar studies with more single-step mutational deficiencies in *C parvum* could be informative regarding mechanisms.

In humans, *C parvum* immunotherapy has had a mixed result. We are not able to give a balanced evaluation, but of the controlled studies available to us, seven (179–185) showed no significant response to *C parvum* therapy against a variety of tumors, which were generally in advanced stages. Treatment was usually combined with chemotherapy or radiotherapy, and *C parvum* was given by a variety of routes, ie, intralymph node, intramuscularly, or subcutaneously. However, eight studies (186–193) did show objective responses in a proportion of the treated groups. Once again a variety of tumors was involved, treatment was usually combined with chemotherapy or surgery, and the vaccine was given intravenously or regionally. Two of these studies were of early (Stage I or II) carcinomas. In general, cures were not reported, the results being either extended survival or remissions and improved quality of life.

These results must be regarded as encouraging but preliminary: clearly, some activity is present but variables are missing. It is difficult to gauge the correct administration regimen when there is no theoretical basis and no monitoring parameter available. Also, there is a marked difference in the adjuvant effects of *C parvum* strains (194). In one study (195) one strain of *C parvum* inhibited metastases from the Lewis lung carcinoma in C57BL mice whereas another strain did not. It is not clear what consideration has been given to *C parvum* strain differences and methods of vaccine preparation.

In cell-free systems, intact *C parvum* vaccine is a potent activator of the APC in human and guinea pig serum (102). In human serum the classical pathway was also activated, but this was due to anti-*C parvum* antibodies in the serum used, whose source was not given. Thore et al (196) concluded that phagocytosis and killing of *C parvum* in normal human serum by human peripheral blood leukocytes is mediated by C3, but that in some cases it is activated by the classical pathway and in others by the alternative pathway.

The majority of the complement-activating effect for human serum is located in the cell wall of *C parvum* and is polysaccharide in nature (197); peptidoglycan, lipid, protein, and nucleic acid do not appear to contribute. Attempts to extract the active moiety (198) produced a teichoic-acid-free polysaccharide with partial APC activating properties.

Complement activation was found in 48% of human cancer patients receiving IV *C parvum* (199); in some activation proceeded via the APC and in others via the classical pathway. Vaccination (SC) of normal human volunteers with *C parvum* significantly elevated cell-mediated (antibody-independent) cytotoxicity against two tumor cell lines (200).

Protein A from *S aureus*

A substantial amount of practical interest has been generated by an ex vivo perfusion procedure involving continuous flow separation of particulate elements from blood, passing the separated plasma over heat- and formalin-fixed *S aureus* (Cowan's type I strain, carrying covalently bonded surface protein A), then recombining the filtered plasma with the formed elements and returning the whole to the patient (201). Most subsequent studies have used separated but immobilized protein A preparations of undefined purity. Some striking regressions have been obtained with cat, dog, and rat tumors (202–205). The results have been less impressive with human patients, perhaps because the volume of blood to be processed is greater, but nevertheless some benefit was regularly observed in approximately 50% of the patients (131,141,206a), most of whom were in an advanced stage of malignant disease.

At first sight this treatment procedure seems radically different from the other regimens described in this section. Indeed, the original rationale was quite unrelated, as it sought to remove circulating immune complexes by means of the high affinity of protein A on the bacterial surface for their IgG. Immune complexes are considered able to block host immune responses against cancer (206b). However, it seems less likely now that this is the mechanism, as the proportion of body fluids treated is rather low (207,131), and strains of *S aureus* that do not present protein A (and even protein A-free soluble extracts from these strains) can be equally effective (135).

In a laboratory model set up to mimic this treatment procedure (131), we found that *S aureus* treatment of serum from B16 melanoma-bearing mice altered the serum so that when it was administered to fresh tumor-bearing mice, there was a highly significant increase in mean survival time. Untreated serum was ineffective. However, it was found that *S aureus* treatment of sera from normal mice and also from rabbits, and from guinea pig and human serum with some manipulation, was equally effective. An active principle could be eluted from protein A columns or *S aureus* treated with serum. Finally, highly active preparations could be obtained without contact with protein A, from human, rabbit, guinea pig, or mouse sera, by serum fractionation procedures designed to purify complement components. The active principle was shown not to be C1 or C1q, but frequently copurified with these components. It was stable at 56° for 30 minutes (148).

A derivative of C3 was suspected from the purification procedures, and taking this to its conclusion, Cooper and Sim (141) were able to show that isolated human and guinea pig C3b and $C3(H_2O)$ or C3u were highly active in a closely related system. Zymosan and isolated CVF had similarly high activity. Although the link could not be proved in this way, it was concluded that the ex vivo *S aureus* perfusion treatment was very likely to be activating the APC and that reintroduction of the activated moieties in the returned plasma was probably responsible for the antitumor effects.

This then brings the theory behind the protein A treatments completely into line with that deduced for the other nonspecific immunopotentiators of Table 4-1. Protein A is a potent activator of the APC as well as the classical pathway of complement (129,130), as indeed are the cell wall components of the nonprotein A-bearing *S aureus* strains (132,133). Protein A probably requires the presence of IgG and forms aggregates resembling immune complexes (208). Treatment with *S aureus* extracts has induced marked hypocomplementemia (135), and C3 has been observed to be deposited on tumor cell walls after protein A perfusion (203). Pain and heat at the tumor site are frequently reported after this treatment, suggesting an inflammatory response.

One of the reports on which the original rationale was based was the presumed abrogation by protein A treatment of a serum-blocking activity against in vitro cytotoxicity of lymphocytes (209). These experiments showed that tumor-specific complement-dependent cytotoxicity was induced by *S aureus* treatment of "blocking" sera, and, curiously, that mixtures of treated and untreated sera still lacked blocking activity. Such a situation is unexpected if the treatment were simply removing blocking substances. Instead, it seems likely that the lymphocytes, already primed for this specific tumor, were being activated by complement components (putatively C3b). Miller et al (210) found that *S aureus* treatment of sera created a heat-stable cytotoxicity for acute myelogenous leukemia cells but not normal peripheral blood cells, a specificity like that of C3b, which is also heat stable. The possible interactions of C3b with these leuko-cytes, or the presence of C3b in the separated IgG fractions in which the activity was found, was apparently not considered.

Other Agents Active in Nonspecific Immunotherapy

Table 4-1 summarizes some properties of the most-studied nonspecific immunopotentiators that have shown antitumor activity in vivo. Many (eg, live BCG) are highly complex in nature and are likely to have multiple effects (resulting from, eg, antigenic determinants in common with tumor antigens, immunogenicity in their own right, toxic components), but at-tention here has been focussed on only three properties: ability to activate the APC in cell-free systems (whether or not the classical pathway is also involved), ability to activate macrophages in vitro and/or in vivo, and some kind of antitumor response in vivo, although active agents do not seem to show antitumor activity in all applications. The gaps in Table 4-1 reflect an inability to trace reference to the datum in question, and in only one case (carboxymethyl pachymaran, 150) has a report been found that an active antitumor agent is inactive in triggering the APC or macro-phages.

The following are some notes on Table 4-1.

Live Vaccine—BCG

BCG is attenuated bovine mycobacteria used for antituberculosis vacci-nation. It was one of the earliest modern agents used for immunopotentia-tion against human cancer, with some successes (1,4). Best results are obtained with live organisms (211) inserted as close to the tumor as possi-ble, the tumor must not be large, there is a sharp dose dependence and the animal must be immunocompetent. Activated macrophages are produced in vitro and in vivo; activation of the APC is to be expected but surpris-ingly does not seem to be recorded earlier than 1980 for any mycobacte-rial fraction or preparations. This deficiency was remedied by Ramana-than et al (101), who showed that *M. bovis* BCG (Glaxo strain), *M. leprae,* and *M. lepraemurium* activated the APC, while *M. bovis* BCG (Pasteur strain) did not.

Killed Whole Bacterial Vaccines

C parvum has been considered in some detail in an earlier section of this chapter. It activates macrophages in vivo and in vitro, activates the APC, and has shown considerable clinical activity. Where information is avail-

Table 4-1. Agents active in vivo in nonspecific immunotherapy against cancer.

Agent	Activation of APC	Activation of macrophages	Antitumor response in vivo
Live Vaccine:			
Mycobacterium tuberculosis (BCG)	(101)	(92,104)	(105,106)
Killed Whole Bacterial Vaccines:			
C parvum	(102,103)	(107,108)	(109)
B abortus	?	(110)	(111)
M tuberculosis			
(Freund's complete adjuvant)	?	(112,113)	(114,115)
P aeruguinosa	?	(116)	(116)
Microbial Cell Wall Fractions:			
Brucella			
—Bru-pel	?	(117–119)	(117–119)
Streptococcus			
—OK 432	(120,121)[a]	122[b]	(123–125)
Mycobacterium			
—Methanol extraction residue	?	(107)	(107)
—Trehalose mycolate (cord factor) in oil	(101)	(126)	(127,128)
—Muramyl dipeptide	?	(95)	(95)
Staphylococcus			
—Protein A	(129,130)[c]	?	(131) (201–206a)
—Cell walls, peptidoglycan	(132,133)	(122)[b]	(134,135)
Saccharomyces			
—Zymosan	(136,137)	(138)	(138–141)
Lipopolysaccharides			
Various gram-negative bacteria	(142–144)	(145,146)	(127,147)
Polysaccharides			
Inulin[d]	(136)	?	(148)
Beta-1,3 glucans			
—lentinan, pachymaran	(149,150)	?	(151–153)
—from zymosan	(137)	(154,155)	(137,154)
Polyanions			
Poly A : U	?	(145)	(156)
Pyran copolymer	(157)	(158)	(158)
Levamisole	(159,160)	(161)	(162)
Specific APC Activators			
C3b	(141)	(25,27,28,163)	(141)
CVF	(60)	?	(141,164)

Note: Numbers in parentheses indicate references.
[a] Cell wall glucan
[b] Streptococcal peptidoglycan
[c] In presence of IgG
[d] Insoluble state

able, other vaccines (eg, *Brucella abortus*, Freund's complete adjuvant, *Pseudomonas aeruginosa*, Table 4-1) are similarly active, except that APC activation (although to be expected) does not appear to be recorded for these three. All preparations are potent immunoadjuvants. As in the case of live vaccines and some cell wall derivatives, their antitumor activity is likely to depend on active subcomponents such as polysaccharides and lipopolysaccharides (see below).

Microbial Cell Wall Preparations

S aureus protein A fractions have been considered earlier. Many bacterial subfractions have been investigated for in vivo antitumor effect, and a substantial number have activity (Table 4-1). They all appear to include intact cell walls or major components of the cell wall, which is rather robust in bacteria and yeast and usually comprises covalently interlinked polysaccharide-peptide moieties. Most of them activate the APC as well as macrophages. Muramyl dipeptide (synthetic *N*-acetylmuramyl-L-alanine-D-isoglutamine), a single-sugar glycopeptide, is the simplest component of mycobacteria that retains full adjuvant activity (94) when administered in Freund's incomplete adjuvant, a water-in-oil emulsion. Encased in liposomes (to direct it to macrophages) but not in free form, muramyl dipeptide activates the macrophages in vivo and in vitro and has substantial antitumor effect in mice (Table 4-1). It does not activate the APC in free solution (101). It would be of considerable interest to know if, in liposomes or in water-in-oil emulsion, muramyl dipeptide was able to activate the APC; conceivably on a phase interface, it could present an array of appropriately aligned saccharides.

Lipopolysaccharides

Lipopolysaccharides (LPS) or endotoxins comprise various complex polysaccharides covalently attached to lipid A, a unique glycophospholipid. They occur in the outer membrane of gram-negative bacteria and provide via their polysaccharide moiety the somatic antigens. The lipid moiety is responsible for the endotoxic activity. LPS is a potent adjuvant and modulator of immune reactions, interacting with many leukocyte types. It is strongly immunogenic. It also has multiple effects in vivo, including release of pyrogens from macrophages, production of interferon, endocrine changes, granulocytosis and proliferation of hemopoietic stem cells, release of vasomotor agents resulting in progressive hypotension and shock, and disseminated intravascular coagulation. LPS is accordingly quite toxic and has not been much used in man, but causes regression of tumors in animals, activates macrophages in vivo and in vitro, and in cell-free systems activates primarily the APC rather than the classical pathway.

The soluble "tumor necrosis factor" produced in the presence of serum by activation of macrophages with LPS (212a) has properties (alpha-glob-ulin glycoprotein—mol wt 150,000) that are tantalizingly close to those of C3b (alpha-2 globulin glycoprotein—mol wt 170,000; ref. 7).

Polysaccharides

A number of high molecular weight polysaccharides, several extracted from edible fungi, have potent, often systemic antitumor effects in vivo (Table 4-1). The beta-1,3 glucans lentinan and pachymaran are linear polyglucoses. Lentinan and the glucan from zymosan are immunoadju-vants but differ from each other and are more selective than LPS. They also activate the APC in vitro and in vivo and activate macrophages in vitro and in vivo. Activation of the APC and of macrophages by many beta-1,3 glucans is correlated with insolubility (155). Inulin is a linear beta-1,2 poly D fructofuranose of about 30 residues (212b). Particulate, but not dissolved, inulin is a potent activator of the APC but not of the classical pathway (136), and particulate, but not dissolved inulin, has antitumor activity in mice (Fig. 4-4). As expected, dissolved inulin did not activate macrophages (155), but unfortunately Seljelid and colleagues did not appear to test the particulate state for this activity.

An attempt to correlate in vitro APC activation and effect against sar-coma-180 in mice among eight related beta-1,3 glucans (150) succeeded in five cases, but two APC activators had no antitumor effect and one effec-tive antitumor agent (the highly soluble carboxymethyl pachymaran) did not activate the APC in vitro. However, it was difficult to reconcile the

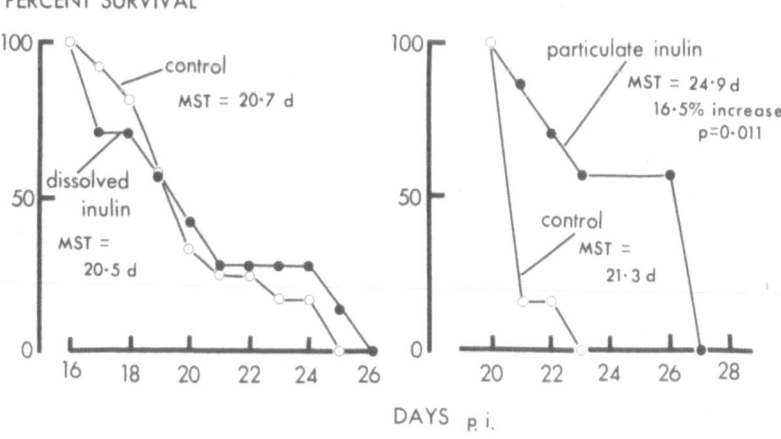

Figure 4-4. Increase of mean survival time (MST) by particulate inulin (5 mg/mouse on day 1, **right**) in C57BL mice after inoculation with melanoma cells, compared with the lack of effect on MST of dissolved inulin (4 mg/mouse on days 1, 4 and 5, **left**) in a similar experiment (148).

differences between the in vivo and in vitro assays with differences in solubility and chemical properties. A comparison of macrophage activation in vivo and in vitro may be illuminating.

Polyanions

Many high molecular weight polyanions, eg, heparin, dextran sulfate, Sephadex, polyacrylic acid, and agarose, will activate both APC and macrophages and are immunopotentiators (25,136,213–215). The anions may be either carboxylate, sulfate, phosphate, or thiophosphate (15). Other polyanions have been shown to activate macrophages and to have antitumor effects in vivo (Table 4-1). Pyran, a copolymer of divinyl ether and maleic anhydride, is a synthetic polyanion, mol wt 23,000, that has a strong antitumor effect. Double-stranded RNAs, either synthetic or from fungi, are adjuvants and activate macrophages: of these poly A : U is a poor inducer of interferon, is less toxic than poly I : C, and more easily explored in vivo. It has moderate antitumor effects, of the same order as poly I : C, probably not mediated via interferon. The structure of both pyran copolymer and double-stranded RNA would suggest that they activate the APC in vitro, and one such report has been traced (157) for pyran copolymer.

Levamisole

Levamisole (2,3,5,6-tetrahydro-6-phenyl imidazo [2,1-*b*] thiazole) is a synthetic antihelminthic that appears to restore immune functions to, but not above, normal levels. It has a moderate but definite antitumor effect in many human and animal applications, activates macrophages in vitro and in vivo, and (somewhat unexpectedly from its chemical structure) activates the APC at low concentrations in vitro.

Specific Activators of the APC

CVF is a classical, specific, and potent activator of the APC. Its antitumor activity in the isolated state (Table 4-1) has considerable significance. CVF activates B cells (216a), but although activated macrophages are also to be expected, they have apparently not been reported.

The molecule C3b is conventionally considered a component rather than an activator of the APC, but, nevertheless, addition of a small amount of C3b to serum has the full effect of any other activator (141), a function that is predictable from the concepts of maintenance of the APC amplification cascade ("tick-over" hypothesis, ref. 8). Its in vivo antitumor activity in the isolated state seems highly significant, as is its ability to activate macrophages to lyse tumor cells in vivo and in vitro.

An Overview of Table 4-1

Where information is available and with one exception, all agents that we have been able to trace as having nonspecific antitumor immunopotentiation in vivo (Table 4-1) are able either to activate the APC directly or to activate macrophages (usually to specific tumor cell cytolysis), an ability that appears to depend on APC activation. Eleven (ie, 50%) of the agents in Table 4-1 (BCG, *C parvum,* streptococcal and staphylococcal cell wall preparations, zymosan, lipopolysaccharides, certain beta-1,3 glucans, pyran copolymer, levamisole, C3b), of rather diverse nature, have been shown to possess all three activities.

This correlation appears to be beyond coincidence. In particular, three antitumor agents (inulin, C3b, and CVF) can be expected to have a quite specific primary effect, namely to activate the APC. It is a tenable thesis, therefore, that the primary antitumor effect of all the agents listed in Table 4-1 is to activate the APC, whether free in plasma or carried by macrophages or other leukocytes.

Clinical Prospects for Deliberate Manipulation of the APC in Human Cancer Patients

From the many reports of APC activators deliberately or accidentally present in the human body, it seems quite clear that clinical manipulation of the APC without gross morbidity is feasible, within certain limits. It has to be established whether or not these limits include those that are clinically useful in the treatment of cancer.

Time of Treatment

According to Mathé (1), an active immunotherapy is best suited for conditions where the tumor burden is very small, ie, for treatment of residual disease. Mathé recommends that it should follow surgery, radiotherapy, and chemotherapy, although a complication may be the possibly slow recovery of the immune system from attenuation by these treatments, as the subject must be immunocompetent. On the other hand, two subsequent reports (188,216b) point out that under certain regimes, immune reactions make a critical contribution to regression of large tumor masses.

Dose

Most studies emphasize the importance of dose, since an overdose can lead to rapid exhaustion of C3 with consequent immunosuppression (1,139). There are some instances where higher doses of APC activators have increased the incidence of tumors (217–219), although in some cases this may be due to blockage of the activator by development of antibody. The immunosuppressive effect of C3 exhaustion may itself constitute a clinical hazard (220), requiring, for example, antibiotic cover. In general, the lowest effective dose seems the most desirable, although this is difficult to define in the absence of a suitable parameter to monitor. If partial depletion of C3 is the aim, then doses could be timed to allow the body to replenish serum levels (about 1 week).

Toxicity

Many reports on toxic effects of immunopotentiating agents are available, and in general these are similar. Frequently, there are chills and fever of variable severity, some nausea, vomiting, headache and confusion "not infrequently," a flu-like syndrome but not anaphylaxis [quoted for *C parvum* (221), a relatively nontoxic preparation], and changes in blood pressure, usually a drop. The toxicity was dramatically controlled by hydrocortisone. A cardiopulmonary toxicity after ex vivo perfusion of plasma over immobilized protein A was controlled essentially by decreasing the dose (222). An extreme toxicity found in a similar study was controlled in the same way (207), but two patients died as a result of respiratory problems. Both had severe pulmonary compromise as a result of their tumors. The possible contribution of enterotoxin was not excluded.

In general, however, toxic problems have not been severe, but there is no satisfactory way of knowing whether the dose has been optimized. Also it is usually not possible to distinguish a toxic effect of APC activation from other effects, especially toxic shock from contaminating endotoxin or enterotoxin. Curry and Morrison (223) conclude that complement activation is insufficient to account for the lethality of endotoxin in mice, but mice are very tolerant of APC activation since relatively huge doses of very pure CVF have no detectable adverse effect on mice, although C3 is explosively exhausted (224a).

There are few studies in humans of administration of substances that solely activate or deplete the APC. However, slight (ca 10%) but significant decreases in titres of serum C3b and total hemolytic complement but not of C4 were observed in 12 volunteers given dissolved inulin to a steady level >260 μg/ml of serum, with no adverse effect reported (224b). Complement activation has also been observed on cellophane membranes after hemodialysis (225). Activation occurred via the APC, and reinfusion of the activated complement caused granulocytes to be attracted to and partially block the pulmonary microvasculature, with demonstrable lung dysfunction (226) and profound but transient neutropenia. The active fragment was C5a. There were respiratory symptoms, chills, and hypotension. In general the symptoms were mild, but the degree of APC activation was not measured. Extensive APC activation in a compromised patient might have severe effects; therefore the progress of activation needs to be monitored. Possibly, a low level of continuous activation is desirable. Serum levels of C3, C3b, C3a, and C5a should be followed. It may also be advisable to have available a supply of the serum anaphylatoxin (C3a, C5a) inactivator, a C-terminal carboxypeptidase (227), if this could be shown to be of benefit. It is not known whether anti-inflammation regimens are counterproductive.

Which Agent?

The choice of agent is probably crucial. It seems important to know whether or not APC activation is the fundamental principle behind the positive results obtained so far; if so, then it is necessary to employ agents that will activate only the APC. Although CVF is very specific and potent, its high cost, low availability, and need for extensive purification rule it out. In addition, it is highly immunogenic (228) and therefore can only be used once. Most microbial agents, in addition to being complex, are likely to have toxic components.

There are several other possibilities. Purified or semi-purified C3 from human or other mammalian sources is isolable in a very few biochemical steps in good yield and can be directly converted to C3u. Alternatively, it may be possible to treat serum in a simple way—eg, with heat to inactivate degradative enzymes followed by ammonium ions at pH 9 to break the thioester bond and thus to create a serum with C3u activity. Administration of serum or serum fractions from nephritic patients screened for presence of serum nephritic factor [which activates the APC by protecting $\overline{C3b,Bb}$ from factors H and I (7)] may be feasible if sufficient donors can be found.

However, the most practical source at the moment appears to be the active polysaccharides, particularly the beta-1,3 glucans, which are highly potent in vivo and among which there is a range of choice. Availability and cost may be a consideration.

Inulin, a 2,1 linear fructosan, is known to activate the APC in the particulate but not dissolved state (136), with the colloidal dimensions being the most effective. A preliminary experiment showing antitumor activity in the particulate but not dissolved state is given in Fig. 4-4. Inulin is very soluble at 60 °C (>10% wt/vol), but is only slightly soluble in the cold and precipitates out quite slowly on cooling. The particulate form dissolves rather slowly at 37 °C, at a rate dependent on crystal type. Consequently it is feasible to work at 37 °C for an extended period with a given concentration either of a solution or a suspension over a range of concentrations.

Inulin has been used in its dissolved state extensively in the past as a glomerular filtration rate index in clinical tests for renal function. A standard is given in the *British Pharmacopoeia,* and the *British Pharmaceutical Codex* (ed 11, 1979) states that inulin (dissolved state) is not degraded by any known mammalian enzyme, has a half-life in the body of about one hour, and has as its only pharmacologic effect an osmotic diuresis when given in large amounts. Its soluble form is consequently nontoxic; the dose is 3 g IV, with continuous drip to maintain this level (approximately 300 μg/mL in blood). Possibly in the particulate state such a dose may have undesirable side effects, but even particulate inulin appears to be virtually nonimmunogenic and to cause no glomerular injury in rabbits (229). Its lack of pharmacologic activity in the dissolved state means that any effect found for the particulate state is (like APC activation) entirely dependent on physical structure and very likely to be due to APC activation alone. It is cheap, easily prepared, and readily available (from dahlia roots, where it is the main storage carbohydrate).

Discussion

In this review we have concentrated on one particular aspect of the immune system, because it had been noticed that the majority of active immunotherapy procedures that have shown clinical effectiveness can be expected to activate complement very early in a chain of resultant events. In particular, our own study (131,141) has shown that several diverse agents, each rather specific for activating the APC, had a pronounced regional antitumor effect on their own. It is significant that "C3b . . . [as] a common factor in many antitumor systems" was commented on some years ago (25), but appears not to have been developed. In general, it is surprising to find how frequently the involvement of complement has been overlooked or misinterpreted, despite the intimate detail in which it is understood.

Concerning specific active immunotherapy, in which particular tumor antigens are used to raise various components of the specific immune response, it may be expected that the classical pathway of complement activation will be prominently involved. However, it is not exclusively so, as IgG complexes can also activate the APC (65,230). In addition, specific antigen is often given with an adjuvant, in which case both classical and alternative pathways will probably be involved since most adjuvants also activate the APC. For reasons of space, and because they seem secondary to our thesis, specific immunotherapy (reviewed in ref. 4) and antibody-dependent cytotoxicity (reviewed in ref. 85) have not been considered here.

Instead we have reviewed aspects of nonspecific active immunotherapy in which APC activation was alone involved, or was the most prominent. No attempt was made at exhaustive coverage; rather, some illustrative examples were selected from a voluminous literature.

We have seen that APC activation and leukocyte activation, particularly of macrophages, appear to be inextricably intertwined in vivo. Arguably, the activated macrophage is the most important component of the antitumor effect of nonspecific immunotherapy. However, target cell lysis in the presence of complement is not necessarily cell-mediated. Because APC activation seems the more general case (and is likely to be the common basic mechanism), it has been the main focus of this review. A more significant point clinically is that APC activation is a parameter that can be manipulated and monitored directly.

Bessis' hypothesis (231) "that there is an antileukemic substance in normal blood" was based on many observations that remissions could occur after transfusion of normal heparinized plasma. Perhaps he was right, and his "antileukemic substance" was actually $\overline{C3b,Bb}$.

Conclusions

We attempted to answer the question: Is there sufficient evidence to implicate APC activation as the most usual primary event in nonspecific active immunotherapy? We believe that the material reviewed in this chapter comprises abundant evidence that this is the case and that APC activation can be proposed to be the specific theoretical ground so far lacking for this treatment modality. To confirm or invalidate such a hypothesis, work needs to be done with highly specific activation of the APC in human and animal models. Several choices are available for such an activator, which should be relatively inexpensive, safe, and easy to use. The parameters of activation (serum C3, C3a, C3b, C5a, and C5a inactivator levels, macrophage and lymphocyte activation, etc) in regional and systemic situations need to be carefully monitored to find the optimum response in particular case presentations. If fine tuning of APC activation does regularly improve the clinical response to levels approaching the best so far observed in nonspecific immunotherapy of cancer, then both science and citizen will indeed be served.

Summary

Activation of the APC is pointed out as the common factor in all sufficiently studied cancer treatments employing nonspecific, active immunotherapy. This chapter outlines the molecular biology of both APC and classical pathway of complement, summarizes the alternative pathway's biologic activities especially in relation to the C3/C5 convertase $\overline{C3b,Bb}$, and its implications in the mechanism of host defense against malignancies, particularly relating to the activated macrophage. The many involvements of the APC in the various agents used for nonspecific active immunotherapy are reviewed, and possible clinical implications outlined. It is concluded that activation of the APC can be proposed as the specific

theoretical basis so far lacking for this treatment modality and that it is
accordingly feasible to attempt to monitor clinical application of this principle by fine-tuning of APC activation in cases of human cancer.

References

1. Mathé G: Active immunotherapy. *Adv Cancer Res* 14:1–36, 1971.
2. Nauts HC, Fowler GA, Bogatko FH: A review of the influence of bacterial
   infection and of bacterial products (Coley's toxins) on malignant tumors in
   man. *Acta Med Scand Suppl* 276:1–103, 1953.
3. Nauts HC: Immunotherapy of cancer by microbial products, in Mizuno D,
   Chihara G, Fukuoka F, Yamamoto T, Yamamura Y (eds): *Host-Defense
   Against Cancer and Its Potentiation.* Baltimore, University Park Press,
   1975, pp 337–351.
4. Hersh EM, Mavligit GM, Gutterman JU, Richman SP: Immunotherapy of
   human cancer. Becker FF (ed): *Cancer,* Vol 6. New York, Plenum Press,
   1977, pp 425–532.
5. Sadler T, Castro JE: Experimental non-specific immunotherapy, in Castro
   JE (ed): *Immunological Aspects of Cancer.* Lancaster, MTP Press, 1978,
   pp 357–384.
6. Müller-Eberhard HJ: Complement. *Ann Rev Biochem* 44:697–724, 1975.
7. Götze O, Muller-Ebherhard, HJ: The alternative pathway of complement
   activation. *Adv Immunol* 24:1–35, 1976.
8. Lachmann PJ: Complement, in Sela M (ed): *The Antigens,* Vol V. New
   York, Academic Press, 1979, pp 283–303.
9. Porter RR, Reid KBM: Activation of the complement system by antibody-
   antigen complexes: the classical pathway. *Adv Prot Chem* 33:1–71, 1979.
10. Muller-Eberhard HS, Schreiber RD: Molecular biology and chemistry of the
    alternative pathway of complement. *Adv Immunol* 29:1–55, 1980.
11. Reid KBM, Porter RR: The proteolytic activation systems of complement.
    Ann Rev Biochem 50:433–464, 1981.
12a. Colten RH: Biosynthesis of complement. *Adv Immunol* 22:67–118, 1976.
12b. Ballow M: Phylogenetics and ontogenetics of the complement system, in
    Good RA, Day SB (eds): *Comprehensive Immunology,* Vol 2. New York,
    Plenum Press, 1977, pp 183–204.
13. Müller-Eberhard HJ: The serum complement system, in Miescher PA, Mül-
    ler-Eberhard HJ (eds): *Textbook of Immunopathology,* ed 2. New York,
    Grune & Stratton, 1976, pp 33–47.
14. Müller-Eberhard HJ: The human complement protein C3: its unusual func-
    tional and structural versatility in host defence and inflammation, in Weigle
    WO (ed): *Advances in Immunopathology.* Miami, Florida, Symp Specialists
    Inc, 1981, pp 141–160.
15. Allison AC: Macrophage activation and nonspecific immunity. *Int Rev Exp
    Pathol* 18:303–346, 1978.
16. Adams DO: Macrophage activation and secretion. *Fed Proc* 41:2193–2197,
    1982.
17. North RJ: The concept of the activated macrophage. *J Immunol* 121:806–
    808, 1978.

18. Karnovsky ML, Lazdins JK: Biochemical criteria for activated macrophages. *J Immunol* 121:809–812, 1978.
19. Cohn ZA: The activation of mononuclear phagocytes: fact, fancy and future. *J Immunol* 121:813–816, 1978.
20. Lohmann-Matthes ML: The macrophage as cytotoxic effector cell, in Schmalzl F, Huhn D, Schaefer HE (eds): *Disorders of the Monocyte Macrophage System*. New York, Springer-Verlag, 1981, pp 49–57.
21. Meltzer MS, Occhionero M, Ruco LP: Macrophage activation for tumor cytotoxicity: regulatory mechanisms for induction and control of cytotoxic activity. *Fed. Proc* 41:2198–2205, 1982.
22. Huber H, Ledochowski M, Michlmayr G: The role of macrophages as effector cells, in Schmalzl F, Huhn D, Schaefer HE (eds): *Disorders of the Monocyte Macrophage System*. New York, Springer-Verlag, 1981, pp 39–48.
23. Schorlemmer, HU, Davies P, Hylton W, Gugig M, Allison AC: The selective release of lysosomal acid hydrolases from mouse peritoneal macrophages by stimuli of chronic inflammation. *Brit J Exp Pathol* 58:315–326, 1977.
24. Schorlemmer HU, Edwards JH, Davies P, Allison AC: Macrophage responses to mouldy haydust, *Micropolyspora faeni* and zymosan, activators of complement by the alternative pathway. *Clin Exp Immunol* 27:198–207, 1977.
25. Schorlemmer HU, Ferluga J, Allison AC: Interactions of macrophages and complement components in the pathogenesis of chronic inflammation, in Willoughby DA, Giroud JP, Velo GP (eds): *Perspectives in Inflammation*. Lancaster, MTP, 1977, pp 191–210.
26. Schorlemmer HU, Bitter-Suermann D, Allison AC: Complement activation by the alternative pathway and macrophage enzyme secretion in the pathogenesis of chronic inflammation. *Immunol* 32:929–940, 1977.
27. Schorlemmer HU, Allison AC: Effects of activated complement components on enzyme secretion by macrophages. *Immunol* 31:781–788, 1976.
28. Schorlemmer HU, Hadding U, Bitter-Suermann D, Allison AC: The role of complement cleavage products in killing of tumor cells by macrophages, in James K, McBride B, Stuart A (eds): *The Macrophage and Cancer*. Edinburgh, Econoprint, 1977, pp 68–77.
29. Schorlemmer HU: The role of complement in the function of the monocyte-macrophage system, in Schmalzl F, Huhn D, Schaefer HE (eds): *Disorders of the Monocyte Macrophage System*. New York, Springer-Verlag, 1981, pp 59–71,
30. Bentley C, Fries W, Brade V: Synthesis of factors D, B and P of the alternative pathway of complement activation as well as of C3 by guinea pig peritoneal macrophages in vitro. *Immunol* 35:971–980, 1978.
31. Huber H, Polley MJ, Linscott WD, Fudenberg HH, Müller-Eberhard HJ: Human monocytes: distinct receptor sites for the third component of complement and for immunoglobulin G. *Science* 162:1281–1283, 1968.
32. Lay WH, Nussenzweig V: Receptors for complement on leucocytes. *J Exp Med* 128:991–1009, 1968.
33. Schnyder J: Biochemical properties of human and murine mononuclear phagocytes and their changes on activation, in Schmalzl F, Huhn D,

Schaefer HE (eds): *Disorders of the Monocyte Macrophage System*. New York, Springer-Verlag, 1981, pp 23–30.

34. Sundsmo, JS: The leukocyte complement system. *Fed Proc* 41:3094–3098, 1982.

35. Burns GF, Cawley JC: The detection of membrane-associated complement components (C3 and C4) on circulating human normal and leukemic leukocytes and on cultured cells with monkey erythrocytes. *Eur J Immunol* 9:791–796, 1979.

36. Ross GP, Polley MJ, Rabellino EM, Grey HM: Two different complement receptors on human lymphocytes. *J Exp Med* 138:798–811, 1973.

37. Nelson RA: The immune adherence phenomenon. An immunologically specific reaction between microorganisms and erythrocytes leading to enhanced phagocytosis. *Science* 118:733–737, 1953.

38. Pepys MB, Butterworth AE: Inhibition by C3 fragments of C3-dependent rosette formation and antigen induced lymphocyte transformation. *Clin Exp Immunol* 18:273–282, 1974.

39. Dukor P, Bianco C, Nussenzweig V: Bone marrow origin of complement-receptor lymphocytes. *Eur J Immunol* 1:491–494, 1971.

40. Dukor P, Hartmann KU: Bound C3 as the second signal for B cell activation. *Cell Immunol* 7:349–356, 1973.

41. Pepys MB: Role of complement in induction of antibody production in vivo. Effect of cobra venom factor and other C3 reactive agents on thymus dependent and thymus independent antibody responses. *J Exp Med* 140:126–145, 1974.

42. Gutierrez C, Vega J, Kreisler M: Antibody independent activation of complement by human peripheral B lymphocytes. *Eur J Immunol* 9:72–76, 1979.

43. Platts-Mills TAE, Ishizaka K: Activation of the alternative pathway of complement by rabbit cells. *J Immunol* 113:348–358, 1974.

44. Sandberg AL, Wahl SM, Mergenhagen SE: Lymphokine production by C3b-stimulated B-cells. *J Immunol* 115:139–144, 1975.

45. Pryjma J, Humphrey JH: Prolonged C3 depletion by cobra venom factor in thymus-deprived mice and its implication for the role of C3 as an essential second signal for B-cell triggering. *Immunol* 28:569–576, 1975.

46. Hugli TE, Müller-Eberhard HJ: Anaphylatoxins: C3a and C5a. *Adv Immunol* 26:1–53, 1978.

47. Stimler NP, Bach MK, Bloor CM, Hugli TE: Release of leukotrienes from guinea pig lung stimulated by C5a *desArg* anaphylatoxin. *J. Immunol* 128:2247–2252, 1982.

48. Goldstein IM, Roos D, Kaplan HB, Weissmann G: Complement and immunoglobulins stimulate superoxide production by human leukocytes independently of phagocytosis. *J Clin Invest* 56:1155–1163, 1975.

49. Kay AB, Austen KF: Chemotaxis of human basophil leucocytes. *Clin Exp Immunol* 11:557–563, 1972.

50. Fernandez HN, Henson P, Otani A, Hugli TE: Chemotactic response to human C3a and C5a anaphylatoxins. I. Evaluation of C3a and C5a leukotaxis in vitro and under simulated in vivo conditions. *J Immunol* 120:109–115, 1978.

51. Snyderman R, Shin HS, Hausman MH: A chemotactic factor for mononuclear leukocytes. *Proc Soc Exp Biol Med* 138:387–390, 1971.

52. Weigle WO, Morgan EL, Goodman MG, Chenoweth DE, Hugli TE: Modu-

lation of the immune response by anaphylatoxin in the microenvironment of the interacting cells. *Fed Proc* 41:3099–3103, 1982.

53. Meuth JE, Morgan EL, DiScipio RG, Hugli TE: Suppression of T lymphocyte functions by human C3 fragments. I. Inhibition of human T cell proliferative responses by a kallikrein cleavage fragment of human iC3b. *J Immunol* 130:2605–2611, 1983.

54. Griffin FM: Opsonization, in Good RA, Day SB (eds): *Comprehensive Immunology,* Vol 2. New York, Plenum Press, 1977, pp 85–113.

55. Ross GD: Structure and function of membrane complement receptors. *Fed Proc* 41:3089–3093, 1982.

56. Wright AE, Douglas SR: An experimental investigation of the role of the body fluids in connection with phagocytosis. *Proc R Soc Lond* 72:357–370, 1903.

57. Griffin FM, Griffin JA, Leider JE, Silverstein SC: Studies on the mechanism of phagocytosis. I. Requirements for circumferential attachment of particle-bound ligands to specific receptors on the macrophage plasma membrane. *J Exp Med* 142:1263–1282, 1975.

58. Griffin JA, Griffin FM: Augmentation of macrophage receptor function in vitro. I. Characterization of the cellular interactions required for the generation of a T-lymphocyte product that enhances macrophage complement receptor function. *J Exp Med* 150:653–664, 1979.

59. Kassel RL, Old LJ, Carswell EA, Fiore NC, Hardy WD: Serum-mediated leukemia cell destruction in AKR mice. *J Exp Med* 138:925–938, 1973.

60. Müller-Eberhard HJ, Fjellström KE: Isolation of the anticomplementary protein from cobra venom and its mode of action on C3. *J Immunol* 107:1666–1672, 1971.

61. Kassel RL, Hardy WD, Day NK: Complement in cancer, in Good RA, Day SB (eds): *Comprehensive Immunology,* Vol 2. New York, Plenum Press, 1973, pp 277–294.

62. Nishioka K, Kawamura K, Hirayama T, Kawashima T, Shimada K: The complement system in tumor immunity: significance of elevated levels of complement in tumor bearing hosts. *Ann NY Acad Sci* 267:303–315, 1976.

63. Carli M, Bucolo C, Pannunzio MT, Ongaro G, Businaro R, Revoltella R: Fluctuation of serum complement levels in children with neuroblastoma. *Cancer* 43:2399–2404, 1979.

64. Rossen RD, Reisberg MA, Hersh EM, Gutterman JU: The C1q binding test for soluble immune complexes: clinical correlations obtained in patients with cancer. *J Nat Cancer Inst* 58:1205–1215, 1977.

65. Gadd KJ, Reid KBM: The binding of complement component C3 to antibody-antigen aggregates after activation of the alternative pathway in serum. *Biochem J* 195:471–480, 1981.

66. Porta C, Villa ML, Clerici E: Immunoadherence and complement in cancer-bearing mice. *Brit J Cancer* 37:23–27, 1978.

67. Kalwinsky DK, Urmson JR, Stitzel AE, Spitzer RE: Activation of the alternative pathway of complement in childhood acute lymphoblastic leukemia. *J Lab Clin Med* 88:745–756, 1976.

68. Olszewski WL, Lukomska B, Engeset A: High concentration of inactivator of C3b in sera of cancer patients—preliminary communication. *Arch Immunol Ther Exp (Warsz)* 30:87–88, 1982.

69. Budowle B, Acton RT, Barger BO, Blackstock R, Crist W, Go RC, Hum-

phrey GB, Ragab, A, Rober M, Vietti T, Dearth J: Properdin factor B and acute lymphocytic leukemia (ALL). *Cancer* 50:2369–2371, 1982.

70. Budowle B, Barger BO, Balch CM, Go RC, Roseman JM, Acton RT: Associations of properdin factor B with melanoma. *Cancer Genet Cytogenet* 5:247–251, 1982.

71. Schreiber RD, Pangburn MK, Medicus RG, Müller-Eberhard HJ: Raji cell injury and subsequent lysis by the purified cytolytic alternative pathway of human complement. *Clin Immunol Immunopathol* 15:384–396, 1980.

72. Budzko DB, Lachmann PJ, McConnell I: Activation of the alternative complement pathway by lymphoblastoid cell lines derived from patients with Burkitt's lymphoma and infectious mononucleosis. *Cell Immunol* 22:98–109, 1976.

73. Daveau M, Fontaine M, Gilbert D: Interactions of the third component of human complement (C3) with tumour cells: evidence for presence of C3b acceptor sites and direct activation of C3 by tumour cells. *Ann Immunol (Paris)* 132C:339–350, 1981.

74. McConnell I, Klein G, Macanovic M, Gorman NT, Raniwalla J: Malignant cells isolated from Burkitt's lymphoma but not other forms of leukemia activate the alternative complement pathway in human serum. *Eur J Immunol* 11:132–135, 1981.

75. McConnell I, Klein G, Lint TF, Lachmann PJ: Activation of the alternative complement pathway by human B cell lymphoma lines is associated with Epstein-Barr virus transformation of the cells. *Eur J Immunol* 8:453–458, 1978.

76. Okada N, Okada H: Activation of complement by spontaneous leukemic cells of AKR mice. *Int J Cancer* 22:282–287, 1978.

77. Shimbo T, Yata J, Okada H: Non-specific activation of complement by leukemic cells. *Int J Cancer* 22:422–425, 1978.

78. Eidinger D, Bello E, Mates A: The heterocytotoxicity of human serum. I. Activation of the alternative complement pathway by heterologous target cells. *Cell Immunol* 29:174–186, 1977.

79. Ferluga J, Schorlemmer HU, Baptisda LC, Allison AC: Cytolytic effects of the complement cleavage product C3a. *Brit J Cancer* 34:626–634, 1976.

80. Alexander P: The function of the macrophage in malignant disease. *Ann Rev Med* 27:207–224, 1976.

81. Fink MA (ed): *The Macrophage in Neoplasia*, New York, Academic Press, 1976.

82. Nathan CF, Murray HW, Cohn ZA: Current concepts: the macrophage as effector cell. *New Engl J Med* 303:622–626, 1980.

83. Adams DO, Snyderman R: Do macrophages destroy nascent tumors? *J Nat Cancer Inst* 62:1341–1345, 1979.

84. Evans R: Macrophage accumulation in primary and transplanted tumours growing in C5-deficient B10.D2/oSn mice. *Int J Cancer* 26:227–229, 1980.

85. Shin HS, Johnson RJ, Pasternack GR, Economou JS: Mechanisms of tumor immunity: the role of antibody and nonimmune effectors. *Prog Allergy* 25:163–210, 1978.

86. Adams DO, Johnson WJ, Marino PA: Mechanisms of target recognition and destruction in macrophage-mediated tumour cytotoxicity. *Fed Proc* 41:2212–2221, 1982.

87. Sharma SD, Piessens WF, Middlebrook G: In vitro killing of tumour cells by soluble products of activated guinea pig peritoneal macrophages. *Cell Immunol* 49:379–383, 1980.

88. Nathan CF: Secretion of oxygen intermediates: role in effector functions of activated macrophages. *Fed Proc* 41:2206–2211, 1982.

89. Conolly K, Kaplan AM: In vivo reduction of tumor cell DNA content by pyran, *Corynebacterium parvum* and *5-Fluorouracil. Fed Proc* 40:761 (Abst.), 1981.

90. Granger DL, Taintor RR, Cook JL, Gibbs JH: Injury of neoplastic cells by murine macrophages leading to inhibition of mitochondrial respiration. *J Clin Invest* 65:357–370, 1980.

91. Ferluga J, Schorlemmer HU, Baptisda LC, Allison AC: Production of the complement cleavage product C3a by activated macrophages and its tumorilytic effects. *Clin Exp Immunol* 31:512–517, 1978.

92. Cleveland RP, Meltzer MS, Zbar B: Tumour cytotoxicity in vitro by macrophages from mice infected with *M. bovis* strain BCG. *J Nat Cancer Inst* 52:1887–1895, 1974.

93. Hibbs JB, Lambert LH, Remington JS: Possible role of macrophage mediated nonspecific cytotoxicity in tumour resistance. *Nat New Biol* 235:48–51, 1972.

94. Ellouz F, Adam A, Clorban R, Lederer E: Minimal structural requirements for adjuvant activity of bacterial peptidoglycan derivatives. *Biochem Biophys Res Commun* 58:1317–1325, 1974.

95. Fidler IJ, Sone S, Fogler WE, Barnes ZL: Eradication of spontaneous metastases and activation of alveolar macrophages by intravenous injection of liposomes containing muramyl dipeptides. *Proc Nat Acad Sci USA* 78:1680–1684, 1981.

96. Orr W, Varani J, Ward PA: Characteristics of the chemotactic response of neoplastic cells to a factor derived from the fifth component of complement. *Am J Pathol* 93:405–422, 1978.

97. Orr FW, Mokashi S, Delikatny J: Generation of a complement-derived chemotactic factor for tumor cells in experimentally induced peritoneal exudates and its effect on the local metastasis of circulating tumor cells. *Am J Pathol* 108:112–118, 1982.

98. Orr FW, Delikatny EJ, Mokashi S, Krepart GV, Stiver HG: Detection of a complement-derived chemotactic factor for tumor cells in human inflammatory and neoplastic effusions. *Am J Pathol* 110:41–47, 1983.

99. Hanna MG, Key ME, Oldham RK: Biology of cancer therapy: some new insights into adjuvant treatment of metastic solid tumors. *J Biol Resp Modif* 2:295–309, 1983.

100. Coley WB: The therapeutic value of the mixed toxins of erysipelas and *Bacillus prodigiosus* in the treatment of inoperable malignant tumors. *Am J Med Sci* 112:251–281, 1896.

101. Ramanathan VD, Curtis J, Turk JL: Activation of the alternative pathway of complement by mycobacteria and cord factor. *Infect Immun* 29:30–35, 1980.

102. McBride WH, Weir DM, Kay AB, Pearce D, Caldwell JR: Activation of the classical and alternative pathways of complement by *Corynebacterium parvum. Clin Exp Immunol* 19:143–147, 1975.

103. Sadler TE, Jones PD, Castro JE, Lampert IA: Effects of intravenous injec-

tion of two different strains of *Corynebacterium parvum* in the mouse. *Brit J Exp Pathol* 60:627–631, 1979.

104. Germain RN, Williams RM, Benacerraf B: Specific and non-specific antitumor immunity. II. Macrophage mediated non-specific effector activity induced by BCG and similar agents. *J Nat Cancer Inst* 54:709–720, 1975.

105. Zbar B, Bernstein ID, Rapp HJ: Suppression of tumor growth at the site of infection with living BCG. *J Nat Cancer Inst* 46:831–839, 1971.

106. Zbar B, Bernstein ID, Bartlett GL: Immunotherapy of cancer: regression of intradermal tumors and prevention of growth of lymph node metastases after intralesional injection of living *M. bovis*. *J Nat Cancer Inst* 49:119–130, 1972.

107. Morahan PS, Kaplan AM: Macrophage activation and antitumor activity of biological and synthetic agents. *Int J Cancer* 17:82–89, 1976.

108. Astry CL, Loose LD, Megirian R: *Corynebacterium parvum* treatment of P388 tumor-bearing mice. I. Lysosomal enzyme levels in adherent peritoneal cells and peritoneal lavage fluid. *J Immunopharmacol* 3:29–47, 1981.

109. Brunda MJ, Mathews HL, Ferguson HR, McClatchy JK, Minden P: Immunotherapy of the guinea pig line-10 hepatocarcinoma with a variety of nonviable bacteria. *Cancer Res* 40:3211–3213, 1980.

110. Berger FM, Fukui GM, Ludwig BJ, Rosselet JP: Increased host resistance to infection solicited by lipopolysaccharides from *Brucella abortus*. *Proc Soc Exp Biol* 131:1376–1381, 1969.

111. Martin A, Toujas L, Le Garrec Y, Dazord L, Amice J: Resistance to tumor graft in mice treated with inactivated *Brucella abortus* cultured in smooth or rough phase. *J Nat Cancer Inst* 62:123–127, 1979.

112. Hibbs JB, Lambert LH, Remington JS: In vitro nonimmunological destruction of cells with abnormal growth characteristics by adjuvant-activated macrophages. *Proc Soc Exp Biol Med* 139:1049–1052, 1972.

113. Keller R: Mechanisms by which activated normal macrophages destroy syngeneic rat tumours in vitro—cytokinetics, non-involvement of T lymphocytes and effect of metabolic inhibitors. *Immunol* 27:285–298, 1974.

114. Hirano M, Sinkovics JG, Schullenberger CC, Howe CD: Murine lymphoma: augmented growth in mice with pertussis vaccine-induced lymphocytosis. *Science* 158:1061–1064, 1967.

115. Hibbs JB, Lambert LH, Remington JS: Adjuvant induced resistance to tumour development in mice. *Proc Soc Exp Biol Med* 139:1053–1056, 1972.

116. Mathé G, Florentin I, Bruley-Rosset M, Hayat M, Bourut C: Heat-killed *Pseudomonas aeruginosa* as a systemic adjuvant in cancer immunotherapy. *Biomedicine* 27:368–373, 1977.

117. Schultz RM, Pavlidis NA, Chirigos MA: Macrophage involvement in the antitumor activity of *Brucella abortus* ether extract against experimental lung carcinoma metastases. *Cancer Res* 38:3427–3431, 1978.

118. Schultz RM, Chirigos MA, Pavlidis NA, Youngner JS: Macrophage activation and antitumor activity of a *Brucella abortus* ether extract, Bru-Pel. *Cancer Treat Rep* 62:1937–1941, 1978.

119. Glasgow LA, Crane JL Jr, Schleupner CJ, Kern ER, Youngner JS, Feingold DS: Activation of reticuloendothelial system macrophages and enhancement of host resistance to a transplantable osteogenic sarcoma in mice by an extract of *Brucella abortus*. *Cancer Treat Rep* 62:1931–1935, 1978.

120. Sakai S, Ryoyama K, Koshimura S, Migita S: Studies on the properties of a streptococcal preparation OK-432 (NSC-B116209) as an immunopotentiator. I. Activation of serum complement components and peritoneal exudate cells by group A streptococcus. *Jpn J Exp Med* 46:123–133, 1976.

121. Inai S, Nagaki K, Ebisu S, Kato K, Kotani S, Misaki A: Activation of the alternative complement pathway by water insoluble glucans of *Streptococcus mutans*. *J Immunol* 117:1256–1260, 1976.

122. Davies P, Page RC, Allison AC: Changes in cellular enzyme levels and extracellular release of lysosomal acid hydrolases in macrophages exposed to Group A streptococcal cell wall substance. *J Exp Med* 139: 1262–1282, 1974.

123. Kimura I, Ohnoshi T, Yasuhara S: Immunotherapy in human lung cancer using a streptococcal agent OK432. *Cancer* 37:2201–2203, 1976.

124. Mickshe M, Kokoschka EM, Sagaster P, Kofler K: Clinical and immunological studies with OK-432 (*Streptococcus pyogenes*) on immunotherapy in cancer patients. *Onkologie* 1:106–111, 1978.

125. Tanemura H, Sakata K, Kunieda T, Saji S, Yamamoto S, Takekoshi T: Influences of operative stress on cell-mediated immunity and on tumor metastasis and their prevention by non-specific immunotherapy: experimental studies in rats. *J Surg Oncol* 21:189–195, 1982.

126. Yarkoni E, Wang L, Bekierkunst A: Stimulation of macrophages by cord factor (trehalose-6,6 dimycolate) and by heat-killed and living BCG. *Infect Immun* 16:1–8, 1977.

127. Ribi E, Granger DL, Milner KC, Strain SM: Tumor regression caused by endotoxins and mycobacterial fractions. *J Nat Cancer Inst* 55:1253–1257, 1975.

128. Yarkoni E, Meltzer MS, Rapp HJ: Tumor regression after intralesional injection of emulsified trehalose-6,6′ dimycolate (cord factor): efficacy increases with oil concentration. *Int J Cancer* 19:818–821, 1977.

129. Stålenheim G, Götze O, Cooper NR, Sjöquist J, Müller-Eberhard HJ: Consumption of human complement components by complexes of IgG with protein A of *Staphylococcus aureus*. *Immunochem* 10:501–507, 1973.

130. Sveen K, Grov A: Induction of leukemotaxis by protein A of *Staphylococcus aureus*. *Acta Pathol Microbiol Scand* 86B: 369–373, 1978.

131. Cooper PD, Masinello GR: Protein A treatment of cancer: activation of a serum component with trans-species anti-B16 melanoma activity. *Int J Cancer* 32:737–744, 1983.

132. Verbrugh HA, Van Dijk WC, Peters R, van Vor Tol ME, Verhoef J: The role of *Staphylococcus aureus* cell-wall peptidoglycan, teichoic acid and protein A in the process of complement activation and opsonization. *Immunol* 37:615–621, 1979.

133. Wilkinson BJ, Kim Y, Peterson PK: Factors affecting complement activation by *Staphylococcus aureus* cell walls, their components and mutants altered in teichoic acid. *Infect Immun* 32:216–224, 1981.

134. Minden P, McClatchy JK, Brunda MJ: Suppression and immunotherapy of the guinea pig line-10 hepato-carcinoma mediated by non-viable *Staphylococcus aureus*. *J Nat Cancer Inst* 61:535–538, 1978.

135. Gordon BR, Matus RE, Saal SD, MacEwen EG, Hurvitz AI, Stenzel KH, Rubin AL: Protein A-independent tumoricidal responses in dogs after extra-

corporeal perfusion of plasma over *Staphylococcus aureus*. *J Nat Cancer Inst* 70:1127–1133, 1983.

136. Götze D, Müller-Eberhard HJ: The C3 activation system: an alternative pathway of complement activation. *J Exp Med* 135:90S–108S, 1971.

137. Glovsky MM, Cortez-Haendchen L, Ghekiere L, Alenty A, Williams DL, Di Luzio R: Effects of particulate beta-1,3 glucan on human, rat and guinea pig complement activity. *J Reticuloendothel Soc* 33:401–413, 1983.

138. Martin DS, Hayworth P, Fugmann RA: Combination therapy with cyclophosphamide and zymosan on a spontaneous mammary cancer in mice. *Cancer Res* 24:652–654, 1964.

139. Bradner WT, Clarke DA, Stock CC: Stimulation of host defence against experimental cancer. I. Zymosan and sarcoma 180 in mice. *Cancer Res* 18:347–351, 1958.

140. Maeda YY, Chihara G: The effects of neonatal thymectomy on the antitumour activity of lentinan, carboxymethyl pachymaran and zymosan and their effects on various immune responses. *Int J Cancer* 11:153–161, 1973.

141. Cooper PD, Sim RB: Substances that can trigger activation of the alternative pathway of complement have anti-melanoma activity in mice. *Int J Cancer* 33:683–687, 1984.

142. Gewurz H, Shin HS, Mergenhagen SE: Interaction of the complement system with endotoxic lipopolysaccharide: consumption of each of the six terminal complement components. *J Exp Med* 128:1049–1057, 1968.

143. Marcus RL, Shin HS, Mayer MM: An alternative complement pathway: C3 cleaving activity not due to C4,2a or endotoxic lipopolysaccharide after treatment with guinea-pig serum; relation to properdin. *Proc Natl Acad Sci USA* 68:1351–1354, 1971.

144. Galanos C, Luderitz O: The role of the physical state of lipopolysaccharides in the interaction with complement. High molecular weight as a pre-requisite for the expression of anti-complementary activity. *Eur J Biochem* 65:403–408, 1976.

145. Alexander P, Evans R: Endotoxin and double stranded RNA render macrophages cytotoxic. *Nat New Biol* 232:76–78, 1971.

146. Gordon S, Unkeless JC, Cohen ZA: Induction of macrophage plasminogen activator by endotoxin stimulation or phagocytosis: evidence for a 2-stage process. *J Exp Med* 140:995–1010, 1974.

147. Yarkoni E, Goren MB, Rapp HJ: Regression of a transplanted guinea pig hepatoma after intralesional injection of a emulsified mixture of endotoxin and mycobacterial sulfolipid. *Infect Immun* 24:357–362, 1979.

148. Cooper PD: unpublished data.

149. Nishioka K: Complement system and tumour immunity, in Mizuno D, Chihara G, Fukuoka F, Yamamoto T, Yamamuro Y (eds): *Host Defense Against Cancer and Its Potentiation*. Baltimore, University Park Press, 1975, pp 83–96.

150. Hamuro J, Hadding U, Bitter-Suermann D: Solid phase activation of alternative pathway of complement by beta-1,3-glucans and its possible role for tumour regressing activity. *Immunol* 34:695–705, 1978.

151. Chihara G, Hamuro J, Maeda YY, Arai Y, Fukuoka F: Fractionation and purification of the polysaccharides with marked antitumour activity, espe-

cially lentinan from *Lentinus edodes* (Berk.) Sing, (an edible mushroom). *Cancer Res* 30:2776–2781, 1970.

152. Hamuro J, Maeda YY, Arai Y, Fukuoka F, Chihara G: The significance of the higher structure of the polysaccharides lentinan and pachymaran with regard to their antitumour activity. *Chem Biolog Interactions* 3:69–71, 1971.

153. Dennert DW, Tucker D: Antitumour polysaccharide lentinan—a T cell adjuvant. *J Nat Cancer Inst* 51:1727–1729, 1973.

154. Mansell PWA, Ichinose H, Reed RJ, Krementz ET, McNamee R, Di Luzio NR: Macrophage mediated destruction of human malignant cells in vivo. *J Nat Cancer Inst* 54:571–576, 1975.

155. Seljelid R, Bögwald J, Lundwall A: Glycan stimulation of macrophages in vitro. *Exp Cell Res* 131:121–129, 1981.

156. Hadden JW, Delmonte L, Oettgen HF: Mechanism of immunopotentiation, in Good RA, Day SB (eds): *Comprehensive Immunology*, Vol 3. New York, Plenum Press, 1977, pp 279–313.

157. Majeski JA, Stinnett JT: Chemoattractant properties of *Corynebacterium parvum* and pyran copolymer for human monocytes and neutrophils. *J Nat Cancer Inst* 58:781–783, 1977.

158. Harmel RP, Zbar B: Tumor suppression by pyran copolymer: correlation with production of cytotoxic macrophages. *J Nat Cancer Inst* 54:989–992, 1975.

159. Di Perri T, Auteri A, Laghi Pasini F, Mattioli F: Biological, chemical and pharmacological induction of the properdin-mediated pathway of complement activation in vitro, in Willoughby DA, Giroud JP, Velo GP (eds): *Perspectives in Inflammation*. Lancaster, MTP, 1977, pp 405–416.

160. Di Perri T, Laghi Pasini F, Capecchi PL, Orrico A, Pasqui AL: Complement-mediated polymorphonuclear leukocyte aggregation in vitro induced by levamisole. *J Immunopharmacol* 4:233–246, 1982.

161. Lima AO, Javierre MQ, da Silva WD, Camara DS: Immunological phagocytosis: effect of drugs on phosphodiesterase. *Experientia* 30:945–946, 1974.

162. Symoens J: Levamisole, an antianergic chemotherapeutic agent: an overview, in Chirigos MA (ed): *Progress in Cancer Research and Therapy*, Vol 2. New York, Raven Press, 1977, pp 1–24.

163. Leijh, PCJ, van den Barzelaar MT, van Zwet TL, Daha MR, van Furth R: Requirement of extracellular complement and Ig for intracellular killing of microorganisms by human monocytes. *J Clin Invest* 63:772–784, 1979.

164. Orbach-Arbouys S, L' Heritier J, Allouche M, Pouillart P: Intense tumour-cell destruction by syngeneic mice: role of macrophage, complement activation and tumour-cell factors. *Brit J Cancer* 36:743–750, 1977.

165. Halpern BN, Prevot AR, Biozzi G, Stiffel C, Mouton D, Morard JC, Bouthillier Y, Decreusefond C: Stimulation of the phagocytic activity of the reticuloendothelial system provided by *Corynebacterium parvum*. *J Reticuloendothel Soc* 1:77–96, 1964.

166. Woodruff MFA, Boak JL: Inhibitory effect of injection of *Corynebacterium parvum* on the growth of tumor transplants in isogenic hosts. *Brit J Cancer* 20:345–355, 1966.

167. Milas L, Gutterman JU, Basic I, Hersh EM, Hunter N, Mavligit GM, Withers HR: Immunoprophylaxis and immunotherapy for a murine fibrosarcoma

with *Corynebacterium granulosa* and *C parvum*. *Int J Cancer* 14:493–500, 1974.

168. Fisher B, Wolmark N, Saffer E, Fisher ER: Inhibitory effect of prolonged *Corynebacterium parvum* and cyclophosphamide administration on the growth of established tumors. *Cancer* 35:134–143, 1975.

169. Sadler TE, Castro JE: Lack of immunological and anti-tumour effects of orally administered *Cornebacterium parvum* in mice. *Brit J Cancer* 31:359–363, 1975.

170. Wilkinson PC, O'Neal GJ, McInroy RJ, Cater JC, Roberts JA: Chemotaxis of macrophages: the role of a macrophage-specific cytotoxin from anaerobic corynebacteria and its relation to immune potentiation in vivo, in Wolstenholme GEW, Knight J (eds): *Immunopotentiation. CIBA Found Symp* 18:120–140, 1973.

171. Ghaffar A, Cullen RT, Dunbar N, Woodruff MFA: Antitumor effect *in vitro* of lymphocytes and macrophages from mice treated with *Corynebacterium parvum*. *Brit J Cancer* 29:199–205, 1974.

172. Ghaffar A, Cullen RT, Woodruff MFA: Further analysis of the antitumour effect *in vitro* of peritoneal exudate cells from mice treated with *Corynebacterium parvum*. *Brit J Cancer* 31:15–24, 1975.

173. Ojo E, Haller O, Wigzell H: *Corynebacterium parvum* induced peritoneal exudate cells with cytolytic activity against tumor cells are non-phagocytic cells with characteristics of natural killer cells. *Scand J Immunol* 8:215–222, 1978.

174. Flad HD, Fink U, Dierich MP: K cell activity of normal and chronic lymphocytic leukaemia lymphocytes: association with lymphocytes bearing receptors for human C3b. *Haematol Blood Transfus* 20:197–202, 1977.

175. Woodruff MF, Whitehead VL, Speedy G: Studies with a spontaneous mouse tumor. I. Growth in normal mice and response to *Corynebacterium parvum*. *Brit J Cancer* 37:345–355, 1978.

176. Moore K, McBride WH: Enhanced FC receptor expression by a sub-population of murine intra-tumour macrophages following intravenous *Corynebacterium parvum* therapy. *Brit J Cancer* 47:797–802, 1983.

177. Astry CL, Loose LD, Megirian R: *Corynebacterium parvum* treatment of P388 tumor-bearing mice. II. Lysosomal enzyme levels associated with P388 tumor cells. *J Immunopharmacol* 3:49–66, 1981.

178. Likhite VV: Suppression of the incidence of death with spontaneous tumours in DBA/2 mice after *Corynebacterium parvum*-mediated rejection of syngeneic tumours. *Nature* 259:397–399, 1976.

179. Barlow JJ, Piver MS, Lele SB: High-dose methotrexate with "RESCUE" plus cyclophosphamide as initial chemotherapy in ovarian adenocarcinoma. A randomized trial with observations on the influence of *Corynebacterium parvum* immunotherapy. *Cancer* 46:1333–1338, 1980.

180. Chahinian AP, Goldberg J, Holland JF, Reisman A, Jaffrey IS, Mandel EM: Chemotherapy versus chemoimmunotherapy with levamisole or *Corynebacterium parvum* in advanced lung cancer. *Cancer Treat Rep* 66:1291–1297, 1982.

181. Cheng VS, Suit HD, Wang CC, Raker J, Kaufman S, Rothman K, Walker A, McNulty P: Clinical trial of *Corynebacterium parvum* (intra-lymph-node and

intravenous) and radiation therapy in the treatment of head and neck carcinoma. *Cancer* 49:239–244, 1982.

182. Clunie GJ, Gough IR, Dury M, Furnival CM, Bolton PM: A trial of imidazole carboxamide and *Corynebacterium parvum* in disseminated melanoma: clinical and immunologic results. *Cancer* 46:475–479, 1980.

183. Drapkin R, Bjornsson S, Naeher C, Higby D, Caracandas J, Wallens WT, Kuberka N, Suh K, Siddiqi N, Henderson ES: Doxorubicin, cisplatin, and *Corynebacterium parvum* in non-small cell bronchogenic carcinoma. *Cancer Treat Rep* 64:1367–1369, 1980.

184. Issell BF, Valdivieso M, Hersh EM, Richman S, Gutterman JU, Bodey GP: Combination of chemoimmunotherapy for extensive non-oat cell lung cancer. *Cancer Treat Rep* 62:1059–1063, 1978.

185. Murray JL, Ishmael DR, Bottomley RH, Grozea PN, Lee ET: Inefficacy of sc *Corynebacterium parvum* in stage I malignant melanoma: preliminary results of a single-institution pilot study. *Cancer Treat Rep* 67:191–192, 1983.

186. Band PR, Jao-King C, Urtasun RC, Haraphongse M: Phase I study of *Corynebacterium parvum* in patients with solid tumors. *Cancer Chemotherap Rep* 59:1139–1145, 1975.

187. Balch CM, Smalley RV, Bartolucci AA, Burns D, Presant CA, Durant JR: A randomized prospective clinical trial of adjuvant *Corynebacterium parvum* immunotherapy in 260 patients with clinically localized melanoma (Stage I): prognostic factors analysis and preliminary results of immunotherapy. *Cancer* 49:1079–1084, 1982.

188. Israel L, Edelstein R, De Pierre A, Dimitrov N: Daily intravenous infusions of *Corynebacterium parvum* in twenty patients with disseminated cancer: a preliminary report of clinical and biologic findings. *J Nat Cancer Inst* 55:29–33, 1975.

189. Kokosche EM, Luger T, Micksche M: Immunochemotherapy in patients with disseminated metastasizing stage III melanoma. Randomized study with methyl-CCNU versus *Corynebacterium parvum* plus methyl-CCNU. *Onkologie* 1:98–103, 1978.

190. Mignot MH, Lens JW, Drexhage HA, von Blomberg BM, Flier VD, Oort J, Stolk JG: Lower relapse rates after neighbourhood injection of *Corynebacterium parvum* in operable cervix carcinoma. *Brit J Cancer* 44:856–862, 1981.

191. McCune CS, Schapira DV, Henshaw EC: Specific immunotherapy of advanced renal carcinoma: evidence for the polyclonality of metastases. *Cancer* 47:1984–1987, 1981.

192. Webb HE, Oaten SW, Pike CP: Treatment of malignant ascitic and pleural effusion with *Corynebacterium parvum*. *Brit Med J* 1:338–340, 1978.

193. Gil J, Badowski A, Orlowski T, Szmigielski S, Ko HL, Jeljaszewicz J, Pulverer G: A 2.5-year follow-up of local immunotherapy of advanced stomach and intestinal adenocarcinoma with *Propionibacterium granulosum*. *J Cancer Res Clin Oncol* 105:98–102, 1983.

194. Smith LH, Woodruff MFA: Comparative effect of two strains of *C parvum* on phagocytic activity and tumour growth. *Nature* 219:197–198, 1968.

195. Jones PD, Sadler TE, Castro JE: Effect of *Corynebacterium parvum* on peripheral blood platelets. *Brit J Cancer* 36:777–782, 1977.

196. Thore M, Löfgren S, Tärnvik A: Oxygen and serum complement in phago-
     cytosis and killing of *Propionibacterium acnes*. *Acta Pathol Microbiol Im-
     munol Scand* (C) 91:95–100, 1983.
197. Webster GF, Nilsson UR, McArthur WP: Activation of the alternative path-
     way of complement in human serum by *Propionibacterium acnes* (*Coryne-
     bacterium parvum*) cell fractions. *Inflammation* 5:165–176, 1981.
198. Webster GF, McArthur WP: Activation of components of the alternative
     pathway of complement by *Propionibacterium acnes* cell wall carbohydrate.
     J Invest Dermatol 1982; 79:137–140.
199. Biran H, Moake JL, Reed RC, Gutterman JU, Hersh EM, Freireich EJ,
     Mavligit GM: Complement activation in vivo in cancer patients receiving
     Corynebacterium parvum immunotherapy. *Brit J Cancer* 34:493–499, 1976.
200. Hokland P, Ellegaard J, Heron I: Immunomodulation by *Corynebacterium
     parvum* in normal humans. *J Immunol* 124:2180–2185, 1980.
201. Bansal SC, Bansal BR, Thomas HL, Siegel PD, Rhoads JE, Cooper DR,
     Terman DS, Mark R: Ex vivo removal of serum IgG in a patient with colon
     carcinoma. *Cancer* 42:1–18, 1978.
202. Jones FR, Yoshida LH, Ladiges WC, Kenny MA: Treatment of feline leuke-
     mia and reversal of FeLV by ex vivo removal of IgG. *Cancer* 46:675–684,
     1980.
203. Terman DS: Tumoricidal responses in spontaneous canine neoplasms after
     extra corporeal perfusion over immobilized protein A. *Fed Proc* 40:45–49,
     1981.
204. Ray PK, Raychaudhuri S, Allen P: Mechanisms of repression of mammary
     adenocarcinomas in rats following plasma adsorption over protein A-con-
     taining *Staphylococcus aureus*. *Cancer Res* 42:4970–4974, 1982.
205. Ray PK, Bandyopadhyay SK: Inhibition of rat mammary tumor growth by
     purified protein A—a potential antitumor agent. *Immunol Commun* 12:453–
     464, 1983.
206a. Ray PK, Clark L, McLaughlin D, Allen P, Idiculla A, Mark R, Rhoads JE,
     Bassett JG, Cooper DR: Immunotherapy of cancer: extra corporeal adsorp-
     tion of plasma-blocking factors using nonviable *Staphylococcus aureus*
     Cowan I, in Beyer JH, Borberg H, Fuchs Ch, Nagel GA (eds): *Plas-
     maphoresis in Immunology*. Basel, Karger, 1982.
206b. Hellström KE, Hellström I: Lymphocyte mediated cytotoxicity and block-
     ing serum activity of tumor antigens. *Adv Immunol* 18:209–277, 1974.
207. Messerschmidt G, Bowles C, Dean D, Parker M, Lester R, Dowling R,
     Holohan T, Osborne L, Schaff BF, McCormack K, Corbitt R, Phillips T,
     Glatstein E, Deisseroth A: Phase I trial of *Staphylococcus aureus* Cowan I
     immunoperfusion. *Cancer Treatment Reports* 66:2027–2031, 1982.
208. Sjöquist J, Stålenheim G: Protein A from *Staphylococcus aureus*. IX. Com-
     plement-fixing activity of protein A-IgG complexes. *J Immunol* 103:467–
     473, 1969.
209. Steele G, Ankerst J, Sjögren HO: Alteration of in vitro anti-tumor activity of
     tumor-bearer sera by absorption with *Staphyloccus aureus* Cowan I. *Int J
     Cancer* 14:83–92, 1974.
210. Miller WJ, Branda RF, Hurd DD, Wachsman W, Nelson NC, Jacob HS:
     Protein A adsorption of acute myelogenous leukemia serum induces in vitro
     blast lysis. *Blood* 59:1344–1347, 1982.

211. Zbar B, Tanaka T: Immunotherapy of cancer: regression of tumours after intralesional injection of living *Mycobacterium bovis*. *Science* 172:271–273, 1971.
212a. Carswell EA, Old LJ, Kassel RL, Green S, Fiore N, Williamson B: An endotoxin-induced serum factor that causes necrosis of tumors. *Proc Natl Acad Sci USA* 72:3666-3670, 1975.
212b. McDonald EJ: The polyfructosans and difructose anhydrides. *Adv Carbohydrate Chem* 2:253–277, 1946,
213. Pillemer L, Schoenberg MD, Blum L, Wurz L: Properdin system and immunity. II. Interaction of the properdin system with polysaccharide. *Science* 122:545–549, 1955.
214. Dukor P, Vasella S, Schläfli E, Perren B, Gisler RH, Dietrich FM, Bitter-Suermann D: Immunopotentiating agents: activity profiles and possible mode of action, in Mizuno D, Chihara G, Fukuoka F, Yamamoto T, Yamamuro Y (eds): *Host Defense against Cancer and Its Potentiation*. Baltimore, University Park Press, 1975, pp 97–111.
215. Johnson E, Seljelid R, Bögwald J, Larm O, Scholander E: Endocytosis of agarose in mouse peritoneal macrophages in vitro. *Scand J Immunol* 15:205–210, 1982.
216a. Dukor P, Schumann G, Gisler RH, Dierich M, König, W, Hadding U, Bitter-Suermann D: Complement dependent B cell activation by cobra venom factor and other mitogens? *J Exp Med* 139:337–354, 1974.
216b. Alexander P: Some immunologically based reactions that can cause the regression of large tumor masses. *Nat Cancer Inst Monogr* 44:105–108, 1976.
217. Herburt PA, Kraemer WH: The possible role of the properdin system in transplantable cancer. The effect of zymosan in transplantable human cancer. *Cancer Res* 16:1048–1052, 1956.
218. Bradner WT, Clark DA: Stimulation of host-defence against cancer. II. Temporal and reversal studies of zymosan effect. *Cancer Res* 19:673–678, 1959.
219. Mitcheson HD, Sadler TE, Castro JE: Single versus multiple human-equivalent dose of *Corynebacterium parvum* in mice: neutralization of the anti-metastatic effect. *Brit J Cancer* 41:407–414, 1980.
220. Gill PG, Morris PJ, Kettlewell M: The complications of intravenous *Corynebacterium parvum* infusion. *Clin Exp Immunol* 30:229–232, 1977.
221. Fisher B, Rubin H, Sartiano G, Eunis L, Wolmark N: Observations following *Corynebacterium parvum* administrations to patients with advanced malignancy. A phase I study. *Cancer* 38:119–130, 1976.
222. Young JB, Ayus JC, Miller LK, Divine GW, Frommer JP, Miller RR, Terman DS: Cardiopulmonary toxicity in patients with breast cancer during plasma perfusion over immobilised protein A. Pathophysiology of reactions and attenuating methods. *Am J Med* 75:278–288, 1983.
223. Curry BJ, Morrison DC: Role of complement in endotoxin initiated lethality in mice. *Immunopharmacol* 1:125–135, 1979.
224. Pepys MB: Role of complement in the induction of immunological responses. *Transplant Rev* 32:93–120, 1976.
225. Craddock PR, Fehr J, Dalmasso AP, Brigham KL, Jacobs HS: Hemodialysis leukopenia. Pulmonary vascular leukotaxis resulting from complement

activation by dialyzer cellophane membrane. *J Clin Invest* 59:879–888, 1977.

226. Craddock PR, Fehr J, Brigham KL, Kronenberg RS, Jacobs HS: Complement and leukocyte-mediated pulmonary dysfunction in hemodialysis. *New Engl J Med* 296–769–774, 1977.

227. Bokisch VA, Müller-Eberhard HJ: Anaphylatoxin inactivator of human plasma: its isolation and characterisation as a carboxypeptidase. *J Clin Invest* 49:2427–2436, 1970.

228. Cochrane CG, Müller-Eberhard HJ, Aiken BS: Depletion of plasma complement *in vivo* by a protein of cobra venom: its effect on various immunologic reactions. *J Immunol* 105:55–69, 1970.

229. Verrouste PJ, Wilson CB, Dixon FJ: Lack of nephritogenicity of systemic activation of the alternative complement pathway. *Kidney Int* 6:157–169, 1974.

230. Nelson B, Ruddy S: Enhancing role of IgG in lysis of rabbit erythrocytes by the alternative pathway of human complement. *J Immunol* 122:1994–1999, 1979.

231. Bessis M: The use of replacement transfusion in disease other than hemolytic disease of the newborn. *Blood* 4:324–337, 1949.

Chapter 5

Role of Carcinoembryonic Antigen Assay in the Management of Cancer

PAUL H. SUGARBAKER

Contents

Introduction

A large number of "biologic markers" have been described for cancer, and these markers are the focus of much ongoing research. These markers may be classified as tumor-associated oncofetal antigens, ectopic hormones, enzymes, and products of tumor or host metabolism. Unfortunately, tumor specificity for nearly all of the tumor markers described to date is quite poor, for the metabolic and immunologic properties of tumor cells closely resemble those of normal cells. There are a large number of individuals in the general population with abnormal tests for a tumor marker caused by nonmalignant conditions. Also, the sensitivity of these tests to detect the presence of malignancy is often low. The small volume of tumor present at the time an early diagnosis is made and an inconsistent production of markers by the same tumor type in different individuals results in a large proportion of false negative tests. Frequent false positive and false negative tests result in a limited use of tumor markers as a screening test for malignancy. However, use of tumor markers in a population of patients known to have cancer has impacted favorably on the management of patients with several types of tumors. Tumor markers have been used as definitive tests through which a clinician can monitor the response of a tumor to therapy and to determining disease recurrence. Decisions to start, continue, or withhold treatment are frequently influenced by serial determinations of the level of tumor marker. In this chapter on carcinoembryonic antigen (CEA) the current clinical use of the tumor marker, CEA, is discussed.

Two oncofetal proteins used as biologic markers of human malignancy have evolved into valuable clinical tools for use in the management of selected patients. CEA and α-fetoprotein (AFP) circulate at high levels during fetal life, but are detectable in only minute amounts in the serum or plasma of normal adults. However, in the neoplastic cell, synthesis of oncofetal proteins may begin again. Tumor cells derived from gut epithelium, a prominent CEA producer in fetal life, may regain their ability to produce CEA in large quantities. Also, tumor cells derived from liver or yolk sac tissue may begin AFP production again. This phenomenon may be consistent with the numerous theories that attribute the carcinogenic process to dedifferentration or regression of cellular processes (1).

Characterization of the CEA Molecule

The original studies by Gold and Freeman were thought to suggest that the CEA antigen was produced only by colon cancer cells and was of uniform molecular structure (2). Molecular weight was estimated at 200,000 and the structure was that of a complex glycoprotein. Further studies by the group in Montreal and others showed CEA production by multiple different tissues; also, the substances that have CEA immunoreactivity consisted of a family of related glycoprotein molecules. The heterogeneity of CEA's molecular structure rests in its carbohydrate moiety, which may vary from 50% to 75% of its composition (3). The terminal carbohydrate structures are also quite variable, particularly with respect to sialic acid (3,4). Also, several different forms are separable by differences in net charge, using ion exchange chromatography or isoelectric focusing (4–6).

The antigenic determinants of CEA were originally thought to reside in the carbohydrate portion of the molecule. However, Vrba and co-workers were unable to competitively inhibit CEA immunoreactivity with a wide variety of carbohydrates (7). As opposed to the variable carbohydrate structure, the protein structure of the CEA molecule seems quite uniform. Terry and co-workers showed a constant sequence of the 24 N-terminal amino acids in several different CEA preparations (4). Arnon and colleagues synthesized the amino terminal peptide of CEA and showed it to have CEA immunoreactivity (8). These data strongly suggest that the internal protein structure of the molecule contains at least part of the antigenic determinants critical for immunoreactivity.

CEA Production and Metabolism

The biologic function of the CEA molecule remains a mystery. Its inconsistent presence in the host with epithelial tumors plus the fact that its production may cease and the malignant process continue makes its production unlikely to be an essential step in the malignant process. CEA, like other embryonic antigens and ectopic hormones, is an epigenetic process not essential to the neoplastic event (9). The degree to which the neoplastic cell machinery reverts to CEA production over and above that produced by normal tissues may be a random, and therefore inconsistent, event.

Only occasionally is CEA detected by immunofluorescent or immunoperoxidase studies to be within cancer cells; usually it is seen accumulating at the cell surface as a glycocalyx (10). CEA at this extracellular site enters the extracellular space, then diffuses into lymphatics and blood capillaries to reach the systemic circulation.

It is well established that CEA is present in many normal as well as malignant tissues; also, alterations in nonmalignant tissue can result in elevated plasma CEA. CEA is present in feces of normal individuals, in normal colonic tissue, in normal liver, and in bile (11–15). The common denominator for increased plasma levels of CEA in the absence of malignancy may be a breakdown in the anatomic barrier between an epithelial surface and its underlying tissues. The structure that must be disrupted to give CEA elevations is probably the epithelial basement membrane. This structure is disrupted in conditions associated with nontumor CEA elevations such as in inflammatory bowel disease, pancreatitis, gastritis, and the bronchitis that accompanies heavy smoking.

Tumors also disrupt the epithelial basement membrane; after invasion, the tumor must release substances it produces in normal or increased amounts into the interstitial fluids and hence into lymphatics and blood. Many colonic tumors have no more CEA in their tissue than does normal colonic epithelium (13–16). However, normal colonic epithelium excretes

CEA into the gut; an invasive adenocarcinoma of the colon lacks this capability.

The other pathophysiologic cause for nontumor CEA elevation is decreased metabolism by the liver. There is strong evidence that CEA degradation and excretion takes plase almost exclusively in the liver (15,17–21). Direct evidence of a prominent role for the liver in CEA metabolism comes from the clinical studies of Lurie and colleagues (22). Patients with elevated CEA levels and biliary tract obstruction from stones were studied both preoperatively and postoperatively. CEA levels returned to normal in patients who had successful relief of biliary obstruction. Recent studies by Lowenstein and co-workers showed that patients with cirrhotic livers excreted less CEA into the duodenal juice, even when plasma CEA levels were elevated (23). From these studies it was clear that decreased excretion of CEA from biliary obstruction or cirrhosis can result in elevated plasma CEA levels.

Nontumor CEA Elevations

Zamcheck and collaborators established through clinical studies that CEA elevations could result from many nontumor disease processes. Alcoholic patients often had CEA levels greater than 2.5 ng/mL but less than 10 ng/mL. Of 88 patients with alcoholic liver disease, 45% had positive CEA tests, whereas none of 14 patients with nonalcoholic liver disease had positive CEA assays (14,24,25).

Numerous other nontumor causes of CEA elevation have been reported: pancreatitis, recent blood transfusion, ulcerative colitis, heavy cigarette smoking, gastritis following partial gastrectomy, and colonic polpys (26–43).

The multiple nontumor causes for elevated CEA may cause a clinician considerable difficulty as he or she seeks to utilize the CEA test in patient management decisions. The following suggestions can be made to assist in differentiating tumor from nontumor CEA elevations. First, the *magnitude* of the elevation is important. CEA elevations in the 2.5 ng/ml to 10 ng/mL range may be from tumor or nontumor. However, nontumor CEA elevations greater than 10 ng/mL are very likely without jaundice and other obvious signs of biliary tract obstruction. Therefore, only patients with moderate CEA elevations (2.5–10 ng/mL range) are those likely to create clinical dilemmas.

Second, in patients with moderate CEA elevations the clinician must make a *search for possible nontumor causes* of CEA elevations (Table 5-1). Hepatic cirrhosis and hepatitis, heavy smoking, and gastrointestinal inflammatory states are the most common causes of these nontumor elevations. Most commonly, as emphasized by Gardner and co-workers, these conditions are usually in an active state when associated with

Table 5-1. Nonmalignant conditions
associated with CEA elevations

	Reference
Hepatic cirrhosis	24,25
Hepatitis	24,25
Heavy smoking	39
Pancreatitis	26
Gastritis	—
Inflammatory bowel disease, especially ulcerative colitis	30,33,37
Uremia	—
Blood transfusion	28

plasma CEA elevations (37). If present in a state of complete remission, it is not safe to assume that they are responsible for an elevated CEA. These clinical entities can usually be identified by a careful medical history and routine laboratory and radiologic tests. Liver function tests including tests for hepatitis antigen are needed. Sugarbaker suggested that routine liver biopsy in all patients undergoing surgery for colorectal cancer should be performed to assist in interpreting postoperative serial CEA assays (44).

Third, to differentiate tumor from nontumor CEA elevation, several *sequential CEA assays* as opposed to individual determinations may be required. If the titer is progressively rising, cancer is the most likely cause; if the serial titers are erratic, with both elevated and normal values, nontumor causes are more common.

The first successful efforts to distinguish between tumor CEA and nontumor CEA elevation on a laboratory basis was recently reported by Lowenstein and colleagues (23). Duodenal juice was collected through a double lumen gastroduodenal (Dreiling) tube and CEA outputs determined for 100 minutes. Normal patients had duodenal CEA outputs of less than 150 ng/min. Six of seven patients with CEA-associated cancers had duodenal outputs of greater than 150 ng/min. Seven of nine patients with benign liver disease or extrahepatic biliary obstruction had normal duodenal CEA outputs. Lowenstein and co-workers suggested that determinations of duodenal juice CEA may assist the oncologist in two ways: (a) It may detect increased CEA production even prior to the occurrence of elevated circulating levels, which may provide a more sensitive CEA assay system than currently available using plasma sampling; (b) determinations of duodenal juice CEA may assist in distinguishing between increased plasma CEA due to increased production (by cancer or inflammatory diseases) and that due to impaired metabolism and excretion due to liver disease.

A second approach to the specificity problem was that taken by Nakamura et al (45). They devised a radioimmunoassay for a CEA-related molecule, CEA-S, which may yield fewer false positive results than CEA. Further comparative studies of CEA and other colon cancer markers are required before the accuracy of these tests are known.

CEA in the Diagnosis of Primary Cancer

Data obtained from screening asymptomatic populations for cancer using the CEA test can be summarized as "too little information too late" (46–50). Unfortunately, the patients with advanced primary tumors in whom a low cure rate is expected generally have CEA levels greater than 2.5 ng/mL, and good prognosis cancers are missed because CEA levels are normal.

McNeil and Adelstein in their studies on the interpretation of laboratory tests show how a laboratory test is "only as good as the patient population in whom it is employed"(49). This explains how CEA can be of little or no value in mass screening for cancer, but of great value for detection of recurrence in a high-risk population such as postoperative colorectal cancer patients (51–56).

Ona and co-workers showed that CEA may be of value when used in a population of patients suspected of having pancreatic cancer (57). They reported that 23 of 27 patients (85%) with pancreatic cancer had elevated CEA levels. The CEA assay was more frequently positive in patients with cancer of the pancreas than was any other diagnostic tests used, including upper gastrointestinal series, hypotonic duodenography, celial arteriography, and percutaneous transhepatic cholangiography. Computerized tomography may be expected to provide a true positive ratio similar to that of CEA in detecting pancreatic cancer (58,59). Also, if CEA levels greater than 10 ng/mL were assumed to indicate liver disease, CEA detected liver metastasis in more patients than did the liver scan.

Occult Gastrointestinal Malignancy

Not infrequently a patient with weight loss, malaise, and other systemic symptomatology suggesting malignancy will present to the physician. Usually radiologic and nuclear medicine studies allow the physician to identify the primary tumor. However, sometimes diagnostic tests do not reveal the expected malignancy. Adenocarcinoma of the small bowel, appendix, or pancreas may escape detection despite the most careful radiologic studies. If this occurs, a markedly elevated CEA level may provide the clue required to make a diagnosis of cancer without further delay. A CEA of 10 ng/mL or above strongly suggests occult malignancy. A confirmed elevation may encourage the surgeon to move to an exploratory laparatomy to diagnose and hopefully treat the occult gastrointestinal tumor.

In summary, CEA tests have not been found to be helpful in screening for cancer or in establishing a diagnosis in the symptomatic patient. An exception to this is the patient with malignancy difficult or impossible to diagnose by conventional radiographic techniques. Pancreatic cancer is the most common occult malignancy whose presence may be signaled by an elevated CEA.

CEA in Assessing Prognosis in Patients with Known Malignancy

Primary Colorectal Cancer

Perhaps the most crucial clinical assessment of a patient with cancer is the initial one made immediately after the diagnosis is established and prior to any definitive therapy. Laurence and co-workers (47), Booth and colleagues (60), and Sugarbaker (61) suggested that CEA tests done at the time of initial patient evaluation were of prognostic value. This was determined retrospectively by correlating preoperative CEA levels with Dukes classification in patients with colorectal cancer (Fig. 5-1). Wanebo and coworkers showed conclusively that recurrence rates were higher in patients with Dukes B and Dukes C lesions who had preoperative levels higher than 5 ng/mL (Fig. 5-2). Also, as the preoperative CEA level increased, the mean time to recurrence decreased as a linear inverse correlation (62,63).

Although preoperative CEA blood tests are prognostic indicators, nevertheless some patients with very large Dukes C, Dukes D, or even meta-

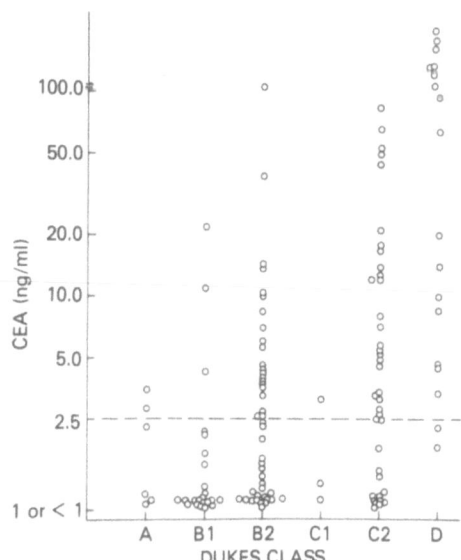

Figure 5-1. Correlation of preoperative CEA level and Dukes stage of patients with large-bowel cancer. Data show that the more advanced the primary cancer, the greater proportion of patients with elevated CEA levels (61).

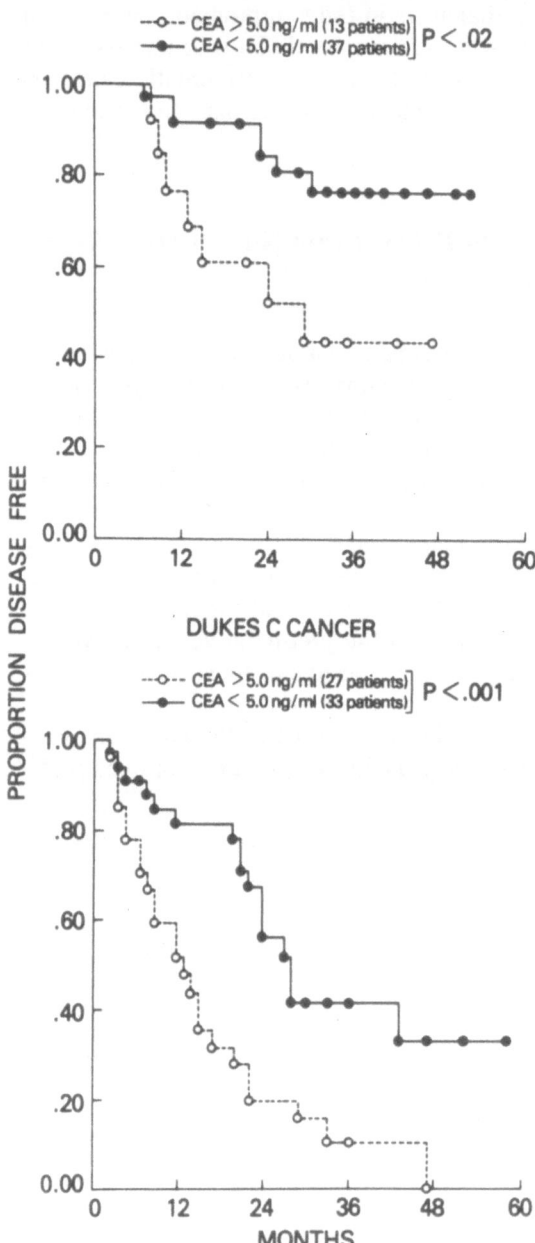

Figure 5-2. Correlation of preoperative CEA level and survival of Dukes B **(top)** or Dukes C **(bottom)** colorectal cancer (62).

static tumors may have normal CEA assays. This is likely due to decreased production or decreased release of CEA by the tumor. Denk and co-workers showed decreased CEA from poorly differentiated tumors (64). Shamberg showed that preoperative plasma CEA levels were statistically significantly related to the degree of tumor differentiation (46). The consistency of this observation is not always appreciated clinically, for primary tumor size also correlates with circulating CEA levels, and poorly differentiated tumor with lesser CEA production tend to be of larger size and to invade more deeply. Consequently, in poorly differentiated tumors, the variables of tumor differentiation and tumor size conflict and therefore tend to nullify each other.

Primary Pancreatic Cancer

CEA has been identified as a prognosticator in several other tumors besides colorectal cancer. Kalser and co-workers found that pancreatic cancer patients with locally unrespectable or metastatic carcinoma had a significantly longer survival if CEA was normal at the time of diagnosis (65).

Primary Breast Cancer

Wang and co-workers showed a relationship between plasma CEA and prognosis in women with breast cancer (66). Patients after mastectomy with CEA levels above 2.5 ng/mL had a significantly ($P < .001$) more rapid recurrence rate than similar patients with CEA levels below this level. At 2 years after mastectomy the disease had recurred in 65% of the patients with CEA greater than 2.5 ng/mL compared with 20% of those with CEA less than 2.5 ng/mL (Fig. 5-3). Haagensen and colleagues and Myers and co-workers both showed a poor prognosis in patients with elevated post-mastectomy CEA levels (67,68). Haagensen and colleagues also showed an increased incidence of tumor recurrence with preoperative CEA levels greater than 3 ng/mL. Tormey and Waalkes noted that patients with metastatic breast cancer with CEA greater than 5 ng/mL prior to treatment had lower response rates and a shorter time to treatment failure than did patients with CEA equal to or less than 5 ng/ml (69).

Bronchogenic Carcinoma

Dent and co-workers reported on the prognostic significance of pretreatment CEA values in patients with bronchogenic carcinoma (70). The use of the CEA assay for diagnostic purposes was somewhat limited, for heavy smokers frequently had elevated CEA levels in the absence of cancer. In groups of nonsmokers, smokers, patients with limited bronchogenic cancer, patients with inoperable cancer, and patients with metastatic cancer, there were different and progressively higher mean CEA

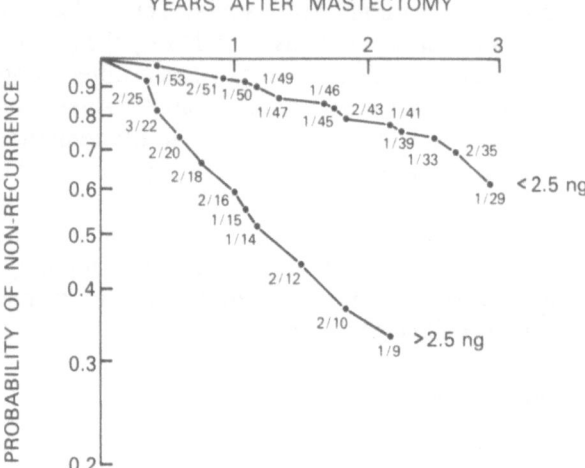

Figure 5-3. Postoperative CEA levels and prognosis in patients with breast cancer. Data show probability of nonrecurrence based on CEA determination taken following mastectomy (66).

values. Concannon and colleagues made the interesting observation that all epidermoid and adenocarcinoma patients in a series of 147 who had pretreatment CEA levels greater than 6 ng/mL died in less than 3 years (Fig. 5-4) (71).

Serial CEA in Monitoring Cancer Therapy

Assessment of the Adequancy of Surgical Removal of a Primary Colon or Rectal Cancer

Serial CEA titers during a period of intensive therapy may also be used as a monitor of the effectiveness of a treatment regimen. After surgical excision of a colorectal cancer, elevated preoperative CEA levels usually fall into the normal range of 2.5 ng/mL or less. Several groups have noted that failure of postoperative CEA values to fall into the normal range is associated with poor prognosis (72–76). In a careful study from the Royal Victoria Hospital, Montreal, colorectal cancer patients were divided into three groups according to their preoperative and postoperative CEA levels (76). Thirty-six patients (group 1) had preoperative and postoperative CEA values less than 2.5 ng/mL. In group 2 (11 patients) elevated preoperative CEA levels fell to less than 2.5 ng/mL postoperatively. Fourteen patients (group 3) had a preoperative CEA greater than 2.5 ng/mL, but the postoperative value failed to decline below 2.5 ng/mL. In group 1, 14% of patients had a recurrence by 19 months postoperatively, in group 2, 18% of

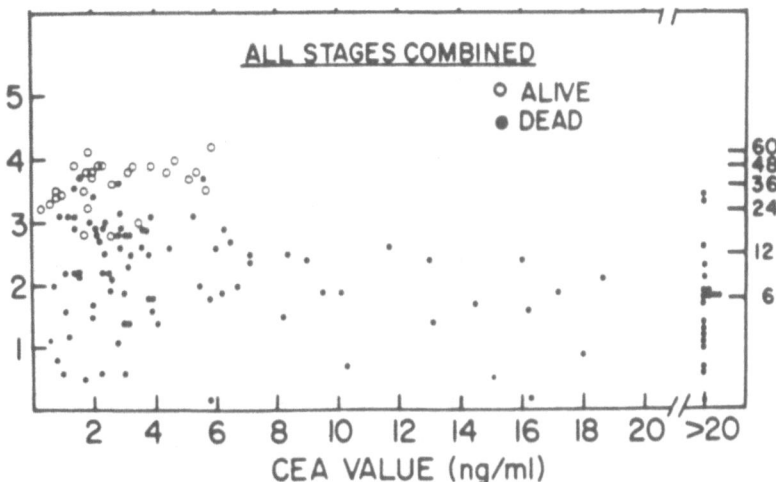

Figure 5-4. Pretreatment CEA levels and survival in patients with bronchogenic carcinoma. In this series of 147 patients with bronchogenic carcinoma, all patients with pretreatment CEA levels greater than 6 ng/mL died in less than 3 years (71).

patients had a recurrence and in group 3, 73% of patients had a recurrence (Fig. 5-5).

Gianola and Sugarbaker compared a variety of tests done postoperatively after resection of a colon or rectal cancer (77). They studied full-lung tomography, liver-spleen scan, computerized tomography of the abdomen, intravenous pyelogram, bone scan, and postoperative CEA assay (Table 5-2). Occult metastases were defined as those that occurred at a particular anatomic site within 1 year of follow-up. Occult metastases for full-lung tomography were in the lungs; for liver/spleen scans they were in the liver. For computerized tomograms they were in the abdominal cavity, abdominal wall, liver, or retroperitoneum. For intravenous pyelogram they were associated with the urinary tract. For bone scan they were within the skeleton, and finally for CEA they were at any site of recurrence. Follow-up of all patients was at least 1 year. Patients included in this study were those thought to be at high risk for recurrence because of lymph node positivity, obstruction, or perforation of the primary tumor. All site-specific recurrences were confirmed by biopsy or radiologic demonstration of an expanding lesion with continued follow-up.

In 53 patients CEA assays were obtained within the first postoperative month after a "curative resection" of a colon or rectal cancer. The preoperative CEA was not considered in this analysis. Eleven patients had postoperative elevations from 2.6–5.0 ng/mL and six had greater than 5.1 ng/mL. In this group of 17 patients with postoperative CEA elevations, 12 had developed recurrent disease. Twelve of the 20 patients with recurrence had elevated postoperative baseline CEA tests (Table 5-2). If the

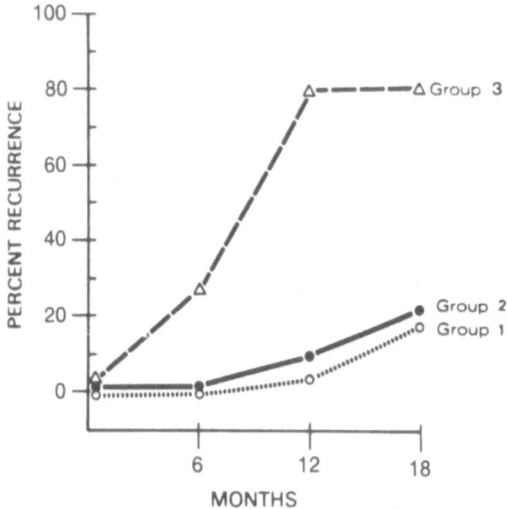

Figure 5-5. Postoperative baseline CEA level and prognosis of colorectal cancer patients. The 36 patients in group 1 have preoperative and postoperative CEA values of less than 2.5 ng/mL. The 11 patients in group 2 had a preoperative CEA value greater than 2.5 ng/mL but postoperative values were all less than 2.5 ng/mL. In the 14 patients in group 3 the preoperative and postoperative values were greater than 2.5 ng/mL. Highly significant differences between those with elevated postoperative CEA levels and normal postoperative CEA levels were observed (76).

CEA test in a patient who has an elevated CEA preoperatively fails to fall within the normal range, this strongly suggests persistent disease. In summary, in this battery of tests CEA appeared to be the most accurate one by which to identify a group of colorectal cancer patients at exceptionally high risk for recurrence following potentially curative surgery.

CEA in Monitoring Response to Radiation Therapy

Vider and colleagues, Sugarbaker and colleagues, and Donaldson and co-workers reported a correlation of CEA levels and the clinical response to radiation therapy (Fig. 5-6) (78–81). These studies showed that CEA titers decreased markedly in patients receiving radiation for colorectal or cervical cancer if the bulk of CEA-producing tumor was within the radiation field. Patients with widespread disease receiving radiation for palliation showed little or no decrease in their CEA level with radiation therapy. The depressed CEA levels in patients receiving potentially curative radiation remain at low levels. A rise was associated with evidence of disease recurrence and indicated either the occurrence or disseminated disease, local treatment failure, or both.

Table 5-2. Comparison of CEA and other diagnostic tests in the detection of occult colorectal cancer

		Sensitivity		
	Total no. patients	No. patients w/site-specific disease	No. positive tests	True positive percentage (number of patients)
Full-lung tomography	52	1	1	(1/1)
Liver/spleen scan	52	9	3	33 (3/9)
Computerized tomogram abdomen	60	15	7	47 (7/15)
Intravenous pyelogram	25	0	0	—
Bone scan	30	0	0	—
Postoperative baseline CEA > 2.5 ng/mL	53	20	12	60 (12/20)

	Specificity		
	No. patients without site-specific disease	No. positive tests	False positive percentage (number of patients)
Full-lung tomography	51	6	12 (6/5)
Liver/spleen scan	43	5	12 (5/43)
Computerized tomogram abdomen	45	5	11 (5/45)
Intravenous pyelogram	25	2	8 (2/25)
Bone scan	30	2	7 (2/30)
Postoperative baseline CEA > 2.5 ng/mL	28	5	18 (5.28)

CEA in Monitoring Response to Chemotherapy

Mulcare and LoGerfo noted good correlations between the pattern of change of serial CEA assays and the patients response to systemic chemotherapy (82). They and other groups emphasized that the CEA test was useful in those cancer patients with elevated CEA in the plasma, but was of no help if the titer was not increased (Fig. 5-7) (82–85).

Herrera and co-workers offer an important *caveat* in interpreting serial CEA values in patients treated with nitrosourea compounds. In these patients they report a tendency of decreased CEA levels regardless of the patient's tumor response to the drug. This could be due to the nitrosoureas producing a diffuse block of cellular activity, including glycoprotein production both at the nucleolus and in the cytoplasm.

In summary, serial CEA assays in patients whose tumors produce an increased level of CEA in the blood can be a valuable monitor of cancer treatment. The adequacy of surgical resection, the likelihood of disease control by radiation therapy, and the response to systemic chemotherapy can be assessed by serial CEA estimations in many patients. Of course, whenever possible, a correlation of serial CEA levels with other clinical assessments should also be made.

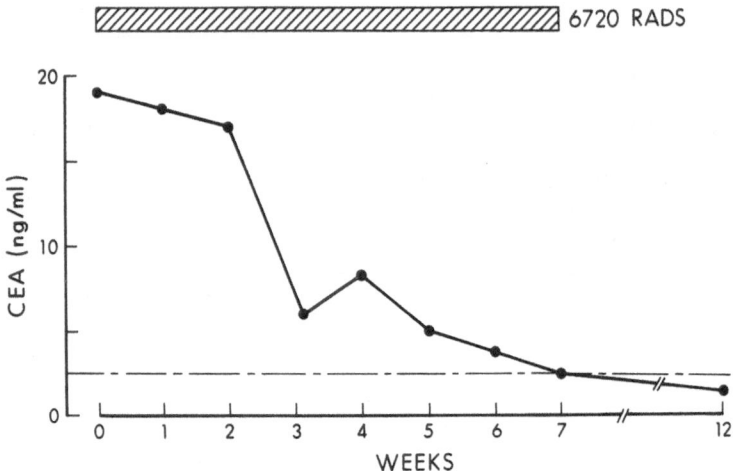

Figure 5-6. CEA as a monitor of radiation therapy. This 60-year-old man had a perineal recurrence of rectal cancer 6 years after an abdominoperineal resection. His workup showed no disseminated disease. He is given 6,720 rads to the pelvis with complete clinical disappearance of his tumor. His urethral obstruction cleared, penile swelling resolved, and the mass resolved. A good correlation of local tumor control and the CEA titer was observed.

CEA in the Detection of Recurrent Colon or Rectal Cancer

Perhaps the most important current use of CEA is as an indicator of early recurrent colorectal cancer and a guide to selected second-look surgery. Usually the rise in CEA associated with disease recurrence is gradually progressive, as illustrated in Fig. 5-8. Occasionally the CEA profile postoperatively is erratic, with multiple elevations that return to the normal range with repeat determinations (Fig. 5-9). This pattern of CEA elevation does not correlate with cancer recurrence. There can be no doubt that CEA is a valuable adjunct to be used in the follow-up of colorectal cancer patients to help detect recurrent disease (86–105).

Sugarbaker, Zamcheck, and Moore studied serial postoperative CEA titers following the surgical removal of a colon or rectal cancer (44). Three types of postoperative profile were recognized: (a) the progressively rising titer associated with recurrence, (b) the stable elevated titer, which may or may not go on to rise, and (c) the titers within the normal range (Fig. 5-10a–c). This study and others suggest that progressively rising serial CEA assays point to recurrent cancer in all patients.

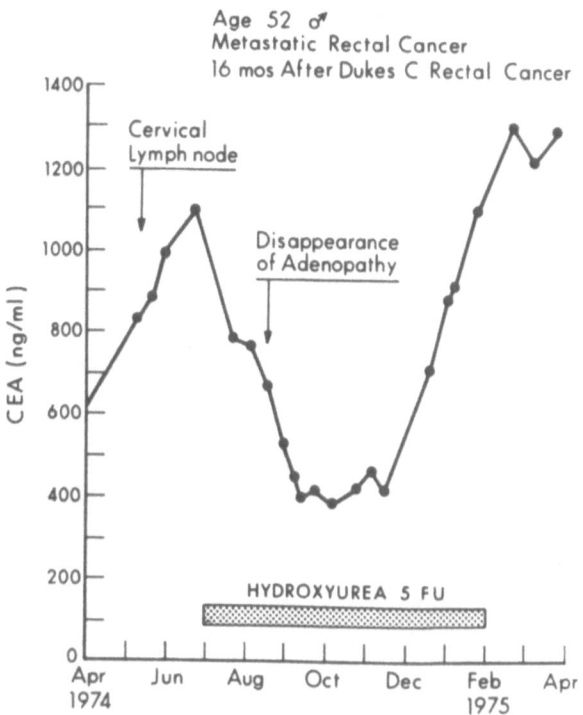

Figure 5-7. CEA as a monitor of cancer chemotherapy. This 52-year-old man had metastatic rectal cancer that occurred 16 months after the resection of a Dukes C rectal cancer. His CEA titers nicely reflect the clinical assessment of his disease after treatment with hydroxyurea and fluroracil (5-FU).

Sugarbaker, Zamcheck, and Moore in their prospective study attempted to compare CEA with physical examination, barium enema, chest x-ray, and liver/spleen scan in the early detection of recurrent cancer. In two-thirds of patients, CEA was the first indication of disease recurrence. The lead time to detection of recurrence by serial CEA over all other diagnostic tests was between 1 and 18 months, with a median of 3 months.

Minton and colleagues at Ohio State University performed serial postoperative CEA assays on 400 colorectal patients. Second-look surgery was indicated for 75 patients because of rising CEA levels. In 59 patients recurrent tumor was found at reexploration, or later. In approximately 60% of patients studied prospectively, repeat excision for cure was reported. Five-year survival in this group of patients was 38% (105). Early detection of recurrent disease and subsequent reoperative surgery does lead to long-term survival in a significant number of patients.

Attiyeh and Stearns performed second-look procedures in 32 colorectal cancer patients based in rising CEA titers (106). Long-term follow-up of

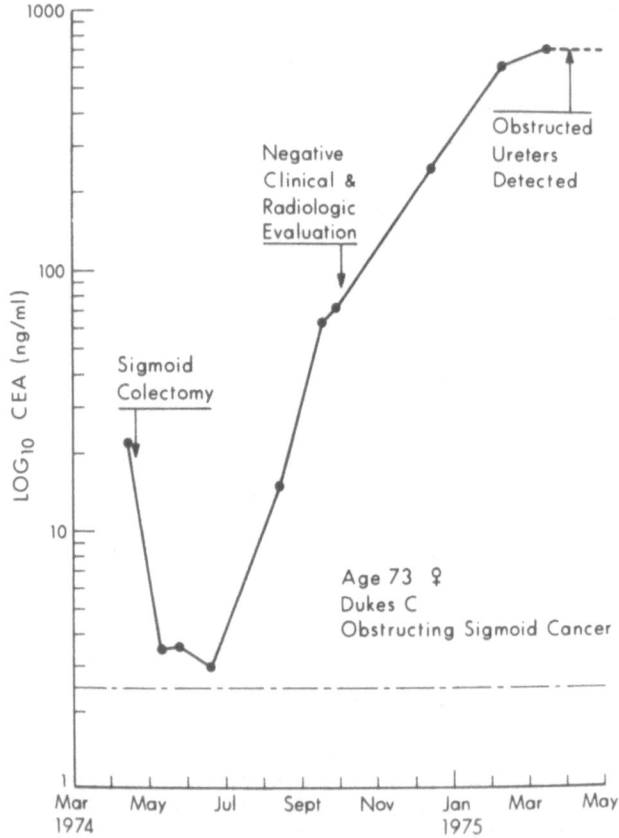

Figure 5-8. Progressively rising CEA titer in patient with recurrent colorectal cancer. This 73-year-old woman had a Dukes C adenocarcinoma obstructing her sigmoid colon. Preoperative CEA of 22 did not fall to within normal range postoperatively. This is associated with a poor prognosis. Over course of next several months her CEA titer rapidly rose. Complete clinical and radiological evaluation gave no evidence of recurrent disease. However, 7 months later an intravenous pyleogram showed her ureters to be obstructed, and she died shortly thereafter. In this patient the CEA signaled recurrent disease approximately 8 months prior to clinical or radiologic manifestations of disease recurrence.

these patients is shown in Fig. 5–11. Approximately one-third of patients may be expected to be cured of their disease by reoperative surgery if early recurrence is detected by CEA tests postoperatively. Further studies of this important problem are required.

Rittgers and colleagues interjected a timely precautionary note regarding transient CEA elevations occasionally seen following resection of colorectal cancer. Nine of 25 patients showed transient elevations without cancer recurrence upon follow-up and close clinical investigation. Trends

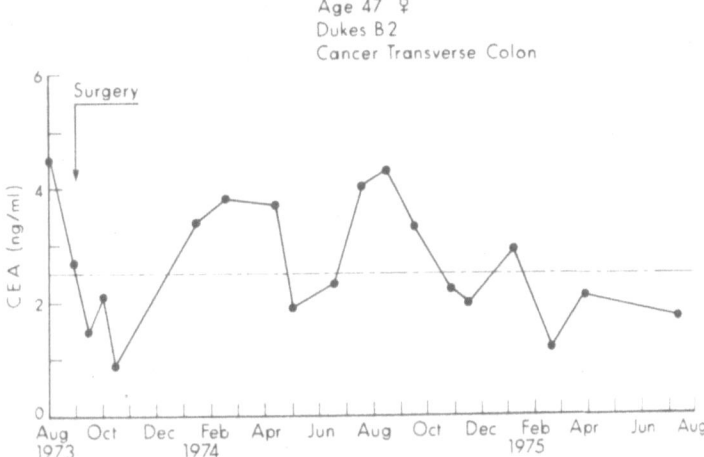

Figure 5-9. Eratic CEA levels associated with a nontumor cause of antigen elevation. This 47-year-old female had Dukes B adenocarcinoma removed from her
transverse colon. Several elevations with eventual decline to within normal range
were noted in her course. She remains free of disease with 10 year follow-up.

in serial CEA titers rather than isolated CEA values must be used, along
with all other clinical and laboratory data available, in making the deci-
sion to perform a second-look surgical procedure (104).

The high percentage of early CEA elevations in patients with hepatic
metastases plus the development of resection techniques to remove liver
metastases but preserve liver parenchyma suggests that salvage of patients with early hepatic metastatic disease may be possible. Successful
resection of metastatic colorectal cancer in the liver, similar to the resection of osteosarcoma in the lungs, may be possible.

Recent data provided by August and colleagues suggest that the earlier
hepatic metastases are detected, the greater the likelihood for a potentially curative hepatic resection (107). Forty-three patients were explored
with the hope of curatively resecting hepatic metastases for a primary
colon or rectal malignancy. In six patients (14%) hepatoduodenal nodes
were found to be involved with metastatic cancer. Four of these patients
had Dukes B primary cancers, and no recurrence was detected at the
resection site or along para-aortic nodes. August and colleagues concluded that malignancy at the hepatoduodenal nodes was most likely
metastases from the hepatic deposits of tumor. They suggest that a "wait
and see attitude" toward hepatic metastases and their subsequent treatment seems unjustified. Delay in the surgical excision of hepatic metastases will lead to more rapid dissemination of disease (metastases from
metastases) and to a lesser number of potentially curative hepatic resec-
tions.

Figure 5-10. Postoperative CEA profiles of patients in follow-up after resection of colon or rectal adenocarcinoma.

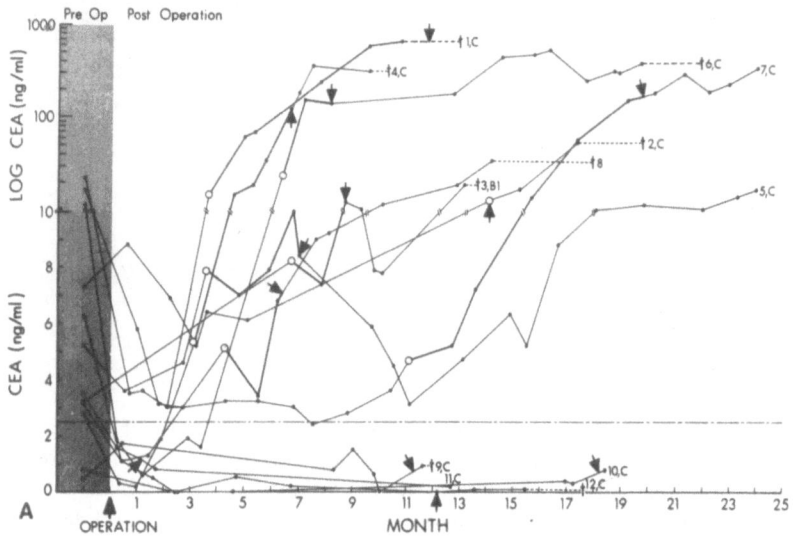

Figure 5-10A. In 12 patients with recurring cancer, 8 showed progressively rising CEA titers. Time at which recurrent cancer became clinically evident is shown by *arrows*. Four of the 12 showed no CEA elevation with recurrent disease. However, in 8 of the 12 patients with recurrence, the CEA titers signaled recurrent disease 3 to 18 months prior to other clinical evidence of disease recurrence.

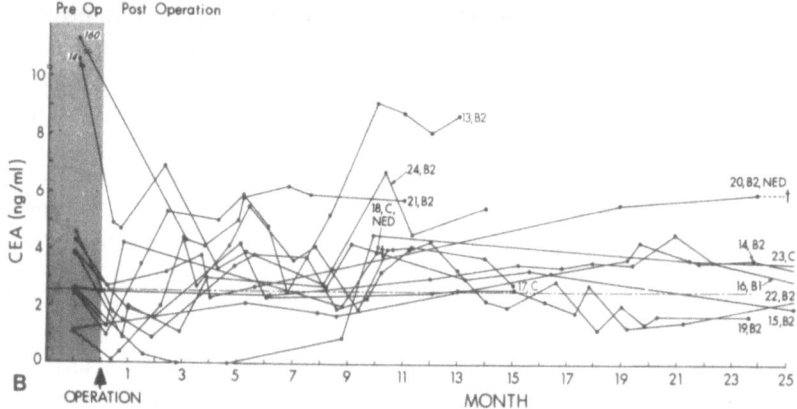

Figure 5-10B. Eleven patients with stable, elevated postoperative CEA titers who did not show recurrent cancer. The CEA titer in patient #13 was associated with hepatitis.

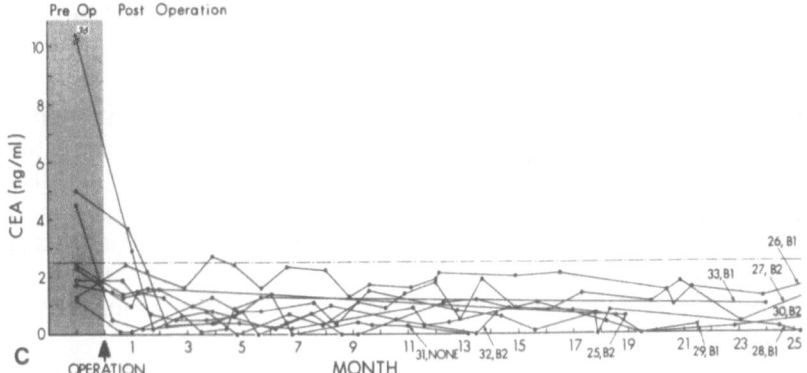

Figure 5-10C. Nine patients, all free of recurrent disease who had CEA titers consistently less than 2.5 ng/mL.

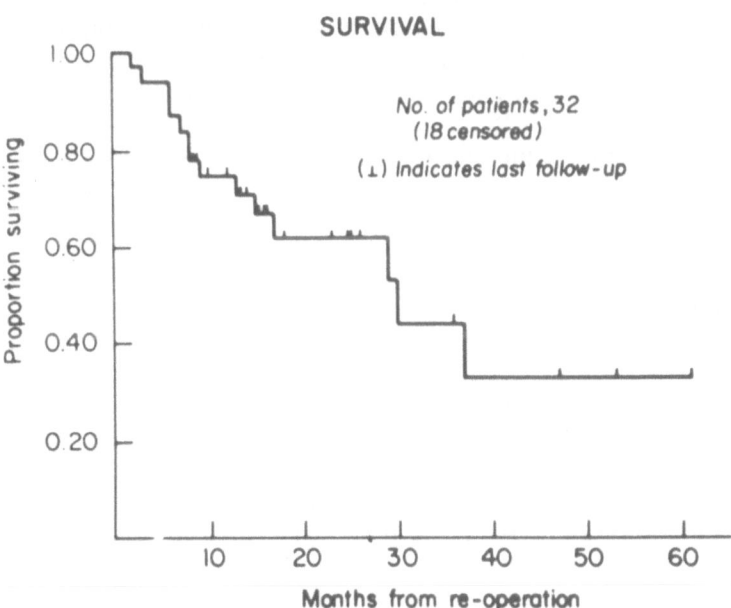

Figure 5-11. Kaplan Myers survival for 32 patients who underwent second-look surgery based on CEA elevations. Resectability in this group of patients was 43%. In approximately one-third of patients long-term survival using this treatment strategy and serial CEA follow-up may be expected (106).

Anti-CEA Antibody in the Localization of Colorectal Cancer Metastases

An interesting use for anti-CEA antibody has recently been developed by Goldenberg and co-workers (108). This group took anti-CEA antibody made in goats, coupled it to radioactive iodine, and after injecting this into cancer patients, performed total-body isotope scans. Tumor location could be demonstrated 48 hours after injection in almost all patients studied. Circulating antigen levels up to 350 μg/mL did not prevent successful tumor imaging. Work using monoclonal anti-CEA for tumor imaging is underway.

CEA in the Detection of Recurrent Breast Cancer

Sugarbaker et al (109) combined the liver scan and CEA as a composite in patients with suspected hepatic recurrence of breast cancer. In this study the composite test was positive if both tests were positive, negative if both tests were negative, and equivocal (further studies indicated) if the results disagreed. The number of false positive scans was markedly reduced by the composite. The false positive rate for the liver scan was 14% and for the CEA assay, 25%; however, there were no false positive composite tests. Similar studies have been reported by McCartney and Hoffer for composites of liver scan plus CEA and of barium enema plus CEA (110,111).

Summary

CEA is a molecule produced by a large number of malignant and benign tissues. Measuring levels of CEA circulating in the blood by radioimmunoassay can be used in the management of cancer patients. Because of high false positive and false negative percentages in normal populations, it has not been useful in screening for malignancy. However, in several types of cancer patients the test has been shown to be of considerable clinical value. Elevated CEA levels indicate a poor prognosis in patients with primary colorectal cancer, primary pancreatic cancer, primary breast cancer, and primary lung cancer. Serial CEA titers obtained following cancer treatments can be used to monitor the therapy. CEA can assess the adequacy of surgical removal of a primary colon or rectal cancer, monitor responses to chemotherapy, and assess response to radiation therapy. The greatest clinical impact of CEA has been in the detection of recurrent colon or rectal cancer following surgical resection of the primary malignancy. Early detection of recurrence, when combined with reoperative second-look surgery, may result in 30% long-term survivors.

References

1. Ray, P.K.: Immune rejection and acceptance phenoma in transplant recipients, tumor hosts and pregnancy. (In) *Immunobiology of Transplantation, Cancer and Pregnancy*, Ray P.K. (ed). New York, Pingamont Press, 1983, p. 409–430.
2. Gold, P., Freedman, S.O.: Demonstration of tumor-specific antigens in human colonic carcinomata by immunologic tolerance and absorption techniques. *J. Exp. Med.* 122:467–481, 1965.
3. Banjo, C., Shuster, J., Gold, P.: Intermolecular heterogeneity of the carcinoembryonic antigen. *Cancer. Res.* 34:2114–2121, 1974.
4. Terry, W. D., Henkart, P.A., Coligan, J.E., *et al:* Structural studies of the major glycoprotein in preparations with carcinoembryonic antigen activity. *J. Exp. Med.* 136:100–129, 1972.
5. Coligan, J.E., Henkart, P.A., Todd, C.W., *et al:* Heterogeneity of the carcinoembryonic antigen. Immunochemistry 10:591–599, 1973.
6. Eveleigh, J.W.: Heterogeneity of carcinoembryonic antigen. *Cancer. Res.* 34:2122–2124, 1974.
7. Vrba, R., Alpert, E., Isselbacher, K.J.: Carcinoembryonic antigen: Evidence for multiple antigenic determinants and isoantigens. *Proc. Natl. Acad. Sci. USA* 72:4602–4606, 1975.
8. Arnon, R., Bustin, M., Calef, E., *et al:* Immunologic cross-reactivity of antibodies to a synthetic undecapeptide analogous to the aminoterminal segment of the carcinoembryonic antigen, with the intact protein and with human sera. *Proc. Natl. Acad. Sci. USA* 73:2123–2127, 1976.
9. Sherbert, G.V.: Epigenetic processes and their relevance to the study of neoplasia. *Advances Cancer Res.* 97:167, 1970.
10. Burton, P., von Kleist, S., Sabine, M.C., *et al:* Immunohistologica localization of carcinoembryonic antigen and nonspecific cross-reacting antigen in gastrointestinal normal and tumor tissues. *Cancer Res.* 33:3299–3302, 1973.
11. Freed, D.J.L., Taylor, G.: Carcinoembryonic antigen in feces. *Br. Med. J.* 1:85–87, 1972.
12. Elias, E.G., Hoyoke, E.D., Chu, T.M.: Carcinoembryonic antigen in feces and plasma of normal subjects and patients with colorectal cancer. *Dis. Colon Rectum* 1:38–41, 1974.
13. Martin, F., Martin, M.S.: Radioimmunoassay of carcinoembryonic antigen in extracts of human colon and stomach. *Int. J. Cancer* 9:641–647, 1972.
14. Khoo, S.K., Warner, N.L., Lie, J.T., *et al:* Carcinoembryonic antigenic activity of tissue extracts: A quantitative study of malignant and benign neoplasms, cirrhotic liver, normal adult and fetal organs. *Int. J. Cancer* 11:681–687, 1973.
15. Molnar, I.G., Vandevoorde, J.P., Gitnick, G.L.: CEA levels in fluids bathing gastrointestinal tumors. *Gastroenterology* 70:513–515, 1976.
16. Dyce, B.J., Haverback, B.J.: Free and bound carcinoembryonic antigen in neoplasms and in normal adult and fetal tissues. *Immunochemistry* 11:423–430, 1974.
17. Schuster, J., Silverman, M., Gold, P.: Metabolism of human carcinoembryonic antigen in xenogeneic animals. *Cancer Res.* 33:65–68, 1973.
18. Primus, F.J., Goldenberg, D.M., Hansen, H.J.: Metabolism of carcinoem-

bryonic antigen (CEA) in a human tumor-hamster model (abstr). *Fed. Proc.* 32:834, 1973.

19. Thomas, P., Heims, P.A.: The hepatic clearance of circulating carcinoembryonic antigen by the mouse. *Biochem. Soc. Trans.* 5:312–313, 1977.

20. Holyoke, E.D., Reynoso, G., Chu, T.: Carcinoembryonic antigen in patients with carcinoma of the digestive tract. In Proceedings of second conference on embryonic and fetal antigens in cancer, p 215. National Technical Information Service, Springfield, VA., US Department of Commerce, 1972.

21. Go, V.L.W., Ammon, H.V., Holtermuller, K.H., *et al:* Quantitation of carcinoembryonic antigen-like activities in normal human gastrointestinal secretions. *Cancer* 36:2346–2350, 1975.

22. Lurie, B.B., Lowenstein, M.S., Zamcheck, N.: Elevated circulating CEA levels in benign extraheptic biliary tract obstruction and inflammation. *JAMA* 233:326–330, 1975.

23. Lowenstein, M.S., Rau, P., Rittgers, R.A., *et al:* CEA in duodenal aspirates of patients with benign and malignant disease: Preliminary observations. *JNCI* 66:803–806, 1981.

24. Moore, T., Dhar, P., Zamcheck, N., *et al:* Carcinoembryonic antigen(s) in liver disease. I. Clinical and morphologic studies. *Gastroenterology* 63:88–94, 1972.

25. Kupchik, J.Z., Zamcheck, N.: Carcinoembryonic antigen(s) in liver disease. II. Isolation from human cirrhotic liver and serum from normal liver. *Gastroenterology* 63:95–101, 1972.

26. Delwiche, R., Zamcheck, N., Marcon, N.: Carcinoembryonic antigen in pancreatitis. *Cancer* 31:328–330, 1973.

27. Sharma, M.P., Gregg, J.A., Lowenstein, M.S., Ona, F.V., Zamcheck, N., Dhar, P.: CEA in the diagnosis of pancreatic cancer. *Cancer* 31:324–327, 1973.

28. Gitnick, G.L., Molnar, I.G.: Carcinoembryonic antigen transmission by blood products. *Cancer* 42:1568–1573, 1978.

29. LoGerfo, P., Krupey, J., Hansen, H.J.: Demonstration of an antigen common to several varieties of neoplasis. Assay using zirconly phosphate gel. *N. Eng. J. Med.* 285:138–141, 1971.

30. Wight, D.G.D., Gazet, J.C.: Carcinoembryonic antigen levels in inflammatory disease of the large bowel. *Proc. Royl. Soc. Med.* 65:967–968, 1972.

31. Moore, T.L., Kantrowitz, P.A., Zamcheck, N.: Carcinoembryonic antigen (CEA) in inflammatory bowel disease. *JAMA* 222:944–947, 1972.

32. Rule, A.H., Straus, E., Vandevoorde, J., *et al:* Tumor associated (CEA reacting) antigen in patients with inflammatory bowel disease. *N. Eng. J. Med.* 287:24–26, 1972.

33. Dilawari, J.B., Lennard-Jones, J.E., MacKay, A.M., *et al:* Estimation of carcinoembryonic antigen in ulcerative colitis with special reference to malignant change. *Gut* 16:255–260, 1975.

34. Morson, B.C., Pang, L.S.C.: Rectal biopsy as an aid to cancer control in ulcerative colitis. *Gut* 8:423–434, 1967.

35. Yardley, J.H., Keren, D.F.: "Precancer" lesions in ulcerative colitis. A retrospective study of rectal biopsy and colectomy specimens. *Cancer* 34:835–844, 1974.

36. Cook, M.G., Path, M.R.C., Golighan, J.C.: Carcinoma and epithelial dysplasia complicating ulterative colitis. Gastroenterology 68:1127–1136, 1975.
37. Gardner, R.C., Feinerman, A.E., Kantrowitz, P.A., et al: Serial carcinoembryonic antigen (CEA) levels in patients with ulcerative colitis. Am. J. Dig. Dis. 23:129–133, 1978.
38. Stevens, D.P., MacKay, I.R.: Increased carcinoembryonic antigen in heavy cigarette smokers. Lancet 1:1238–1239, 1973.
39. Alexander, J.C., Silverman, N.A., Chretien, P.G.: Effect of age and cigarette smoking on carcinoembryonic antigen levels. J. Am. Med. Assoc. 235:1975–1979, 1976.
40. Pulimood, B.M., Knudsen, A., Coghill, N.F.: Gastric mucosa after partial gastectomy. Gut 17:463–470, 1976.
41. Doos, W.G., Wolff, W.I., Shinya, H., et al: CEA levels in patients with colorectal polyps. Cancer 36:1996–2003, 1975.
42. Alm, T., Wahren, B.: Carcinoembryonic antigen in hereditary adenomatosis of the colon and rectum. Scan. J. Gastroenterol. 10:875–879, 1975.
43. Guirgis, H.A., Lynch, H.T., Harris, R.E., et al: Carcinoembryonic antigen (CEA) in the cancer family syndrome. Cancer 42:1574–1578, 1978.
44. Sugarbaker, P.H., Zamcheck, N., Moore, F.D.K.: Assessment of serial carcinoembryonic antigen (CEA) in postoperative management of colon and rectal cancer. Cancer 38:2310–2315, 1976.
45. Nakamura, R.M., Plow, E.F., Edgington, T.S.: Current status of carcinoembryonic antigen (CEA) and CEA-S assays in the evaluation of neoplasm of the gastrointestinal tract. Ann. Clin. Lab. Sci. 8:4–10, 1978.
46. Dykes, P.W., King, J.: Progress report: Carcinoembryonic antigen. Gut 13:1000–1013, 1972.
47. Laurence, J.J.R., Stevens, U., Bettelheim, R., et al: Evaluation of the role of plasma carcinoembryonic antigen (CEA) in the diagnosis of gastrointestinal, mammary and bronchial carcinoma. Br. Med. J. 3:605–609, 1972.
48. Concannon, J.P., Dalbow, M.H., Frich, J.C.: Carcinoembryonic antigen (CEA) plasma levels in untreated cancer patients with metastatic disease. Radiology 108:191–193, 1973.
49. McNeil, B.J., Adelstein, J.: Determining the value of diagnostic and screening tests. J. Nucl. Med. 17:349–448, 1976.
50. Joint National Cancer Institute of Canada/American Cancer Society Investigation, a collaborative study of a test for carcinoembryonic antigen (CEA) in the sera of patients with carcinoma of the colon and rectum. Can. Med. Assoc. J.107:25–33, 1972.
51. March, J.P., Jaeger, P.H., Bertholet, M.M., et al: Detection of recurrence of large bowel carcinoma by radioimmunoassay of circulating carcinoembryonic antigen (CEA). Lancet 2:535–540, 1974.
52. MacKay, A.M., Patel, S., Carter, S., et al: Role of serial plasma CEA assays in detection of recurrent and metastatic colorectal carcinoma. Br. Med. J. 4:382–385, 1974.
53. Herrera, M.A., Chu, T.M., Holyoke, E.D.: Carcinoembryonic antigen (CEA) as a prognostic and monitoring test in clinically complete resection of colorectal carcinoma. Ann. Surg. 183:5–9, 1976.
54. Martin, E.W., James, K.K., Hurtubise, P.E., et al: The use of CEA as an

early indicator for gastrointestinal tumor recurrence and second-look procedures. *Cancer* 39:440–446, 1977.

55. Ratcliffe, J.G., Wood, C.B., Burt, R.W., *et al:* Patterns of change in carcinoembryonic antigen (CEA) levels in patients developing recurrent colorectal cancer. Sixth Meeting of the International Research Group for Carcinoembryonic Proteins held in Marburg/Lahn, W. Germany 17–21 Sept., 1978.

56. Martin E.W., Cooperman, M., Carey, L.C., *et al:* Sixty second-look procedures indicated primarily by rise in serial CEA. Thirteenth Annual Meeting Association for Academic Surgery, November 1979.

57. Ona, F., Zamcheck, N., Dhar, P., *et al:* Carcinoembryonic antigen (CEA) in the diagnosis of pancreatic cancer. *Cancer* 31:324–327, 1973.

58. Sheedy, P.F., Stephens, D.H., Hattery, R.R.: Computed tomography in the evaluation of patients with suspected carcinoma of the pancreas. *Radiology* 124:731–740, 1977.

59. Stanley, R.J., Sagel, S.S., Levitt, R.G.: Computed tomographic evaluation of the pancreas. *Radiology* 124:715–720, 1977.

60. Booth, S.N., Jamison, G.G., King, J.P.G., *et al:* Carcinoembryonic antigen in the management of colorectal carcinoma. *Br. Med. J.* 4:183–187, 1974.

61. Sugarbaker, P.H.: Carcinoma of the colon—Prognosis and operative choice. *Curr. Probl. Surg.* 18:755–802, 1981.

62. Wanebo, H.J., Rao, B., Pinsky, C.M., *et al:* Preoperative carcinoembryonic antigen level as a prognostic indicator in colorectal cancer. *N. Eng. J. Med.* 299:448–457, 1978.

63. Goslin, R., Steele, G., MacIntyre, J., *et al:* The use of preoperative plasma CEA levels for the stratification of patients after curative resection of colorectal cancer. *Ann. Surg.* 192:747–751, 1980.

64. Denk, H., Tappeiner, G., Eckerstorfer, R., *et al:* Carcinoembryonic antigen (CEA) in gastrointestinal and extragastrointestinal tumors and its relationship to tumor cell differentiation. *Int. J. Cancer* 10:262–272, 1972.

65. Kalser, M.H., Barkin, J.S., Redlhammer, D., *et al:* Circulating carcinoembryonic antigen in pancreatic carcinoma. *Cancer* 42:1468–1471, 1978.

66. Wang, D.Y., Bulbrook, R.D., Hayward, J.C., *et al:* Relationship between plasma carcinoembryonic antigen and prognosis in women with breast cancer. *Eur. J. Cancer* 11:615–618, 1975.

67. Haagensen, D.E., Kister, S.J., Vandervoord, J.P., *et al:* Evaluation of carcinoembryonic antigen as a plasma monitor for human breast carcinoma. *Cancer* 42:1512–1519, 1978.

68. Myers, R.E., Sutherland, D.J., Meakin, J.W., *et al:* Carcinoembryonic antigen in breast cancer. *Cancer* 42:1520–1526, 1978.

69. Tormey, D.C., Waalkes, T.P.: Clinical correlation between CEA and breast cancer. *Cancer* 42:1507–1511, 1978.

70. Dent, P.G., McCulloch, P.B., Wesley-James, O., *et al:* Measurement of carcinoembryonic antigen in patients with bronchogenic carcinoma. *Cancer* 42:1484–1491, 1978.

71. Concannon, J.P., Dalbow, M.H., Hodgson, S.E., *et al:* Prognostic value of preoperative carcinoembryonic antigen (CEA) plasma levels in patients with bronchogenic carcinoma. *Cancer* 42:1477–1483, 1978.

72. Dhar, P., Moore, T., Zamcheck, N., *et al:* Carcinoembryonic antigen (CEA)

in colonic cancer. Use in preoperative and postoperative diagnosis and prognosis. *J. Am. Med. Assoc.* 221:31–35, 1972.

73. LoGerfo, P., Herter, F., Hansen, J.G.: Tumor-associated antigen in patients with carcinoma of the colon. *Am. J. Surg.* 123:127–131, 1972.

74. Livingston, A.S., Hampson, L.G., Schuster, J., et al: Carcinoembryonic antigen in the diagnosis and management of colorectal carcinoma. *Arch. Surg.* 109:259–264, 1974.

75. Sorokin, J.J., Sugarbaker, P.H., Zamcheck, P.M., et al: Serial carcinoembryonic antigen assays. Use in detection of cancer recurrence. *J. Am. Med. Assoc.* 228:49–53, 1974.

76. Oh, J.H., MacLean, L.D.: Prognostic use of preoperative and immediate postoperative carcinoembryonic antigen determinations in colonic cancer. *Can. J. Surg.* 20:64–67, 1977.

77. Gianola, F.J., Sugarbaker, P.H., Dwyer, A., et al: Detection of occult metastases in patients with primary colorectal cancer diseases of the colon and rectum (in press).

78. Vider, M., Kashmiri, R., Hunder, L., et al: Carcinoembryonic antigen (CEA) monitoring in the management of radiotherapeutic patients. *Oncology* 30:257–272, 1974.

79. Vider, M., Kashmiri, R., Meeker, W.R., et al: Carcinoembryonic antigen (CEA) monitoring in the management of radiotherapeutic and chemotherapeutic patients. *Am. J. Roentgenol.* 124:630–635, 1975.

80. Sugarbaker, P.H., Bloomer, W.D., Corbett, E.D., et al: Carcinoembryonic antigen (CEA) monitoring of radiation therapy for colorectal cancer. *Am. J. Roentgenol.* 127:641–644, 1976.

81. Donaldson, E., Van Nagell, J.R., Wood, E.G., et al: Carcinoembryonic antigen in patients with radiation therapy for invasive squamous cell carcinoma of the cervis. *Am. J. Roentgenol.* 127:829–831, 1976.

82. Mulcare, R., LoGerfo, P.: Tumor associated antigen in chemotherapy of solid tumors. *J. Surg. Oncol.* 4:407–417, 1972.

83. Herrea, M.A., Chu, T.M., Holyoke, E.D., et al: CEA monitoring of palliative treatment for colorectal carcinoma. *Ann. Surg.* 185:23–30, 1977.

84. Young, V.L., Kashmiri, R., Hazen, R., et al: Usefulness of serial carcinoembryonic antigen (CEA) determinations in monitoring chemotherapy. *South. Med. J.* 69:1274–1276, 1976.

85. Mayer, R.J., Garnick, M.B., Steele, G.D., et al: Carcinoembryonic antigen (CEA) as a monitor of chemotherapy in disseminated colorectal cancer. *Cancer* 42:1428–1433, 1978.

86. Rieger, A., Wahren, B.: CEA levels at recurrence and metastases: Importance for detecting secondary disease. *Scand. J. Gastroent.* 10:869–874, 1975.

87. Herrera, M.A., Chu, T.M., Holyoke, E.D.: Carcinoembryonic antigen (CEA) as a prognostic and monitoring test in clinically complete resection of colorectal carcinoma. *Ann. Surg.* 183:5–9, 1976.

88. Wanebo, H.J., Stearns, M., Schwartz, M.K.: Use of CEA as an indicator of early recurrence and as a guide to a selected second-look procedure in patients with colorectal cancer. *Ann. Surg.* 188:481–493, 1978.

89. Minton, J.P., James, K.K., Hurtubise, P.E., et al: The use of serial carcinoembryonic antigen determinations to predict recurrence of carcinoma of

the colon and the time for a second-look operation. *Surg. Gynecol. Obstet.* 147:208–210, 1978.

90. Minton, J.P., Martin, E.W., Jr.: The use of serial CEA determinations to predict recurrence of colon cancer and when to do a second-look operation. *Cancer* 42:1422–1427, 1978.

91. Beatty, J.D., Romero, C., Brown, P.W., *et al:* Clinical value of carcinoembryonic antigen. Diagnosis, prognosis, and follow-up of patients with cancer. *Arch. Surg.* 114:563–567, 1979.

92. Martin, E.W., Cooperman, M., King, G., *et al:* A retrospective and prospective study of serial CEA determinations in the early detection of recurrent colon cancer. *Am. J. Surg.* 137:167–169, 1979.

93. Cohen, A.M., Wood, W.C.: Carcinoembryonic antigen levels and an indicator for reoperation in patients with carcinoma of the colon and rectum. *Surg. Gynecol. Obstet.* 149:22–26, 1979.

94. Steele, G., Jr., Zamcheck, N., Wilson, R., *et al:* Results of CEA-initiated second-look surgery for recurrent colorectal cancer. *Am. J. Surg.* 139:544–548, 1980.

95. Gray, B.N., Walker, C., Barnard, R.: Value of serial carcinoembryonic antigen determinations for early detection of recurrent cancer. *Med. J. Aust.* 1:177–178, 1981.

96. Persijn, J.P., Hart, A.A.M.: Prognostic significance of CEA in colorectal cancer: A statistical study. *J. Clin. Chem. Clin. Biochem.* 19:1117–1123, 1981.

97. Wedell, J., Meier Zu Eissen, P., Luu, T.H., *et al:* A retrospective study of serial CEA determinations in the early detection of recurrent colorectal cancer. *Dis. Col. Rect.* 24:618–621, 1981.

98. Tate, H.: Plasma CEA in the post-surgical monitoring of colorectal carcinoma. *Br. J. Cancer* 46:323–330, 1982.

99. Szymendera, J.J., Nowacki, M.P., Szawlowski, A.W., *et al:* Predictive value of plasma CEA levels: Preoperative prognosis and postoperative monitoring of patients with colorectal carcinoma. *Dis. Col. Rect.* 25:46–52, 1982.

100. Staab, H.J., Anderer, F.A., Hornung, A., *et al:* Doubling time of circulating CEA and its relation to survival of patients with recurrent colorectal cancer. *Br. J. Cancer* 46:773–781, 1982.

101. Koch, M., Washer, G., Gaedke, H., *et al:* Carcinoembryonic antigen: Usefulness as a postsurgical method in the detection of recurrence in Dukes stages B_2 and C colorectal cancers. *JNCI* 69:813–815, 1982.

102. Finlay, I.G., McArdle, C.S.: Role of carcinoembryonic antigen in detection of asymptomatic disseminated disease in colorectal carcinoma. *Br. Med. J.* 286:1242–1244, 1983.

103. Carlsson, U., Stewenius, J., Ekelund, G., *et al:* Is CEA analysis of value in screening for recurrences after surgery for colorectal carcinoma? *Dis. Col. Rect.* 26:369–373, 1983.

104. Rittgers, R.A., Steele, G., Zamcheck, N., *et al:* Transient carcinoembryonic antigen (CEA) elevations following resection of colorectal cancer: A limitation in the use of serial CEA levels as an indicator for second-look surgery. *JNCI* 61:315–318, 1978.

105. Minton, P.: Second-look surgery in colon and rectal cancer patients with rising CEA (submitted for publication).

106. Attiyeh, F.F., Stearns, M.W.: Second-look laparotomy based on CEA elevations in colorectal cancer. *Cancer* 47:2199–2125, 1981.
107. August, D.A., Sugarbaker, P.H., Schneider, P.D.: Lymphatic dissemination of hepatic metastases: Implications for the follow-up and treatment of patients with colorectal cancer. *Cancer* (in press).
108. Goldenberg, D.M., Deland, F., Kim, E., *et al:* Use of radiolabeled antibodies to carcinoembryonic antigen for the detection and localization of diverse cancers by external photoscanning. *N. Eng. J. Med.* 298:1384–1388, 1978.
109. Sugarbaker, P.H., Beard, J.O., Drum, D.E.: Detection of hepatic metastases from cancer of the breast. *Am. J. Surg.* 133:531–535, 1977.
110. McCartney, W.H., Hoffer, P.B.: Carcinoembryonic antigen assay: An adjunct to liver scanning in hepatic metastases detection. *Cancer* 42:1457–1462, 1978.
111. McCartney, W.H., Hoffer, P.B.: The value of carcinoembryonic antigen as adjunct to the radiological colon examination in the diagnosis of malignancy. *Radiology* 110:325–328, 1974.

Chapter 6

Active Specific Immunotherapy as an Adjunct to the Treatment of Metastatic Solid Tumors: Present and Future Prospects

MARC E. KEY, HERBERT C. HOOVER, JR., AND MICHAEL G. HANNA, JR.

Contents

Introduction

Surgery remains the most effective therapy for the majority of solid tumors, offering the best possibility of cure or palliation in most circumstances. Further improvements in surgical techniques are unlikely to produce vastly improved cure rates because anatomically defined limits have already been reached for the excision of most tumors (1). Adjuvant chemotherapy and radiation therapy play relatively minor roles in the treatment of cancer because tumors develop resistance to the therapy or because dosages are limited by toxicity considerations (2). Thus, new strategies for the treatment of metastatic solid tumors are desperately needed (3).

This need has spurred a decade-long struggle to implement biologic therapy as an adjunct to standard cancer treatment. In current terminology, immunotherapy is considered to be a subcategory of biologic therapy, with two general forms: nonspecific and specific. In nonspecific immunotherapy, a biologic response modifier (biologic or chemical) is administered in an attempt to activate general host defense systems to restrict the growth of tumors. In specific immunotherapy, vaccines of tumor cells or tumor cell fractions are administered to the host to augment or induce host response to tumor-associated antigens (TAAs).

Immunotherapy gained popularity as a treatment in the 1960s because of data from experimental tumor models that indicated that both specific stimulation of the immune system with antigen-bearing tumor cells and nonspecific stimulation with bacteria, viruses, or other adjuvant-type compounds could enhance the immune response in animals and prevent recurrence of, or delay growth of, experimentally transplanted tumors. Since immunotherapy was most effective against small tumor burdens, investigators began to study immunotherapy as a possible treatment for minimal residual disease. These studies were based on the premise that treatment of animals with minimal residual disease would be analogous to postsurgical treatment of cancer in humans. However, this analogy was frequently stretched beyond the limits of sound logic in that immunotherapy was often begun within a day or two of the tumor transplant. Such artificially induced foci of tumor cells were unlikely to be representative of the well-vascularized metastases of a cancer patient. Given the variability of clinical presentation, it is not surprising that randomized trials of immunotherapy, often based on artifactual tumor models, did not succeed in reducing the incidence of recurring cancer.

The vast majority of past clinical trials of immunotherapy have used primarily nonspecific methods. Most agents utilized in these experimental trials stimulate the reticuloendothelial system. These agents also produce tumoricidal macrophages after in vitro and in vivo activation. This nonspecific tumoricidal activity is of interest to immunotherapists because it is different from the classical immune response. The question of whether tumor cells are antigenic or whether cancer patients can respond to tumor antigens is unimportant in nonspecific immunotherapy. Furthermore, macrophages are widely distributed throughout the body and infiltrate virtually all types of solid malignancies (4). Although nonspecific immunotherapy and macrophage activation have shown some promise in animal models, especially when animals were given less than the minimum lethal dose of tumor cells (5), macrophage activation in cancer patients has been less effective (6). The most striking examples of tumor regression occurred when BCG was directly injected into cutaneous malignant melanomas (7,8). Unfortunately, this procedure has limited applicability for inaccessible visceral metastases.

In this chapter, we discuss some of the issues implicit in the rationale for active specific immunotherapy and review recent experimental and clinical findings that indicate, in contrast to the earlier immunotherapy trials mentioned above, that this mode of therapy may play an adjunctive role in the treatment of cancer in the future.

Aspects of Tumor Biology Pertinent to the Rationale of Active Specific Immunotherapy

Antigenicity of Tumors

The exquisite specificity of the immune system, as opposed to the generalized toxicity of standard chemotherapy or radiation therapy, makes active specific immunotherapy a desirable approach. Implicit in the rationale for this therapy is the existence on tumor cells of distinct tumor antigens that are not expressed or are expressed to a lesser extent on normal cells. These TAAs must be available on the tumor cell surface to serve as effective sites for antibody-mediated or cell-mediated destruction. The assumption that human tumors are antigenic is founded largely on the extensively documented findings that TAAs are present on chemically and virally induced tumors in animals (9–11). Whether the antigenicity of these experimentally induced tumors implies the existence of comparable antigens in naturally occurring human tumors is presently a subject of major controversy (12–15).

Tumor transplantation studies in animals have convincingly demonstrated the presence of TAAs that can function as strong transplantation antigens. However, these techniques cannot be used in studies with humans. To circumvent this limitation, various in vitro assays have been devised to study potential antitumor immune response in humans. However, currently these assays have not succeeded in elucidating the role of the immune response in host resistance to cancer (16).

The demonstration of tumor-specific immunoglobulin in the serum or in tumors of certain cancer patients provides a more convincing argument for the existence of TAAs in human tumors. Although the presence of antibody is by no means universal, its presence has been demonstrated in a sufficiently diverse population of cancer patients to suggest that this is not an infrequent occurrence (17,18). Recent studies by Jessup et al (*personal communication*) have shown that humoral immunity to autologous tumor is significantly boosted in patients treated by specific immunization with their own tumor cells. Thus, the presence of antibody in some cancer patients, but not in others, may reflect the degree to which these patients have been sensitized to their tumors rather than to any inherent deficiency in the antigenicity of the tumors themselves.

Recent technologic developments using murine monoclonal antibodies have allowed preliminary characterization of the surface of tumor cells at the molecular level. In particular, various molecular components of human malignant melanoma cells have been identified that are restricted to, or preferentially expressed on, malignant cells (19,20). For these components to be exploited for specific immunization, they must be shown to be antigenic in the host of origin. This antigenicity has not yet been demonstrated. Whether some of these unique determinants may ultimately prove to be the elusive TAAs remains to be determined.

A more direct approach to the identification and categorization of potentially antigenic molecular determinants on the surface of human tumor cells would be with monoclonal antibodies of human origin, or even better, with monoclonal antibodies derived from cancer patients. Recently Haspel et al (21) reported the development of stable clones of human B lymphocytes that produce tumor-specific monoclonal antibody. These clones were derived from peripheral blood lymphocytes of colorectal cancer patients who were specifically immunized against their tumor (22). Of the 30 monoclonal antibodies developed, 16 showed preferential binding to tumor cell surface antigens. In contrast to murine monoclonal antibodies, human monoclonal antibodies may be appropriate probes for the isolation and characterization of TAAs relevant to human cancer. These recent advances in the field of monoclonal antibody technology suggest that tumor cells possess unique molecular determinants that are quantitatively or qualitatively different from corresponding determinants on normal tissue. Furthermore, at least some of these unique determinants are immunologically recognized in the host of origin (21) and thus are, by definition, TAAs.

Immunogenicity of Tumor-Associated Antigens

Presumably the presence of unique antigenic determinants on tumor cell surfaces is the minimum requirement for immunologic rejection; however, their presence in itself does not guarantee that such immune responses can, in fact, occur. Experimental data on immunologic rejection of cancer in animals suggest that such rejection is rare and usually occurs only after extensive immunologic manipulation. Is it possible that human cancers can be similarly controlled by appropriate immunologic manipulation? The central hypothesis underlying all attempts at specific immunotherapy is that this will ultimately prove to be the case.

This hypothesis, however, has been viewed by some investigators as an unwarranted extension of laboratory findings with little relevance to naturally occurring neoplasms (12,13). For example, some studies using tumor transplantation techniques have been unable to demonstrate the immunogenicity of a wide variety of naturally occurring mouse (23) and rat (24) tumors. These results were in sharp contrast to earlier studies, which showed that experimentally induced animal tumors were highly immunogenic as defined by the ability of immunized mice to reject subsequent transplants of tumor tissue (9–11). According to Hewitt and co-workers

(12,13,23), these results imply that experimental tumors frequently express artifactual immunogenicity imposed on them by viral antigens, strong chemical carcinogens, or histocompatibility differences between tumor and host and that these expressions of immunogenicity bear little relevance to the situation encountered with naturally occurring malignancies.

To address the question of immunogenicity of naturally occurring tumors experimentally, several points must be considered: (a) New tumor models must be developed that minimize the potential problem of artifactual immunogenicity as discussed by Hewitt (12,13,23). (b) Tumors in different species of laboratory animals must be investigated before the results can be extrapolated to all naturally occurring tumors. (c) In any given tumor model, the best available methodology must be used for attempting immunization to putative TAAs. Using a systematically developed immunization protocol, we recently tested four guinea pig leukemias with diverse backgrounds for immunogenicity in their syngeneic host (25). Two of these leukemias were appropriate models for the assessment of immunogenicity because of their recent origin and unknown (natural) etiology, whereas two other leukemias could be classified as experimental and prone to artifactual immunogenicity (Table 6-1). Regardless of etiology, appropriately immunized guinea pigs were capable of rejecting challenges with leukemia cells up to 100 to 1,000 times the minimum lethal dose (Table 6-2). These studies clearly demonstrated that naturally occurring malignancies of recent origin could induce protective levels of immunity by appropriate immunologic manipulation and suggested that similar immunologic manipulation may be of some benefit in the treatment of naturally occurring cancers in man as well.

The importance of the optimum immunization procedures used in these immunogenicity studies must not be underestimated. These procedures were developed for inducing immunity to the syngeneic Line 10 (L10) hepatocarcinoma in the relatively carcinogen-resistant, inbred strain 2 guinea pig. The guinea pig model has received less attention than mouse and rat tumor models, which have been at the center of the controversy

Table 6-1. Characteristics of leukemias of strain 2 guinea pigs.

Leukemia	Type	Etiology	Year of origin	Transplant generation	Colony of origin[a]	Present colony	In vitro passage
L$_2$C	B Cell	Unknown	1953	unknown	NCI	FCRF	None
L76	B Cell	Unknown	1976	4th	FCRF	FCRF	None
K77	B Cell	TPA-induced[b]	1977	2nd	FCRF	FCRF	None
KSL	B Cell	Unknown	1979	4th	FCRF	FCRF	None

[a] NCI, National Cancer Institute's colony during 1953; FCRF, National Cancer Institute's colony maintained at the Frederick Cancer Research Facility.
[b] TPA = 12-0 tetradecanoylphorbol-13-acetate.
  Data taken in part from (25).

Table 6-2. Immunogenicity of leukemias of strain 2 guinea pigs.

Group	Vaccine	Challenge dose	No. survivors/ total	Median survival time (days)
1	None	10^4	0/5	33
2	None	10^5	0/5	27
3	K77 alone	10^4	2/5	106
4	K77 alone	10^5	0/5	93
5	K77 + BCG	10^4	5/5[a]	>207
6	K77 + BCG	10^5	5/5[a]	>207
7	None	10^4	0/5	28
8	None	10^5	0/5	24
9	L76 alone	10^4	0/5	31
10	L76 alone	10^5	0/5	24
11	L76 + BCG	10^4	5/5[a]	>207
12	L76 + BCG	10^5	5/5[a]	>207
13	None	10^5	0/5	25
14	None	10^6	0/5	21
15	L_2C alone	10^5	0/5	27
16	L_2C alone	10^6	0/5	20
17	L_2C + BCG	10^5	5/5[a]	>207
18	L_2C + BCG	10^6	5/5[a]	>207
19	None	10^5	0/5	139
20	None	10^6	0/5	121
21	KSL alone	10^5	0/5	144
22	KSL alone	10^6	0/5	122
23	KSL + BCG	10^5	4/5[b]	>321
24	KSL + BCG	10^6	2/5	123
25	KSL alone (×6)[c]	10^5	0/3	150
26	KSL + BCG (×6)	10^5	3/3	>247
27	None	10^6	0/5	122
28	KSL + CFA[d]	10^6	2/10	158

[a] Value significantly different from untreated control (P = .0040; Fisher's exact test, 1-tailed).
[b] Value significantly different from untreated control (P = .0238; Fisher's exact test, 1-tailed).
[c] Received a total of six vaccinations rather than the standard three vaccinations.
[d] Received 0.1 mL of complete Freund's adjuvant (CFA) in place of BCG.
   Data taken in part from (25).

about the relevance of animal models to human cancer (12,13). However, our recent studies have underscored the utility of the guinea pig tumor model: We have demonstrated the potential immunogenicity of the transplantable L10 hepatocarcinoma for development of effective cell-mediated immunity in tumor-bearing guinea pigs (26–31) and have demonstrated the practical translation of the immunization procedures developed in the model to clinical treatment of human colorectal cancer (22). A major factor in the success of these studies was the use of optimum immunization procedures.

In summary, the important question that must be asked with regard to the potential of immunologic intervention in malignant disease is not whether naturally occurring tumors are immunogenic under normal, untreated conditions, but rather whether they are potentially immunogenic.

Immunologic Heterogeneity of Tumors

The concept of tumor progression implies that tumors are composed of populations of cells that continually give rise to mutant cells, a few of which may gain an advantage over others and predominate under selective conditions of growth, thus resulting in a markedly heterogeneous tumor. The heterogeneous nature of tumors also extends to include antigenic or immunogenic variability among different tumor cell subpopulations (32–41). The importance of the concept of immunologic heterogeneity to the problem of tumor recurrence and metastases is illustrated by the studies of Pimm and Baldwin (35), who showed that tumors recurring at the site of excision of a primary tumor were immunologically distinct from the primary tumor. Other studies have shown that tumor cells within metastases also may contain antigens different from those of cells of the primary tumor, or may have completely lost some antigens (32,37,38).

The presence of immunologic heterogeneity within a tumor has profound implications for the practical application of specific immunotherapy in the treatment of cancer patients. Potentially, the continual pressures of an immune attack could eliminate the predominating antigenic subpopulations, allowing the expansion of minor subpopulations of antigenic variants or the development of new antigenic variants (40). Indeed, should this be the case, even under the best of conditions, specific immunotherapy would not be curative.

Several experimental protocols utilizing animal models to assess the feasibility of specific immunotherapy as a relevant method of a cancer treatment have yielded encouraging results (26,42–47). These studies, however, like other studies with experimental animal tumors, use transplantable tumors, which may not be analogous to primary tumors. For example, it has been suggested that primary or early-passage tumors may exhibit marked immunologic heterogeneity, but that this heterogeneity is lost as a consequence of repeated in vivo passage (48). The significance of such immunologic variability, or the lack thereof, must be taken into account in the design and evaluation of immunotherapy models using transplantable tumors.

In our studies of active specific immunotherapy using the guinea pig L10 hepatocarcinoma model, we have found that poorly immunogenic variants of the parental L10 tumor occasionally emerge following treatment of tumor-bearing guinea pigs with active specific immunotherapy (49). These tumors grow progressively and eventually kill their host despite aggressive immunotherapy. Yet, despite these occasional failures, immunotherapy was successful in curing most guinea pigs. These results suggest that specific immunotherapy may still be successfully applied even to tumors in which immunologic heterogeneity exists.

Recent studies have shown that two highly metastatic variants of a transformed hamster cell line were nonimmunogenic by classical immunization and rechallenge experiments. However, immunization with the parent cell line afforded complete protection from challenge with either metastatic variant (50). Thus, although the metastatic variants had lost the ability to immunize (loss of immunogenicity), they, nevertheless, retained antigenicity as demonstrated by immunization with the parent tumor line. The finding that metastases, even poorly immunogenic metastases, are susceptible to immune rejection after immunization with the parent tumor is encouraging for the practical application of immunotherapy. This finding would indicate that a patient's primary tumor could serve as the source of immunogen for immunizations targeted for metastases.

Even if potentially effective strategies for specific immunotherapy are developed, it is unclear how antigenic heterogeneity of tumor cell subpopulations will influence the practical application of this treatment (41,51). If antigenic heterogeneity represents primarily quantitative differences among tumor cell subpopulations, as suggested by our own as well as other studies (39,49,52), then the effectiveness of immunotherapy will be proportional to the strength of the immune response elicited by immunization. If qualitative differences in TAAs exist among tumor subpopulations, as suggested by several studies (32,39,40), then the effectiveness of immunotherapy in eradicating metastasis after immunization with the primary tumor will depend on the degree to which the individual subpopulations are represented within the primary tumor. On the whole, the antigenic repertoire of the individual metastatic clones would be expected to be represented in the primary tumor. However, if, by a process of tumor progression, metastases develop antigenic subpopulations that are completely distinct from those of the primary tumor, then immunotherapy by itself would not be curative. Nevertheless, immunotherapy combined with other treatments, each acting by a different mechanism and each selecting a different spectrum of resistant clones, could interact synergistically in the eradication of tumor. For example, we have recently shown that immunotherapy significantly enhances the therapeutic effects of subsequent chemotherapy (53,54). Therefore, even in tumors that are weakly immunogenic or that demonstrate antigenic heterogeneity, combination active specific immunotherapy plus chemotherapy may be able to eradicate the residual tumor cells that resist immunotherapy alone.

Some of the clinical failures of active specific immunotherapy that have been attributed to the existence of antigenic heterogeneity within tumors may, in fact, be the results of suboptimal methods of immunization. The immunogenic potential of many tumors or tumor cell clones may be below the threshold for natural stimulation of the immune system. Tumor antigens, however, like many other weak antigens that are unable to stimulate immune responses by themselves, often stimulate potent immune responses when administered with adjuvants (26,43,55,56). The weakly antigenic L10 tumor, for example, induces little immunity when inactivated tumor cells alone are used for immunization, but therapeutic levels of immunity are obtained when these cells are injected with any one of several adjuvants under restrictive regimens (26,43,57). Thus, the failures of active specific immunotherapy in some studies may be related to numerous different factors, ranging from technical and methodological problems associated with vaccination, to the induction of tumor-related immunosuppression, or to the selection of antigenic variants.

Immunologic heterogeneity within a primary tumor has profound implications for researchers studying immunologic interactions within tumors, as well as for clinicians attempting to treat cancer patients with specific immunotherapy. Only with rational translation of sound basic research to the clinical setting will we be able to answer definitively the question of whether specific immunotherapy can succeed in the face of immunologic diversity within tumors. On the other hand, it is also premature to assume that this diversity will automatically doom specific immunotherapy to failure.

Experimental Studies of Active Specific Immunotherapy in the Guinea Pig Tumor Model System

A major contribution to understanding the principles of active specific immunotherapy has been the development and biologic characterization of adequate experimental models that fulfill the requirements for studying effective immunotherapy of established tumors.

Studies have previously demonstrated that a transplanted, syngeneic L10 hepatocarcinoma established in the skin of inbred guinea pigs (strain 2) regressed, and regional metastases were eliminated after intratumoral injections of adequate doses of viable BCG (58). In the course of this reaction, systemic tumor immunity developed. Further studies showed that this immunity was effective in eradicating both regional and systemic malignancies (27).

This intratumoral model of immunotherapy is limited by the fact that many clinical tumors are not accessible to direct injection. Consequently, the guinea pig hepatocarcinoma model was modified to make it more relevant to the clinical situation. A BCG-L10 tumor cell vaccine was developed that successfully stimulated systemic tumor immunity in strain 2 guinea pigs. A series of studies (26,28–31,59,60) demonstrated that BCG admixed with tumor cells could induce a degree of systemic tumor immunity that could eliminate a small disseminated tumor burden (Table 6-3) when the vaccine was carefully controlled for such variables as the num-

Table 6-3. Survival of guinea pigs after immunotherapy of established metastases.

Vaccination schedule (days after tumor injection)	Survival of guinea pigs (%)	Size of pulmonary metastases (day measured)
No vaccinations	0	
1, 7, 14	70	<5 cells (day 1)
4, 11, 18	65	5–10 cells (day 4)
7, 14, 21	40	0.1–0.2 mm (days 7 to 10)
10, 17, 24	20	0.35–0.5 mm (days 21 to 24)

Note: Inbred strain 2 guinea pigs were given intravenous injections of 10^6 syngeneic L10 hepato-carcinoma cells. Each animal subsequently received two intradermal injections of 10^7 BCG admixed with viable but nontumorigenic L10 cells that had been exposed to x-rays (20,000 rads) and one injection of irradiated L10 cells alone. The data are pooled from three experiments (a total of 45 guinea pigs per group). Data taken in part from (53).

ber of tumor cells (10^7 optimal), the ratio of viable BCG organisms to tumor cells (1:1), the maintenance of metabolically viable tumor cells, and the vaccination regimen (3 vaccines, 1 week apart). Most prior clinical trials of tumor vaccines have used either nonviable (metabolically inactive) autologous tumor cells or allogeneic (tissue culture) tumor cells, both found to be totally ineffective in the guinea pig model.

Using the L10 hepatocarcinoma as a model tumor system, we investigated some mechanisms by which tumors evade host defense systems. These studies suggested that the anatomic characteristics of the developing tumor foci restrict various aspects of the host-tumor interaction. These restrictions may protect tumors not only from immunotherapy but from other forms of treatment as well (61,62). Recent studies have shown that blood-borne antitumor antibodies do not penetrate uniformly into all growing areas of solid tumors, but are restricted to those areas of the tumor that are highly vascularized or hemorrhagic (62). Presumably other blood-borne substances, such as chemotherapeutic agents, encounter similar barriers, which limit their access to portions of the tumor. In vitro studies have shown that the penetration of drugs into avascular tumor spheroids of 0.25 mm diameter is poor (63), and in vivo studies have shown that solid tumors as small as 1 mm in diameter frequently contain areas that are poorly vascularized (64). These characteristics of microscopic metastatic foci may not only limit the effectiveness of immune effector components and cytotoxic drugs, but in the case of the latter, may increase the chance for selection of drug-resistant tumor populations because some cells are exposed to subtherapeutic amounts of the drug. In this way, solid tumor nodules may serve as pharmacologic sanctuaries, allowing even drug-sensitive tumor cells to continue to grow. The resultant continued growth of the tumor could lead to the conclusion that the tumor is drug-resistant.

These findings suggest that a successful therapeutic approach might be a process that would both disrupt these anatomic barriers and deliver cytotoxic agents to the tumor(s). One host response that potentially could achieve the first goal is an induced cell-mediated hypersensitivity reaction analogous to delayed-cutaneous hypersensitivity (DCH) but occurring at distant (micrometastatic) sites. This immune-mediated hypersensitivity, followed by delivery of blood-borne toxic substances to tumors, could be more effective than either therapy alone.

To explore this issue, morphologic studies were undertaken in the guinea pig L10 tumor model. These studies revealed that host cell-mediated hypersensitivity reactions occurred at sites of pulmonary metastases in immunized guinea pigs (53,61). These nodules were infiltrated by a predominantly mononuclear cell population made up of lymphocytes and cells of the macrophage-histiocyte series. This infiltration disrupted the typical compact architecture of the tumor foci (Figs. 6-1,6-2).

The nature of the anatomic alterations in metastatic nodules was explored further by use of an anti-L10 monoclonal antibody (D3) as a probe to assess vascular permeability within tumors (54). This tumor-specific monoclonal antibody was injected intravenously into untreated and vaccinated tumor-bearing guinea pigs at a time determined histologically to be the peak of cell-mediated hypersensitivity reaction in the metastatic nodules. The D3 monoclonal antibody was chosen because of its ability to bind to a tumor-associated antigen and to remain localized at the site of extravasation for extended periods of time (62). After injection of the D3 antibody, an immunoperoxidase staining technique was used to localize monoclonal antibody within metastases. Morphometric analysis of antibody distribution showed that significantly more antibody accumulated in tumors of vaccinated guinea pigs than in comparable tumors of untreated guinea pigs (Table 6-4). These findings suggested that a treatment strategy

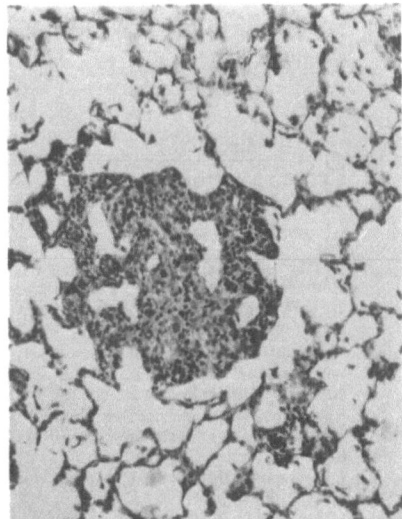

Figure 6-1. Metastatic L10 tumor nodule in lung of guinea pig seven days after first vaccination (14 days after tumor challenge). Nodule is being infiltrated by mononuclear cells (hematoxylin and eosin, ×250). Figure taken from (53).

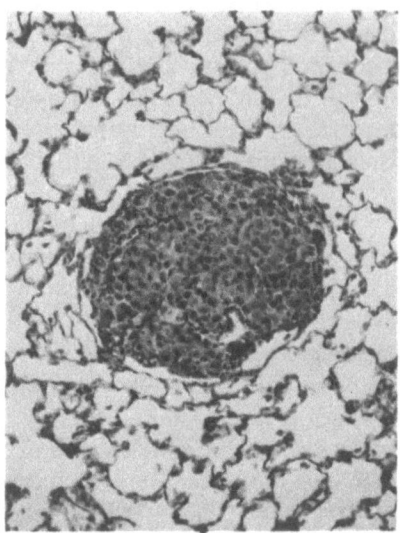

Figure 6-2. Metastatic nodule in lung of control guinea pig 21 days after intravenous injection of L10 cells. Nodule (diameter, 0.35 mm) has numerous mitotic figures and is highly vascularized. There is no evidence of host cell-mediated inflammation (hematoxylin and eosin, ×250). Figure taken from (53).

that combined active immunotherapy with the intravenous delivery of cytotoxic substances, such as chemotherapeutic agents, monoclonal antibodies, or immunoconjugates, might be more effective than any single approach.

To test this hypothesis we challenged strain 2 guinea pigs intravenously with 10^6 L10 cells (100 times the minimum lethal dose). The median survival was 56 days. Treatment with therapeutic doses of cyclophos-

Table 6-4. Vascular patterns and permeability in pulmonary metastases of the L10 hepatocarcinoma after immunotherapy and chemotherapy.

Tumor source[a]	% of tumor positive for D3 antibody[b]	Average distance[c] between tumor cells and blood vessels (μm)
Untreated controls	8 ± 12[d]	58 ± 19
Vaccine-treated g.p.	63 ± 16[d]	32 ± 14[e]
Chemotherapy-treated g.p.	31 ± 23[d]	ND[f]

[a] Guinea pigs (g.p.) bearing pulmonary L10 tumors received no further treatment (untreated controls), received immunotherapy on days 10, 17, and 24 (vaccine-treated g.p.) or received cyclophosphamide on day 31 (chemotherapy-treated g.p.). Values are mean ± SD for a total of 10 untreated tumors, 8 vaccine-treated tumors, and 10 chemotherapy-treated tumors.

[b] D3 antibody was injected intravenously on day 31 in untreated and vaccinated g.p. and on day 38 in chemotherapy-treated g.p. Lungs were removed 24 h later, and distribution of D3 antibody in the pulmonary metastases was analyzed.

[c] Distances were measured on photographic enlargements of tumors.

[d] All three values are significantly different from each other ($P < .01$, Duncan's multiple range test).

[e] Significantly different from untreated controls ($P = .008$, Student's t-test).

[f] ND = not done.

Data taken in part from (54).

phamide (150 mg/kg) 1, 31, or 45 days after tumor cell injection resulted in no cures, but increased median survival times of the animals (Table 6-5). Survival of guinea pigs treated with immunotherapy followed by chemotherapy at the time of peak inflammatory disruption of metastases was significantly greater than that of animals treated with immunotherapy or chemotherapy alone (53,54).

When animals with L10 tumors were given combined immunotherapy and chemotherapy, the number of long-term survivors obtained was highly dependent on the timing of chemotherapy relative to immunotherapy (Table 6-5). In these studies, treatment was always delayed to day 10, regardless of whether immunotherapy or chemotherapy was the initial treatment, because by day 10, tumor-bearing animals were relatively unresponsive to single-modality treatment, and significant macroscopic tumor burdens were present. The best therapeutic results were achieved when chemotherapy was given ten days after the third immunization. Cyclophosphamide given at this time in conjunction with prior immunotherapy significantly increased the survival of tumor-bearing animals over that seen with immunotherapy alone (Table 6-5). In contrast, cyclophos-

Table 6-5. Effect of combined immunotherapy and chemotherapy on survival of guinea pigs bearing L10 tumors.[a]

Treatment		No. survivors/ total	Percentage	Significance[d]	
				Comparison with controls	Comparison with animals receiving immunotherapy alone
Immunotherapy[b]	Chemotherapy[c]				
None	None	0/15	0	—	0.042
None	Cyclophosphamide, day 1	0/15	0	—	0.042
None	Cyclophosphamide, day 31	0/15	0	—	0.042
None	BCNU, day 1	0/15	0	—	0.042
Days 10,17,24	None	5/15	33	0.042	—
Days 10,17,24	Cyclophosphamide, day 31	28/38	74	<0.001	0.011
Days 10,17,24	BCNU, day 31	9/15	60	<0.001	0.032
Days 20,27,34	Cyclophosphamide, day 10	3/15	20	0.224	0.427
Days 20,27,34	None	2/15	13	0.483	0.214

[a] Pulmonary L10 tumors were initiated on day 0 by the intravenous injection of 1×10^6 tumor cells.
[b] Immunotherapy was initiated on day 10 or 20 and consisted of three vaccinations spaced 1 week apart. The first two injections contained an admixture of 10^7 BCG and 10^7 L10 tumor cells. The third injection contained 10^7 L10 tumor cells alone.
[c] Chemotherapy was single intraperitoneal injection of either 150 mg/kg cyclophosphamide or 10 mg/kg BCNU.
[d] By Fisher's exact test, 2-tailed.
   Data taken in part from (54).

phamide administered at a later time did not result in increased survival of tumor-bearing animals (data not shown). Furthermore, when cyclophosphamide therapy was initiated on day 10 followed by immunotherapy (even though a significant reduction of tumor burden must have resulted from the chemotherapy), the survival was no better than with immunotherapy alone.

In each of these groups, some animals were killed on day 45 after tumor inoculation, and their lungs were removed and examined for evidence of macroscopic surface tumor colonies. Again, guinea pigs treated with immunotherapy followed by chemotherapy had significantly fewer pulmonary tumor foci than did untreated guinea pigs or guinea pigs given either immunotherapy or chemotherapy alone (Table 6-6).

The survival rate of tumor-bearing animals given immunotherapy followed by sublethal doses of N,N-bis(2-chloroethyl)-N-nitrosourea (BCNU) was also two times greater than that of animals given immunotherapy alone (53). These findings showed that strategically timed chemotherapy, combined with immunotherapy, can effectively double the number for survivors attainable with immunotherapy alone. Furthermore, we found that the synergistic effects obtained by combining immunotherapy with chemotherapy were not drug-specific, as evidenced by similar results obtained with BCNU. This suggested that other chemotherapeutic agents, in addition to those tested, probably would prove effective in similar protocols.

There are several possible explanations of how cytotoxic drugs work when administered after immunotherapy: (a) Tumor cells killed by drug therapy could shed tumor antigens, boosting the immune response. (b) The tumor burden could be reduced, or tumor-specific suppressor cells could be eliminated, allowing for more efficient expression of the immune

Table 6-6. Effect of combined immunochemotherapy on the number of pulmonary tumor nodules in L10 tumor-bearing guinea pigs.

Treatment[a]	Mean number lung nodules[b] on day 45	Range
None	48 ± 9	42–59
Immunotherapy alone	23 ± 7[c]	16–29
Chemotherapy alone	26 ± 11[c]	14–36
Immunotherapy & chemotherapy	1 ± 2[d]	0–4

[a] All animals received 10^6 L10 tumor cells intravenously on day 0. Animals received no further treatment or were treated with immunotherapy alone beginning on day 10, with cyclophosphamide alone (150 mg/kg) on day 31, or with the combination of immunotherapy and cyclophosphamide chemotherapy.
[b] Animals were killed and their lungs were fixed for 18 h in Bouin's solution. The macroscopically observable tumor colonies were counted (N = 3 animals/group).
[c] Value is significantly different from the untreated group ($P < .05$, Student's t-test).
[d] Value is significantly different from all other groups ($P < .01$, Student's t-test).
  Data taken in part from (54).

response. (c) Antitumor drugs could render tumor cells more susceptible to immune lysis. (d) Conversely, the immune reaction could injure tumor cells and make them more susceptible to chemotherapy. One additional mechanism by which tumor immunity may enhance chemotherapy is the disruption of the normal anatomic architecture of the metastatic lesions by the immune reaction. Our data are more consistent with the last mechanism. These reactions would not only significantly reduce tumor mass, but would also expose surviving tumor cells to blood-borne elements, which in our studies include cytotoxic drugs. The observation that chemotherapy was most effective in curing guinea pigs when given at the time of the peak inflammatory disruption of the tumor nodules suggests that these immunologic reactions create a transient state of vulnerability in the surviving tumor cells. Thus, the exploitation of the inflammatory disruption of anatomic barriers combined with strategically integrated chemotherapy may be useful in the design of future therapy trials in man.

Clinical Studies of Active Specific Immunotherapy

Except for skin cancer, colorectal cancer is now the most prevalent cancer affecting both sexes in the United States. Over 125,000 new cases are reported each year with nearly 60,000 deaths (65). Resection remains the only effective treatment with the exception of radiation therapy, which sometimes can control rectal tumors in their early stages. However, patients with transmural extensions of tumor and metastasis to five or more regional lymph nodes have a 5-year survival rate of only 9.1% when treated by surgery alone (66). Adjuvant radiation therapy for rectal cancer can lower the incidence of local recurrence of tumor but does not control systemic metastasis, the cause of death in many of these patients. Since adjuvant chemotherapy has shown no dramatic influence on survival rates (67), an effective systemic adjuvant is clearly needed.

Over the past 3 years we have translated the results of our experiments with the guinea pig model of active specific immunotherapy into a prospectively randomized, controlled clinical trial of therapy for colorectal cancer in humans (22). Two questions were asked: (a) Can DCH to autologous tumor cells be boosted by immunotherapy, and (b) can active specific immunotherapy improve the disease-free interval and/or survival when used as an adjuvant to surgery? Primary tumors were removed by standard surgical techniques and were enzymatically dissociated and cryopreserved by techniques that maintain cell viability (Fig. 6-3). Adjacent normal colon mucosa was processed similarly. Patients with transmural extension of tumor or nodal metastases were randomized into groups receiving no further treatment or receiving immunotherapy. Skin testing with irradiated, autologous tumor cells and mucosa cells was done 3 weeks postoperatively before immunotherapy began. Immunized patients

210   Marc E. Key, Herbert C. Hoover, Jr., and Michael G. Hanna, Jr.

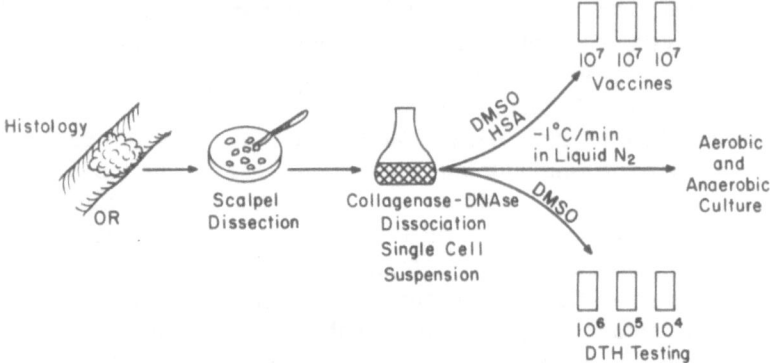

Figure 6-3. Procedures for preparation and use of vaccine and DCH test material from colorectal cancer patients. Figure taken from (22).

received one intradermal vaccination weekly for 2 weeks of 10^7 irradiated, autologous tumor cells and 10^7 BCG and one vaccination of 10^7 irradiated, autologous tumor cells alone in the third week. Skin tests were repeated at 6 weeks, 6 months, and 1 year postvaccination. To date, 40 patients have participated in the trial. Immunized patients demonstrated a significant boost in the DCH response to their autologous tumor cells (Fig. 6-4). Control patients did not react significantly to tumor or mucosa cells at any test period. Reactivity to tumor cells diminished at 6 months and 1 year but continued to be significantly elevated over control values. Histologic analysis of positive skin-test sites revealed marked perivascular infiltrates suggestive of cell-mediated hypersensitivity. The Mantel-Haenszel analysis of the clinical follow-up data [mean follow-up of 22 months (4 months to 37 months)] revealed a significantly improved disease-free status of the immunized patients ($P < .01$); however, further follow-up is necessary before any conclusions can be made. With respect to survival, 0 of 20 treatment patients had died whereas 4 of 20 control patients had died. We conclude that active specific immunotherapy for colorectal cancer can effectively boost reactivity to TAAs.

The early results of our trial with regard to disease-free interval and survival in the immunized versus control group are quite encouraging. The following conclusions can be made: (a) Adequate viable tumor cells for an autologous vaccine can be obtained from nearly all Dukes stages B to D colorectal cancer patients. (b) The procedures for vaccine preparation can be conducted in the clinic by trained personnel, such as nurses and technicians. (c) Toxicity is minimal. (d) Acceptance by patients is excellent. (e) Increased immunoreactivity to autologous tumor cells is evident in immunized patients. (f) No adverse effects of autologous tumor cell immunization have been found; specifically, there is no evidence of immune-mediated enhancement of tumors. The last point is extremely

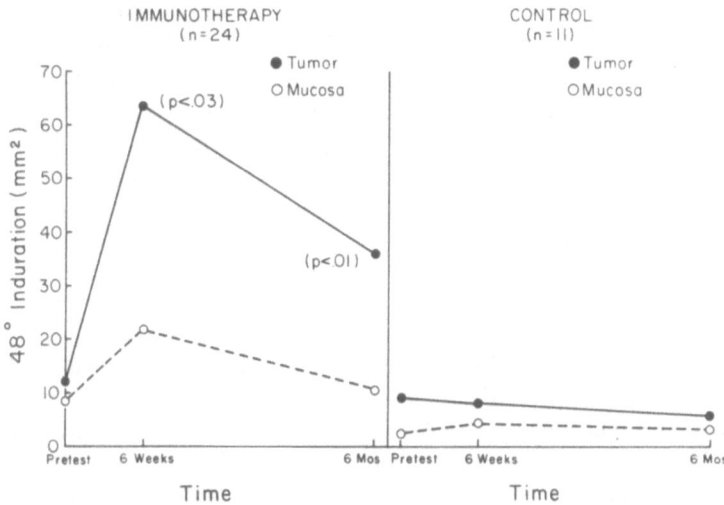

Figure 6-4. DCH response to tumor and mucosa cell preparations in autologous tumor cell immunized (**A**) and nonimmunized patients (**B**). Mean 48-h induration are (mm²) plotted for tumor and mucosa cell preparations. Statistical significance was determined by a paired *t*-test for differences in means (2-tailed). The differences between 48-h induration of tumor and mucosa were statistically significant at 6 weeks (*P* < .03) and 6 months (*P* < .01) in the treated patients. Figure taken from (22).

important as much of the past concern regarding active specific modulation of immunity in cancer patients emanated from anticipated results suggesting immune-mediated enhanced growth of tumors.

Future Prospects for Active Specific Immunotherapy

Although the therapeutic effectiveness of active specific immunotherapy in colorectal cancer patients is suggested by the preliminary data, it is unlikely that the optimal vaccination and treatment protocols have been achieved. These early successes should be viewed as an indication of the therapeutic effect that can ultimately be expected given optimization of all aspects of treatment. For example, our efforts at developing therapeutic tumor vaccines have concentrated primarily on vaccine preparation and administration. Another equally important aspect of immunization is the capacity of the host to respond adequately to potentially immunogenic tumor vaccines. Cancer patients frequently display varying degrees of generalized or specific immunosuppression. Throughout this discussion we have avoided mentioning specific immune tolerance toward tumors and the potential effect that this might have on immunotherapy. This omission reflects our limited understanding of the problem of specific immune tolerance as it applies to the human cancer patient. There is evidence for the existence of specific suppressor cells in several experimental tumor systems (68–70). Whether suppressor cells contribute to the escape of human cancer from immunologic control is unknown. If a significant role for suppressor cells in human cancer is established, then methods must be developed to counteract their adverse effects.

Recent studies with monoclonal antibodies suggest that these reagents may be useful for the specific elimination in vivo of targeted lymphocyte populations. For example, recent studies by Granstein et al (71) have shown that tumor suppressor cells could be eliminated in vivo by treatment of mice with monoclonal antibodies directed against a subregion of the major histocompatibility complex expressed on T-lymphocyte suppressor cells. Another approach for the elimination of specific lymphocyte subpopulations is by active immunization of the host with in vitro expanded lymphocyte subpopulations corresponding to the in vivo subpopulations targeted for elimination (72). The development of these or similar methods for specific lymphocyte depletion may ultimately provide the means for manipulating lymphocyte populations in vivo.

Drug-induced elimination of suppressor cells is another approach under current investigation (71,73). The immunopotentiating effects of cyclophosphamide have long been known and have been extensively documented (74). In addition, cyclophosphamide has been shown to reverse tolerance induced by many kinds of antigens, including, in some cases, tolerance established to autologous tissue antigens (75). The action of cyclophosphamide in reversing the tolerant state or in augmenting immune responses has frequently been attributed to its preferential cytotoxic action on immunoregulatory suppressor cells. Thus, the administration of cyclophosphamide to cancer patients prior to immunotherapy may prove beneficial in promoting a more vigorous immune response to tumor vaccine. In our guinea pig studies, DCH responses to tumor after immunotherapy were significantly enhanced by prior treatment with cyclophosphamide. In a similar study, Berd et al (76) showed enhancement of DCH responses to autologous tumor in cyclophosphamide-treated cancer patients.

Finally, incorporation into the vaccine of an appropriate immunologic adjuvant can frequently provide the stimulus necessary to break tolerance to certain antigens. Most effective in this respect are the BCG-based adjuvants. Humphrey and Turk (77) showed that guinea pigs made tolerant to albumin or human gamma globulin can have their tolerance broken by immunization with the antigen incorporated into complete Freund's adjuvant. Whether tumor-specific tolerance in cancer patients can be similarly manipulated is unknown. However, in our studies of immunotherapy in colorectal cancer patients, immunization with tumor cells plus

BCG significantly increased DCH responses to autologous tumor, suggesting that if a prior state of immunologic unresponsiveness existed, this therapy was at least partially effective in reversing this deficiency.

If specific immunotherapy is to develop into an effective and efficient method of cancer treatment, methods must be devised to facilitate the process of vaccine preparation. Current techniques used in our laboratory involve preparation of specific tumor vaccines for each individual patient. Surgically obtained primary tumors must be enzymatically dissociated, irradiated, and cryopreserved under exacting conditions. Seemingly unimportant deviations from established protocol have rendered vaccines useless in the guinea pig model. The translation of these techniques to the clinic on even a small scale has proved cumbersome at best. Perhaps the second generation of immunotherapy can employ techniques utilizing monoclonal antibodies both to identify classes of antigens on tumor cell surfaces and to aid in antigen purification. If antigens can be identified that are common to classes of tumors and are immunogenic in patients, then perhaps patients could be treated with standard vaccines made for their type of tumor rather than by custom-made vaccines.

The same monoclonal antibody technology that is currently being used to identify TAAs on the surface of tumor cells could also be used in the large-scale isolation and purification of TAAs. The availability in large quantities of highly purified TAA may aid in the production of vaccines against weakly immunogenic tumors. However, not all of the molecular structures on tumor cells that are recognized by murine monoclonal antibodies are immunogenic in the tumor-bearing host or can function as tumor-rejection antigens. For monoclonal antibody technology to be applicable to purification of appropriate antigens for use in immunotherapy, techniques must be developed that allow the identification of the relevant TAAs responsible for tumor rejection. One step in this direction would be through the use of human monoclonal antibodies rather than murine monoclonal antibodies. Immunization of patients with autologous tumor cells in our active specific immunotherapy protocol has provided a unique source of sensitized lymphocytes from which several stable clones of B cells have been developed (21). Furthermore, many of these clones secrete antibodies that react preferentially with colon cancer tissue. These tumor-specific monoclonal antibodies should be useful as probes to isolate and characterize TAA relevant to immunity in human cancer.

One final area of investigation critical to the continued development of specific immunotherapy is the use of immunotherapy in conjunction with conventional and experimental modes of cancer treatment. Recent results in the guinea pig L10 tumor model have shown that chemotherapy acts synergistically with immunotherapy in the eradication of pulmonary micrometastases if a precise sequence of immunotherapy and chemotherapy are followed (53,54). Investigations into the mechanisms for this synergistic interaction suggest that immune components break down the normal anatomic and vascular barriers in solid tumors, allowing greater access of blood-borne chemotherapeutic agents to the tumor cell.

Immunotherapy in combination with more experimental forms of therapy may also be effective. The use of monoclonal antibodies for therapy of solid tumors is an area of current investigation. Several studies in other tumor systems have shown that monoclonal antibodies alone or conjugated to toxic substances can be effective in the treatment of cancer (78,79). One distinct advantage of combining active specific immunotherapy with monoclonal antibody serotherapy is the potential for immunotherapy to break down anatomic and vascular barriers of solid tumors, allowing the entry of monoclonal antibodies into previously inaccessible portions of the tumor.

The encouraging experimental results obtained with combined immunotherapy and chemotherapy in the guinea pig model form the basis for trial therapy implementing this new approach in the clinic. Such a trial in colon cancer is just beginning under the auspices of the Eastern Cooperative Oncology Group (ECOG) with seven institutions. Patients with positive regional lymph nodes are randomly assigned postoperatively to a control group (no further treatment) or to the experimental group who receive a course of active specific immunotherapy with an autologous tumor cell-BCG vaccine followed by eight cycles of fluorouracil (5-FU) chemotherapy. It will be 2 or 3 years before data are available from this trial.

The cumulative evidence from numerous studies of experimental cancer in animals suggests that cancer is subject to immunologic control. However, after more than a decade of trying, this goal has yet to be realized in the treatment of human cancer. With rapid advances in such diverse fields as monoclonal antibody technology with its implications for studying the tumor cell surface at the molecular level, to molecular genetics with its ability to analyze malignant transformation at the level of the gene, new discoveries into the biology of cancer are occurring almost daily. This rapid proliferation of information, taken together with our growing experience with immunotherapy, will undoubtedly form the basis for the development of new and creative strategies for the treatment of cancer in the future.

References

1. DeVita VT. The relationship between tumor mass and resistance to chemotherapy: Implication for surgical adjuvant treatment of cancer. *Cancer* 57:1209–1220, 1983.
2. Salman SE, Jones SE, eds. *Adjuvant Therapy of Cancer, III.* New York: Grune and Stratton, 1981.

3. Hanna MG Jr, Key ME, Oldham RK. Biology of Cancer Therapy: Some new insights into adjuvant treatment of metastatic solid tumors. *J Biol Response Modifiers* 2:295–309, 1983.
4. Key ME. Macrophages in cancer metastases and their relevance to metastatic growth. *Cancer Metastasis Reviews* 2:75–88, 1983.
5. Fidler J, Sone S, Fogler WE, Barnes L. Eradication of spontaneous metastases and activation of alveolar macrophages by intravenous injection of liposomes containing muramyl dipeptide. *Proc Natl Acad Sci USA* 78:1680–1684, 1981.
6. Terry WD, Rosenbert SA, eds. *Immunotherapy of human cancer*. New York: Elsevier/North Holland, 1982.
7. Mastrangelo MJ, Berd D. Immunotherapy with microbial products. In *Immunological Approaches to Cancer Therapeutics*. New York, John Wiley and Sons, 1982, pp 75–106.
8. Rosenberg SA, Rapp H, Terry W, et al. Intralesional BCG therapy of patients with primary stage I melanoma. In *Proceedings of the Second International Conference on the Immunotherapy of Cancer,* Bethesda, MD, 1980.
9. Gross L. Intradermal immunization of mice against a sarcoma originated in an animal of the same line. *Cancer Res* 3:326–333, 1943.
10. Foley EJ. Antigenic properties of methylcholanthrene-induced tumors in mice of the strain of origin. *Cancer Res* 13:35–37, 1953.
11. Prehn RT, Main JM. Immunity to methylcholanthrene-induced sarcomas. *J Natl Cancer Inst* 18:769–778, 1957.
12. Hewitt HB. Animal tumor models and their relevance to human tumor immunology. *J Biol Response Modifiers* 1:107–119, 1982.
13. Hewitt HB. Second point: Animal tumor models and their relevance to human tumor immunology. *J Biol Response Modifiers* 2:210–216, 1983.
14. Herberman RB. Counterpoint: Animal tumor models and their relevance to human tumor immunology. *J. Biol Response Modifiers* 2:39–46, 1983.
15. Herberman RB. Second counterpoint: Animal tumor models and their relevance to human tumor immunology. *J Biol Response Modifiers* 217–226, 1983.
16. Herberman RB, Oldham RK. Cell-mediated cytotoxicity against human tumors: Lessons learned and future prospects. *J Biol Response Modifiers* 2:111–120, 1983.
17. Witz IP. Tumor-bound immunoglobulins: In situ expressions of humoral immunity. *Adv Cancer Res* 25:95–141, 1977.
18. McCoy JP, Hofheintz DE, Abb NG, Nordquist S, Haines HB. Tumor-bound immunoglobulin in human gynecologic cancers. *J Natl Cancer Inst* 63:279–282, 1979.
19. Dippold WG, Lloyd KO, Houghton AN, et al. Human melanoma antigens defined by monoclonal antibodies. In *Hybridomas in Cancer Diagnosis and Treatment*. New York, Raven Press, 1982, pp 173–182.
20. Reisfeld RA, Morgan AC, Bumol TF. Production and characterization of a monoclonal antibody to human melanoma associated antigen. In *Hybridomas in Cancer Diagnosis and Treatment*. New York, Raven Press, 1982, pp 183–186.
21. Haspel MV, Hoover HC, McCabe RP, Pomato N, Hanna MG Jr. Human colon cancer: Generation of tumor specific human monoclonal antibodies. *PROC. A.A.C.R.* 25:236, 1984.

22. Hoover HC Jr, Surdyke M, Dangel RB, Peters LC, and Hanna MG Jr. Delayed cutaneous hypersensitivity to autologous tumor cells in colorectal cancer patients immunized with an autologous tumor cell-Bacillus Calmette Guérin vaccine. *Cancer Res* 44:1671–1676, 1984.
23. Hewitt HB, Blake ER, Walder AS. A critique of the evidence for active host defense against cancer based on personal studies of 27 murine tumors of spontaneous origin. *Brit J Cancer* 33:241–259, 1976.
24. Middle JG, Embleton MJ. Naturally arising tumors of the inbred WAB/NOT rat strain. II. Immunogenicity of transplanted tumors. *J Natl Cancer Inst* 76:637–643, 1981.
25. Key ME, Brandhorst JS, Hanna MG Jr. More on the relevance of animal tumor models: Immunogenicity of transplantable leukemias of recent origin in syngeneic strain 2 guinea pigs. *J Biol Response Modifiers* 3:359–365, 1984.
26. Hanna MG, Peters LC, Fidler IJ. The efficacy of BCG-induced tumor immunity in guinea pigs with regional and systemic malignancy. *Cancer Immunol Immunother* 1:171–177, 1976.
27. Hanna MG, Peters LC. Immunotherapy of established micrometastases with a Bacillus Calmette Guérin tumor cell vaccine. *Cancer Res* 38:204–209, 1978.
28. Hanna MG, Brandhorst JS, Peters LC. Active-specific immunotherapy of residual micrometastases: An evaluation of sources, doses and ratios of BCG with tumor cells. *Cancer Immunol Immunother* 7:165–173, 1979.
29. Peters LC, Hanna MG. Active-specific immunotherapy of established metastases: Effect of cryopreservation procedures on tumor cell immunogenicity in guinea pigs. *J Natl Cancer Inst* 64:1521–1525, 1980.
30. Peters LC, Brandhorst JS, Hanna MG Jr. Preparation of immunotherapeutic autologous tumor cell vaccines from solid tumors. *Cancer Res* 39:1353–1360, 1979.
31. Hoover HC, Peters LC, Brandhorst JS, Hanna MG. Therapy of spontaneous metastases by an autologous tumor vaccine. *J Surg Res* 30:409–415, 1981.
32. Byers VS, Johnston JO. Antigenic differences among osteogenic sarcoma tumor cells taken from different locations in human tumors. *Cancer Res* 37:3173–3183, 1977.
33. Faraci RP. In vitro demonstration of altered antigenicity of metastases from a primary methylcholanthrene-induced sarcoma. *Surgery* 76:469–473, 1974.
34. Killion JJ. Immunotherapy with tumor cell subpopulations. I. Active, specific immunotherapy of L1210 leukemia. *Cancer Immunol Immunother* 4:115–119, 1978.
35. Pimm MV, Baldwin RW. Antigenic differences between primary methylcholanthrene-induced rat sarcoma and post-surgical recurrences. *Int J Cancer* 20:37–43, 1977.
36. Prehn RT. Analysis of antigenic heterogeneity within individual 3-methylcholanthrene-induced mouse sarcomas. *J Natl Cancer Inst* 45:1039–1045, 1970.
37. Sorg C, Bruggen J, Seibert E. Membrane-associated antigens of human malignant melanoma cells. *Cancer Immunol Immunother* 3:259–271, 1978.
38. Sugarbaker EV, Cohen AM. Altered antigenicity in spontaneous pulmonary metastases from an antigenic murine sarcoma. *Surgery* 72:155–161, 1972.

39. Miller FR, Heppner GH. Immunologic heterogeneity of tumor cell subpopulations from a single mouse mammary tumor. *J Natl Cancer Inst* 63:1457–1463, 1979.
40. Olsson L, Ebbesen P. Natural polyclonality of spontaneous AKR leukemia and its consequences for so-called specific immunotherapy. *J Natl Cancer Inst* 62:623–627, 1979.
41. Miller FR. Intratumor immunologic heterogeneity. *Cancer Metastasis Reviews* 1:319–334, 1982.
42. Baldwin RW, Pimm MV. BCG immunotherapy of pulmonary growth from intravenously transferred rat tumour cells. *Brit J Cancer* 27:48–54, 1973.
43. Bartlett GL, Zbar B. Tumor-specific vaccine containing *Mycobacterium bovis* and tumor cells: Safety and efficacy. *J Natl Cancer Inst* 48:1709–1726, 1972.
44. Bomford R. Active specific immunotherapy of mouse methylcholanthrene-induced tumors with *Corynebacterium parvum* and irradiated tumor cell. *Brit J Cancer* 32:551–557, 1975.
45. Kreider JW, Bartlett GL, Boyer C, Purnell DM. Conditions for effective Bacillus Calmette-Guérin immunotherapy of post-surgical metastases of 1376A rat mammary adenocarcinoma. *Cancer Res* 39:987–992, 1979.
46. Likhite VV. Rejection of mammary adenocarcinoma cell tumors and the prevention of progressive growth of incipient metastases following intratumor permeation with killed *Bordetella pertussis*. *Cancer Res* 34:2790–2794, 1974.
47. Likhite VV. Rejection of tumors and metastases in Fisher 344 rats following intratumor administration of killed *Corynebacterium parvum*. *Int J Cancer* 14:684–690, 1974.
48. Denton PM, Syme MO. Observations on the changing behavior of AKR mouse lymphomas serially transplanted in the strain of origin. *Immunology* 15:371–380, 1968.
49. Key ME, Hanna MG Jr. Antigenic heterogeneity of the guinea pig Line 10 hepatocarcinoma. Implications for active specific immunotherapy. *Cancer Immunol Immunother* 12:211–215, 1982.
50. Teale DM, Rees RC, Clark A, Potter CW. Properties of a Herpesvirus transformed hamster cell line: Immunogenicity of sublines of high and low metastatic potential. *Int J Cancer* (in press).
51. Kerbel RS. Implications of immunological heterogeneity of tumours. *Nature* 280:358–360, 1979.
52. Fuji H, Michich E. Selection for high immunogenicity in drug-resistant sublines of murine lymphomas demonstrated by plaque assay. *Cancer Res* 35:946–952, 1975.
53. Hanna MG Jr, Key ME. Immunotherapy of metastases enhances subsequent chemotherapy. *Science* 217:367–369, 1982.
54. Key ME, Brandhorst JS, Hanna MG Jr. Synergistic effects of active specific immunotherapy and chemotherapy in guinea pigs with disseminated cancer. *J Immunol* 130:2987–2992, 1983.
55. Hawrylko E, Mackaness GB. Immunopotentiation with BCG. III. Modulation of the response to a tumor-specific antigen. *J Natl Cancer Inst* 51:1677–1682, 1973.
56. Scott MT. Potentiation of the tumor-specific immune response by *Corynebacterium parvum*. *J Natl Cancer Inst* 55:65–72, 1975.

57. McLaughlin CA, Schwartzman SM, Horner BC, Jones GH, Moffatt JG, Nestor JJ, Tegg D. Regression of tumors in guinea pigs after treatment with synthetic muramyl dipeptides and trehalose dimycolate. *Science* 208:415–416, 1980.
58. Hanna MG Jr, Zbar B, Rapp HJ. Histopathology of tumor regression after intralesional injection of *Mycobacterium bovis. J Natl Cancer Inst* 48:1441–1455, 1972.
59. Key ME, Hanna MG Jr. Mechanism of action of BCG-tumor cell vaccines in the generation of systemic tumor immunity. I. Synergism between BCG and L10 tumor cells in the induction of an inflammatory response. *J Natl Cancer Inst* 853–861, 1981.
60. Key ME, Hanna MG Jr. Mechanism of action of BCG-tumor cell vaccines in the generation of systemic tumor immunity. II. Influence of the local inflammatory response on immune reactivity. *J Natl Cancer Inst* 67:863–869, 1981.
61. Hanna MG Jr, Peters LC. Morphologic and functional aspects of active specific immunotherapy of established pulmonary metastases in guinea pigs. *Cancer Res* 41:4001–4009, 1981.
62. Key ME, Bernhard MI, Hoyer LC, Foon KA, Oldham RK, Hanna MG Jr. Guinea pig line 10 hepatocarcinoma model for monoclonal antibody serotherapy: In vivo localization of a monoclonal antibody in normal and malignant tissues. *J Immunol* 130:1451–1457, 1981.
63. West GW, Weichselbrum R, Little TB. Limited penetration of methotrexate into human osteosarcoma spheroids as a proposed model for solid tumor resistance to adjuvant chemotherapy. *Cancer Res* 40:3665–3668, 1980.
64. Gullino PJ. Angiogenesis and oncogenesis. *J Natl Cancer Inst* 61:639–643, 1978.
65. Siverberg E. Cancer statistics. *CA* 33:9, 1983.
66. Copeland EM, Miller LD, Jones RS. Prognostic factors in carcinoma of the colon and rectum. *Am J Surg* 116:875–880, 1968.
67. Gastrointestinal tumor study group: Adjuvant therapy of colon cancer—results of a prospectively randomized trial. *N Eng J Med* 310:737–743, 1984.
68. Fujimoto S, Green MI, Sehon AH. Regulation of the immune response to tumor antigen. I. Immuno-suppressor cells in tumor-bearing hosts. *J Immunol* 116:791, 1976.
69. Fisher MS, Kriphe ML. Systemic alteration induced in mice by ultraviolet light irradiation and its relationship to ultraviolet carcinogenesis. *Proc Natl Acad Sci USA* 74:1688–1692, 1977.
70. North JR. Cycloposphamide facilitated adoptive immunotherapy of an established tumor depends on elimination of tumor-induced suppressor T cells. *J Exp Med* 55:1063–1074, 1982.
71. Granstein RD, Parrish JA, McAuliffe DJ, Waltenbaugh C, Greene MI. Immunologic inhibition of ultraviolet radiation—induced tumor suppressor cell activity. *Science* 224:615–617, 1984.
72. Cohen IR, Ben-Nun A, Holoshitz J, Maron R, Zerubavel R. Vaccination against autoimmune disease with lines of autoimmune T lymphocytes. *Immunol Today* 4:227–230, 1983.
73. Berd D, McGuire HC, Mastrangelo MJ. Immuno-potentiation by cyclophosphamide and other cytotoxic agents. In *Immunomodulating agents.* New York, Marcel Dekker, 1983.

74. Turk JL, Parker D. Effect of cyclophosphamide on immunological control mechanisms. *Immunol Rev* 65:99–113, 1982.
75. Yoshida S, Nomoto K, Himeno K, et al. Immune response to syngeneic or autologous testicular cells in mice. I. Augmented delayed footpad reactions in cyclophosphamide-treated mice. *Clin Exp. Immunol.* 38:211–217, 1979.
76. Berd D. McGuire H, Mastrangelo MJ. Augmentation of delayed-type hypersensitivity to tumor-associated antigens by treatment with autologous tumor cell vaccine preceeding cyclophosphamide. *Proc Am Soc Clin Oncol* 2:56, 1983.
77. Humphrey JH, Turk JL. Immunological corresponsiveness in guinea pigs. *Immunology* 4:301, 1961.
78. Foon KA, Bernhard MI, Oldham RK. Monoclonal antibody therapy: Assessment by animal tumor models. *J Biol Resp Modif* 1:277–304, 1982.
79. Ritz J, Schlossman SF. Utilization of monoclonal antibodies in treatment of leukemia and lymphoma. *Blood* 59:1–11, 1982.

Index

(*cont.*)

in opsonization, 134, 135
sera levels of, in cancer, 135
CEA, *see* Carcinoembryonic antigen
Calcitonin, 100, 101
Cancer; *see also* Tumor
bestatin effect on, 19–21
breast
primary, 175
recurrent, 186
bronchogenic, 175–176
chemotherapy for, *see*
Chemotherapy
colorectal
clinical studies of immunotherapy
for, 209–211
metastatic, 186
primary, 173–175
recurrent, 180–185
complement in, 135–137
direct cytotoxicity of, 136
indirect cytotoxicity of, 136–137
tumor cell chemotaxis and, 137
variations in sera level of,
135–136
diagnostic tests for, *see* Diagnostic
tests for cancer
gastrointestinal, 172–173
heterogeneity of cells in, 35–36
immune parameters with, 103–112
nonspecific, in vitro assays,
104–107
nonspecific, in vivo assays,
107–108
serial testing of, 112
tumor-associated, in vitro assays,
108–111
tumor-associated, in vivo assays,
111–112
immune process in, 31–36
evaluation of, 36
heterogeneity of effector cells,
33–35
heterogeneity of tumor cells,
35–36
lymphokines in tumor-bearing
hosts, 35
in vitro and in vivo relevance of
effector cells, 31–33

leukemia
BCG for, 21–22
complement levels in, 135–136
immunofluorescent tests for, 102
immunogenicity of
tumor-associated antigens of,
199, 200
metastatic
colorectal cancer, 186
cryosurgery effect on, 72
immunologic heterogeneity of
tumors in, 201–203
immunotherapy for, 195–214
from surgery, 69, 70–71
whole body irradiation effects on,
42
modulation of biologic response in,
9–10
pancreatic, 172, 175
radiotherapy for, *see* Radiotherapy
surgical therapy for, *see* Surgery
tumor markers for, 167–168
Carcinoembryonic antigen
antibodies to, 186
antigenic determinants of, 169
in biliary obstruction, 170
in blood transfusion, 170, 171
in breast cancer
primary, 175
recurrent, 186
in bronchogenic carcinoma,
175–176
characterization of, 168–169
in colorectal cancer
metastatic, 186
primary, 173–175
recurrent, 180–185
detection of, 169
in diagnosis of cancer, 172–173
in gastritis, 170, 171
in gastrointestinal malignancy,
occult, 172–173
in hepatic cirrhosis and hepatitis,
170–171
metabolism of, 169–170
for monitoring cancer therapy,
176–179
chemotherapy, 179
radiotherapy, 178

K
K cells, 49

L
Lawrence transfer factor, 68
Lentinan, 145
Leukemia
  BCG for, 21–22
  complement levels in, 135–136
  immunofluorescent tests for, 102
  immunogenicity of tumor-associated
    antigens of, 199, 200
Leukocyte adherence inhibition tests,
  111
Leukocyte migration inhibition tests,
  111
Levamisole, 18, 63, 146
Levan, 18, 64
Lipopolysaccharides, 18, 144–145
Lithium carbonate, 64
Lymph nodes
  regeneration of, after radiotherapy,
    39
  removal of, effect on immune
    system, 43
Lymphocytes
  alternative pathway of complement
    interaction with, 133
  antigen contact with, 32
  B lymphocytes
    alternative pathway of
      complement interaction with,
      133
    blastogenic responses of, 106
    chemotherapy effects on, 49
    radiotherapy effects on, 13–14,
      37, 39–40, 45–46
    as suppressor cells, 33
  cyclophosphamide effects on,
    48–49
  differentiation of populations of,
    105
  elimination of, via monoclonal
    antibodies, 212
  helper cells
    in antitumor immunity, 31–32
    chemotherapy effects on, 15
    radiotherapy effects on, 11, 12

proliferative assays of, 106–107,
  110–111
radiation effects on, 37
suppressor, see Suppressor cells
T, see T lymphocytes
transfer of, thoracic duct, 62
Lymphokines
  in antitumor immunity, 31–32
  assays of, 35
  as indicators of sensitization to
    tumor antigen, 35

M
M protein, 100
Macrophage activating factor, 4–5
Macrophage electrophoretic mobility
  test, 98–99
Macrophages
  activation of, 4–5
    alternative pathway of
      complement in, 132–133
  in antitumor immunity, 31
  chemotaxis of
    in cancer, 35, 72
    protein inhibition of, 104
  cytotoxicity of, 136–137
    antigen-independent, 3–5
  radiation effects on, 38
  as suppressor cells, 33
Mannosulfan, 59
Mercaptopurine, 48
Metastasis
  colorectal cancer, 186
  cryosurgery effect on, 72
  immunologic heterogeneity of
    tumors in, 201–203
  immunotherapy for, 195–214
    antigenicity of tumors and,
      197–198
    clinical studies of, 209–211
    future prospects for, 211–214
    in guinea pig tumor model
      system, 203–209
    tumor immunologic heterogeneity
      and, 201–203
    tumor-associated antigen
      immunogenicity and, 198–201